THE
POLITICS
OF
MEDICAL
ENCOUNTERS

THE
POLITICS
OF
MEDICAL
ENCOUNTERS

HOW PATIENTS
AND DOCTORS
DEAL WITH
SOCIAL PROBLEMS

HOWARD WAITZKIN

YALE UNIVERSITY PRESS
NEW HAVEN AND LONDON

Published with assistance from the foundation
established in memory of Amasa Stone Mather of the
Class of 1907, Yale College.

Parts of chapters 1–4 and 11 appeared as preliminary versions
in the *International Journal of Health Services, Journal of Health
and Social Behavior,* and *Medical Care.*

Designed by Suzanne G. Bennett
Set in Palatino type by
Keystone Typesetting Inc., Orwigsburg, Pennsylvania.
Printed in the United States of America by
Vail-Ballou Press, Binghamton, New York.

Library of Congress Cataloging-in-Publication Data
Waitzkin, Howard.
    The politics of medical encounters : how patients
and doctors deal with social problems / Howard Waitzkin.
        p.   cm.
    Includes bibliographical references and index.
    ISBN 0-300-04949-8 (cloth)
        0-300-05511-0 (pbk.)
    1. Social medicine.   2. Physician and patient.   I. Title.
RA418.W347   1991
610.69′6—dc20   90–45611
                        CIP

A catalogue record for this book is available from
the British Library.

The paper in this book meets the guidelines for
permanence and durability of the Committee on
Production Guidelines for Book Longevity of the
Council on Library Resources.

10   9   8   7   6   5   4   3   2

For Stephany . . .
she showed the ways

On the whole, my interrogations make me think of a surgeon who sews up his incision without removing the tumor. . . .

Other people's sufferings have been affecting me this way lately; my mind is full of their stories, my dreams are live with them, and though no two are the same, they are all of the same kind: I strongly suspect that those of my acquaintances who manage to live day after day with equanimity are sleight-of-hand artists.

—George Konrád, *The Case Worker*

CONTENTS

PREFACE

This book concerns the interactions and relationships of patients and doctors. Having been both a patient and a doctor, I hold a benign view of each party: I believe that patients seek assistance for concrete problems and that doctors genuinely want to help. Yet patient and doctor meet within a social context that is difficult and complicated. Medicine sometimes, but only rarely, involves a straightforward technical solution to a simple technical problem. In the intimacy of the doctor-patient relationship, social problems arise and get dealt with, often in ways that are unwitting and unintended. One irony, a central theme of this book, is that, by helping patients in little ways, doctors may reinforce the big social problems that keep people distressed and unhappy.

The project really began when, as a teenager, I witnessed my grandfather's dying. I loved his humor amid the sadnesses of poverty, and I admired his tenacity as a worker and political organizer. His liver cancer, I later learned, probably developed because of the toxic solvents that he used in his work as a housepainter. As he was dying, his doctors maintained a circle of lies and distortions that left him confused and dispirited. Other well-meaning members of my family cooperated in these communicative maneuvers, all intended to keep up his morale and our family's ability to function.

This searing experience had much to do with my later decision to enter medicine and my interest in doctor-patient communication. Influenced by the social sciences, I began a long-term study of barriers to communication, especially those deriving from the differences in class background, education, race, sex, and age between doctors and patients. The research went well, generating financial support, publications, and media attention. As the work became more successful, however, I grew more dissatisfied. After more than a decade of studying tapes and transcripts of talk between doctors and patients, I became more and more convinced that the traditional and largely quantitative methods that our research group was using simply were not adequate to the task. That is, while we could say a great deal about communication, and especially about barriers to communication, we were missing important elements of what was happening in the encounters.

Specifically, what was said and what was left unsaid often seemed to encourage patients' acquiescence to difficult conditions that they experienced in their everyday lives. Some doctors were much more inclined than others to discuss these difficulties openly with their patients, but the result was almost always the same anyway: social conditions remained intact while the patient, with the benefit of medical advice, adjusted.

Doctors frequently made statements to their patients that reproduced some of the dominant ideologies of our society or that controlled patients' behavior in other ways that were consistent with mainstream expectations. While doctors and patients varied widely in their communication skills, the doctors all seemed well motivated to help their patients. Yet, even in the most technical encounters, messages of ideology and social control would arise. Such messages rarely appeared to reflect a conscious consideration of their implications by either participant in the dialogue. This observation was a troubling one, since ideologic language and social control seemed to occur among "good" doctors, "bad" doctors, and patients with various degrees of communicative ability, all of whom were trying to do their best under the circumstances. At the personal level, this realization was even more troubling, since my own behavior as a primary-care physician—one who values both technical competence and interpersonal skill—differed little from that of the doctors I was studying.

Coping with these dissatisfactions required a great deal of theoretical and methodological shifting of gears. Medical ideology and social control demanded a critical theory of discourse that could convincingly interpret what happens in medical encounters. Such a theory also, I hoped, would be relevant to professional-client communication in general. What was needed was a method to select, present, and analyze the content of communication in such a way that it would permit review and appraisal by others. Theory and method both required excursions far afield from those research techniques traditionally and narrowly applied to medical or other professional communication. Standards of clinical practice and political "praxis" also required some attempt to suggest progressive directions of change. This book is one step in this process of trying to break new ground.

A NOTE ON HOW THE BOOK IS ORGANIZED
AND HOW IT MIGHT BE READ

At the outset, some words about the book's organization and suggestions about reading it may help. Part I presents the project's theoretical underpinnings and methodologic approach. In chapters 1 and 2, I discuss the contradictions of the helping professions and review prior theoretical work that pertains to the problem of ideologic reproduction and social control in medicine. In chapter 3, influenced by literary criticism in the humanities, I examine more concretely the theoretical problem of analyzing doctor-patient communication as a text and offer a new critical theory of medical discourse. Developing a methodology that is appropriate to study specific medical communications is the goal of chapter 4. I have tried to prepare Part I so that readers who are less theoretically or methodologically inclined can skim or skip from the end of chapter 1 to the beginning of chapter 5 without losing the thread of the arguments. Medical professionals, some of whom may not enjoy all the book's critical comments about doctor-patient communication, might gain solace from the sympathetic account that I offer in chapter 1 concerning the predicament of clinicians. Researchers who have studied medical discourse with quantitative techniques or with nonquantitative methods (for instance, in the fields of sociolinguistics, conversation analysis, and discourse analysis) will probably be interested in the critical and self-critical account of my own and others' work that appears toward the end of chapter 2 and in chapter 4, even if they do not agree with all the views presented there.

In Part II (chapters 5 through 9), I analyze how medical discourse deals with a series of problematic areas: work, family life, and gender roles; aging; self-destructive behavior, especially substance use; and emotional disturbance. In chapter 10, I look at the characteristics of the negative case, in which ideologic reproduction and social control do not seem to occur. These chapters apply the theoretical and methodologic approaches developed in Part I to transcripts of actual doctor-patient encounters.

The problems of medical discourse that appear in Part II create a tension that centers on the question of how doctor-patient communication might be improved. I delay trying to answer this question until Part III, when in conclusion I suggest some directions of reform and point out the study's implications for change in both professional-client relationships and society.

A NOTE ON THE AVAILABILITY
OF ORIGINAL TRANSCRIPTS

Readers who wish to review the transcripts of the seventeen encounters discussed in chapters 5 through 9 may obtain them as a microfilmed appendix from University Microfilms International, Research Abstract Number LD01797, 300 North Zeeb Road, Ann Arbor, Michigan 48106; phone (800) 521–0600.

ACKNOWLEDGMENTS

Money, encouragement, and the cooperation of others played important parts in helping to complete this book. In pursuing my work, I was fortunate to receive financial assistance from the National Center for Health Services Research (grant HS–02100), the Robert Wood Johnson Foundation, the National Endowment for the Humanities (FA–22922), the Fulbright Program, the Academic Senate Committee on Research of the University of California, Irvine (uci), and the National Institute on Aging (1 F32 AG05438). During a span of many years, John Stoeckle, Elliot Mishler, Sam Bloom, Vic Sidel, and members of the primary-care research discussion group at uci gave me constructive suggestions about the study of doctor-patient communication. Stephany Borges, J. Hillis Miller, Mark Poster, Leslie Rabine, John Carlos Rowe, and particularly Theron Britt helped in my attempts to negotiate the terrain of progressive critical theory in the humanities; they deserve thanks but not responsibility for my use of their advice. At various times, Eric Beller, Linda Blum, Theron Britt, Sandra Chapek, Elaine Daunhauer, Mike Dunham, Bob Fitzgerald, Terry Fried, Annie Johnson, Carl Mons, D. C. Peoples, Georgia Taylor, Jacqueline Wallen, and Barbara Waterman contributed to this project through research assistance, technical help, and moral support. Seeing some value in this work, Sandra Dijkstra and Kathy Goodwin extended themselves to represent me as literary agents. At Yale University Press, Gladys Topkis, Stacey Mandelbaum, and Tom May did wonderful editorial work. I, of course, am indebted to the patients and doctors who participated in the study. Most of all, I hope Stephany Borges knows my gratitude for all she lovingly has given.

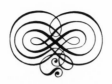

ONE
THE
MICROPOLITICS
OF
MEDICINE

CHAPTER 1

INTRODUCTION
HOW PATIENTS AND DOCTORS DEAL
WITH SOCIAL PROBLEMS

THREE MEDICAL ENCOUNTERS

- A man comes to his doctor several months after a heart attack. He is depressed. His period of disability payments will expire soon, and his union is about to go on strike. His doctor tells him that he is physically able to return to work as a radial drill operator and that working will be good for his mental health. The doctor also prescribes an antidepressant and a tranquilizer.
- A woman visits her doctor because of irregularities in her heart rhythm. She complains that palpitations and shortness of breath are interfering with her ability to do housework. The doctor checks an electrocardiogram while she exercises, changes her cardiac medications, and congratulates her in her efforts to maintain a tidy household.
- A man goes to his doctor for a premarital blood test. The doctor questions him closely about his drinking problem, his smoking, his job as a netmaker for fishermen, his family, and his plans for married life. Then the doctor encourages attendance at Alcoholics Anonymous and orders tests of liver function, in addition to the premarital blood test that the patient requested.

In approaching a physician for help, a patient brings not only a physical problem but also a social context. This context includes relationships at work, in the family, and in the wider community. A patient's experience of physical problems is inseparable from the wider social context in

3

which these problems occur. Pain and pathology afflict more than the body. Instead, somatic processes become troublesome also as they affect and are affected by a person's life experience.

Under these circumstances, patients' expectations of their doctors often include much more than a physical diagnosis and treatment. Based on what they explicitly say, the three patients above—whose interactions were recorded as part of a study that I will describe later—seem to want the following responses that go beyond those of technical medicine. The man recovering from a heart attack would like disability certification for a longer period of time, so that he can continue to receive benefits while his union is on strike. The woman suffering from cardiac symptoms seeks a way to cope with the physical demands of her housework. The man with an alcohol-abuse problem would simply like a blood test for a marriage license, and it is not clear that he welcomes attention to the alcohol issue.

In response to these patients, and from a traditional medical perspective, what are some of a doctor's options? After listening to the concerns of the patient who faces returning to a problematic work situation after a heart attack, the physician could extend the patient's disability certification for a longer period of time or could try to reduce the emotional distress that the patient is experiencing about this contextual problem. In choosing the latter course, this particular doctor prescribes two mood-altering drugs and counsels the patient that returning to work will benefit his mental health. For the woman worried about the impact of cardiac symptoms on housework, the doctor could respond with technical adjustments of medication or with emotional reassurance about her contextual concerns. Indeed, the doctor does use both of these options in addressing the issues that the patient presents. In response to the alcoholic patient's request for a premarital blood test, the physician could choose to explore or ignore the patient's contextual situation. Although this particular patient's request is quite modest, the doctor initiates a lengthy interrogation and list of suggestions about alcohol abuse.

The patients and doctors in these three encounters seem to accept the social context as given. Aside from asking how long the period of disability will last, neither the patient nor the doctor in the first encounter questions whether an eventual return to work is appropriate, and the financial insecurities arising from an uncertain work situation escape attention. In the second encounter, the patient and the doctor do not examine expectations concerning housework or explore changes in family roles to ease the patient's physical responsibilities. Although the participants in the third encounter discuss alcohol abuse at great length, they do not deal with the problems the patient faces in finding a steady job or with how the patient's family situation contributes to his difficulties with alcohol.

In short, *criticism* of the social context remains absent from these encounters. The patients and doctors do not examine critically the contextual sources of personal distress. Apparently seeing little room for basic change in context, these patients and doctors talk about adjustments that will help the patients continue to function in their usual and customary social roles. Potentially relevant modifications in social setting do not arise as topics for discussion.

There may be several reasons why these patients and doctors do not examine the social context critically. First, and most obviously, to do so can become emotionally upsetting. Because change might prove difficult, patients and doctors may fear that discussing contextual problems in any depth would create needless frustration and conflict. Lack of social support for a person seeking change also may inhibit such discussion.

Second, the possibility of physicians' working to improve contextual sources of distress is often overlooked in professional training. Few primary-care practitioners learn to spend much time on contextual concerns in routine doctor-patient encounters. While some medical training programs teach principles of counseling, family therapy, and so forth, these techniques usually involve referrals to other professionals. Such referrals are often difficult to arrange, because of finances, cultural barriers, or patients' reluctance to consult mental health professionals. In any case, these techniques rarely encourage basic changes in patients' contextual arrangements.

A third reason not to examine context involves doctors' own perception that their role is necessarily a limited one. From this viewpoint, a critical discussion of patients' social context goes beyond what doctors should reasonably be expected to do. Because many doctors recognize that delving into the social context of a patient can involve areas of life where they hold little special competence, they frequently feel more comfortable dealing with technical rather than contextual concerns. This reluctance to "medicalize" social problems is consistent with a common perception that medical professionals already have entered nontechnical areas more than they should.

For these reasons among others, criticism of context usually falls outside the realm of what is expected in medicine. In most medical encounters, the presence or absence of contextual criticism is not consciously considered. If doctors and patients view the social context critically, they typically do not perceive that their encounter is an appropriate place to express such criticisms. Nevertheless, since contextual issues frequently enter medical discourse anyway, the *lack* of criticism may help maintain social sources of distress and suffering.

HEALTH PROFESSIONALS' APPROACH
TO CONTEXTUAL PROBLEMS

Like other professionals, doctors usually try to help people in need. Patients come to doctors with a variety of problems—some physical, some psychological, and some social. One of the challenges that doctors face in practice concerns how to respond appropriately to the spectrum of issues that patients present. Humanistically oriented doctors often pride themselves on their ability to elicit the psychological and social components of patients' concerns. Moreover, doctors usually believe that they can assist with such difficulties, or at least that they should try to do so.

Despite practitioners' good intentions, the medical profession and the health-care system as a whole have not exactly escaped negative comment, especially in the United States.[1] Observers have claimed that doctors are overly concerned with making money, exert too much professional dominance over the conditions of practice, do not show enough humanistic concern for patients, spend too little effort on communication, do not try hard enough to improve access for the poor and for minorities, accept expensive technologies and drugs uncritically, cause needless suffering through the harmful ("iatrogenic") impact of their actions, police themselves inadequately to assure high standards of quality, and so forth. Critics of the health-care system point to the lack of access to needed services as the most serious of the system's many defects. For instance, the United States and the Republic of South Africa remain the only two economically developed countries without national health programs that assure universal entitlement to basic medical care. Although people with wealth or private insurance policies can obtain the most technologically advanced services, more than 40 million U.S. citizens face barriers to access because they lack either private or public insurance. The well-known high costs and inefficiencies of the health-care system also have become ever harder to tolerate.

Although such defects of professional motivation and the health-care system are important, they are not the main concerns here. Let us acknowledge these difficulties and accept what is likely a reasonable assumption—that, despite variability in personal motivation and despite the inadequacies of the health-care system, most doctors genuinely do want to help their patients. The question here is how well-meaning doctors, working within the constraints of current realities, deal with patients' contextual problems.

Several institutional contexts regularly become troublesome enough to appear in doctor-patient conversations. First, medical discourse mediates workers' participation in economic production. Patients frequently discuss work-related problems with doctors, as in the first encounter above. These problems involve stress, occupational accidents or illnesses requiring professional evaluation and certification, symptoms that derive from occupational hazards, and nonoccupational illnesses or symptoms that interfere with patients' ability to work. Doctors respond to these contextual difficulties, for instance, by offering advice, ordering tests, prescribing medications, writing notes to employers, and providing certificates for insurance companies. Some of these responses lead to patients' changing jobs, becoming unemployed, or entering periods of "disability." The criteria that doctors use in such decisions, however, are seldom straightforward. Doctors' mediation of workers' roles in economic production remains a problematic component of medical encounters.

Family life is a second institutional context that creates a problem for medicine. Difficulties in family relationships frequently enter conversations between patients and doctors. These difficulties may pertain to gender-role behavior, as in the case of the second patient. The patterning of women's roles creates tensions concerning housework, child care, work outside the home, and many other issues. Such issues have received wide attention, but usually not in terms of how medicine mediates these tensions. The concerns about family life and sexuality that men bring to their doctors are often different from those brought by women. Furthermore, family problems change during various stages of the life cycle. The special difficulties of the elderly, for example, arise frequently in medical encounters. How does medical discourse handle the contextual problems of family life, gender roles, sexuality, and aging? The ways that doctors and patients confront these issues of the family, and what alternative approaches might be feasible, remain little known or discussed.

A third contextual sphere involves "deviant" activities and emotional problems that derive from social conditions. Doctors often are privy to information about patients' most private experiences. Sometimes these activities deviate from mainstream expectations about appropriate behavior. Sexuality and its variations frequently come to doctors' attention. Doctors deal with patients' use or abuse of substances like alcohol, tobacco, prescription medications, and other drugs that lead to physical addiction. Moreover, a substantial part of medical practice involves discussions of emotional problems, including depression, anxiety, psychological disorders related to organic diseases, and stress. These emotional troubles typically arise from contextual difficulties in work, in the family, or in the community. The social context can become crucial as doctors try to deal with personal "vices," addictions, self-destructive behavior, and emotional distress.

When contextual issues arise in medical discourse, messages of ideology and social control often appear as well. Ideology involves the ideas and doctrines of a certain social group. Social control refers to the ways that a society achieves adherence to norms of appropriate behavior. In the next chapter I define ideology and social control in more depth; for now it is enough to say that doctors, implicitly or explicitly, may convey messages of ideology and social control when they confront contextual issues in encounters with patients.

The three encounters noted at the beginning of this chapter show how ideology and social control typically occur in medicine. For instance, when a man is reluctant to return to work after an illness, a doctor expresses the ideologic notion that work is beneficial for mental health; the communication fosters social control as it encourages the patient's return to work. Similarly, when a doctor helps a woman who has trouble doing housework because of cardiac symptoms, the doctor subtly reinforces the idea that housework is desirable and that her participation in it should continue. If a man hears strong advice from his doctor about appropriate behaviors in marriage, family life, drinking, and smoking, the patient carries away the idea that deviance in these areas is undesirable.

Doctors' messages of ideology and social control arise within sincere, but usually uncritical, attempts to help people cope with contextual problems. Such messages guide patients gently into behaviors that are consistent with traditional expectations about work, the family, and other social roles. By speaking this way, and by not criticizing the social context, doctors reinforce unspoken notions about what constitutes a healthy lifestyle. Moreover, especially in remarks about self-destructive behaviors like smoking, drinking, drug abuse, and dangerous recreational activities (which increasingly include sexual activities), doctors convey notions about prevention. Such notions of preventive medicine, whose benefits appear straightforward, often lead patients to act in ways that are socially less troublesome. In short, through messages of ideology and social control, and through lack of contextual criticism, health professionals subtly direct patients' actions to conform with society's dominant expectations about appropriate behavior.

THE PROBLEM OF CONSENT
AND THE MICROPOLITICS OF MEDICINE

Ideology and social control in medical encounters also pertain to the problem of consent. Why do people consent to social patterns that they find oppressive and that make them unhappy? For many reasons, we accept parts of our lives that cause us grief. In the late twentieth century, obvious and familiar tyrannies remain with us. They range from the threat of nuclear holocaust, which colors daily life, to dictatorial regimes that survive around the world. "Democratic" governments maintain sophisticated domestic policing institutions, while they intervene in foreign countries to protect economic and political interests. Equally oppressive and familiar is the persistence of discrimination based on race, sex, age, and handicap.

Yet more subtle mechanisms also win consent to the status quo. Television, radio, movies, newspapers, and magazines convey stabilizing images and ideologies of desirable behavior. Schools and families reinforce these principles. Such noncoercive institutions have become more important than coercive arrangements for winning consent on a long-term basis, since they lead to internalization of stability and control at the level of individual consciousness.[2]

The helping professions play a part in this scenario. Doctors, lawyers, social workers, psychologists—these and other well-meaning professionals—assist their clients in dealing with the everyday realities of social life. Clients either continue their way of life or make changes, with professional guidance. Such advice helps people get along in the world. By turning to professionals, many people feel that they can become healthier, more content, more productive, or at least better able to cope.

Professional-client encounters are not the only way that order is achieved in society, but they are one way. When patients present problems that have roots in the social context, doctors generally offer some form of assistance but rarely express contextual criticism. Efforts to change contextual sources of unhappiness currently are not expected outcomes of doctor-patient encounters, even when physical problems derive in large part from the social context. By easing the physical or psychological impact of these difficulties, or by influencing patients' behavior through messages of ideology and social control, medical discourse helps gain patients' consent to social conditions. Medicine's impact in achieving consent, of course, is merely one of its many achievements. Moreover, other institutions may be more important than medicine in winning a population's acquiescence to current social arrangements. Nevertheless, the subtle part that medicine plays in the scenario of consent is probably more pervasive than usually recognized.

Seen in this light, doctor-patient encounters become micropolitical situations that reflect and support broader social relations, including social class and political-economic power. The participants in these encounters seldom recognize their micropolitical situation on a conscious level. To some degree, doctors and patients may experience frustration when contextual concerns arise and when they feel that their attempts to deal with them remain unsatisfactory. Yet even this discomfort is rarely mentioned as doctors and patients talk.

A contradiction therefore arises in the doctor-patient relationship. While most health professionals doubtless want to help their patients, the micropolitics of medical encounters limit doctors' capacities to respond to their patients' contextual difficulties. The contradiction between the professional commitment to help and medicine's limited ability to deal with contextual problems is a subtle one that rarely gains attention in medical encounters. A similar contradiction predictably arises in other "helping professions," such as social work, psychology, and law.[3]

Such micropolitics of medicine and similar helping professions have become apparent during the late twentieth century, especially in the United States and some other advanced capitalist nations. At earlier times and in other places, the characteristics of doctor-patient encounters have appeared quite different. Likewise, the future will probably produce new kinds of medical micropolitics. In short, the discourse described here remains a historically specific phenomenon, rather than a universal and unchanging one. The medical mediation of social problems, as it occurs in contemporary North America, need not stay always and everywhere the same, and this is a cause for hope.

In this chapter, I have asked how health professionals deal with social problems. Illustrating with three doctor-patient encounters, I have focused on the social context that patients bring with them when they seek help from physicians. Criticism of the social context is unlikely to arise in medical discourse. On the other hand, messages of ideology and social control become apparent, usually without reaching doctors' and patients' conscious awareness. Encounters with doctors help patients consent to social conditions, by softening the physical or psychological effects of contextual problems, or by encouraging adherence to customary expectations about desirable behavior. Doctor-patient encounters thus tend to become micropolitical situations that do not typically foster change in contextual sources of patients' difficulties. Documenting how these processes occur in actual encounters is one of my goals in later chapters of this book.

Such a vision of medical discourse inevitably raises questions of reform. If doctor-patient encounters currently do not address contextual problems very well, how could things go better? The reform of medical discourse should begin to resolve the contradiction between medicine's intent to help and its limited capacity to modify social context. Such improvements, I will argue, demand radically different professional-client relationships, as well as basic changes in society. A reformed medical discourse would deal with contextual difficulties, but without further increasing doctors' power and the medicalization of nonmedical problems. After considering current examples of medical discourse, I offer in the book's concluding chapter some suggestions for short-range and long-range reform. But first, it will be helpful to think further about the medical encounter from a theoretical point of view.

CHAPTER 2

THEORETICAL
APPROACHES
TO MEDICAL
ENCOUNTERS

Why look at medical encounters from a theoretical point of view?

More than a quarter of a century ago, the sociologist C. Wright Mills analyzed the relationships between "personal troubles" and "social issues." Mills pointed out that the troubles a person experiences arise in the context of broader social problems. According to Mills, an individual's difficulties are almost always interconnected with structures in society, although these links may not be obvious on the surface. Mills argued that an important goal for people concerned with social problems—those with what he called "the sociological imagination"—is to clarify how personal troubles and social issues relate to one another.[1]

In the intimacy of the medical encounter, patients present to their doctors a variety of personal troubles. From Mills' perspective, these troubles often have roots in social issues that go beyond the individual level. Yet the social issues themselves tend not to receive critical attention in conversations between patients and doctors. In trying to help their patients, doctors often find ways that patients can adjust to troubling social conditions.

Seen from this vantage point, medical encounters are "micro-level" processes that involve the interaction of individuals. These interpersonal processes, however, occur in a social context, which is shaped by "macro-level" structures in society. For example, when patients and doctors discuss problems at work, they take their bearings from the organization of work in the society, social expectations about work, social class relations pertaining to work, and so forth. Similarly, when problems pertaining to family life arise in medical encounters, the conversation must deal in some way with such issues as women's and men's roles in the family, expectations about reproduction and the maintenance of households, and social patterns affecting children, elderly people, and individuals at different stages of the life cycle. Patients also raise other kinds of social problems when they talk with their doctors, and macro-level structures in the society shape the context of those problems as well.

One challenge for social theory has been to clarify how macro-level social structures and micro-level processes affect one another. Many schools of thought have dealt with this theoretical challenge. Some theorists have argued for the importance of macro-level structures like social class and political power in determining what happens in interpersonal processes at the micro level. Others have claimed that micro-level processes are primary, and that macro-level structures emerge only as a reflection (similar terms include "integration," "aggregation," "gloss," "repetition," and "transformation") of micro-level processes occurring routinely in everyday life. A compromise position holds that macro-level structures profoundly influence interpersonal processes, but that micro-level processes cumulatively reinforce social structures at the macro level as well.[2]

In this chapter, I do not hope to resolve this theoretical debate, but rather to explore how the macro and micro levels impinge on each other in the single institutional sphere of medicine. When patients and doctors talk with each other about social problems, their words have much to do with the social order around them. Structures of society help generate the specific social context in which patients and doctors find themselves. The talk that occurs in medical encounters also may reinforce broader social structures. In exploring the interconnections between personal troubles and social issues, and between the micro and macro levels, I first build on the work of prior theorists to deal with the issue of medical ideology. I then examine social control by professionals in their encounters with clients. Afterward, I ask how the language of medical encounters pertains to the social context of medicine.

MEDICAL IDEOLOGY

Ideology, while difficult to define simply, is in general an interlocking set of ideas and doctrines that form the distinctive perspective of a social group. Through such ideas and doctrines, ideology represents—on an imaginary level—individuals' relationship to the real conditions of their existence.[3] This imaginary quality of ideology, which patterns how individuals perceive and interpret their experiences, contributes to ideology's impact in society. As it helps shape a population's perceptions and interpretations, ideology can achieve a most profound effect on social life.

One of this book's central concerns involves ideology in medical encounters. As a macro-level structure in society, ideology impinges on patients and doctors as part of their social context. At the micro level of interpersonal interaction, elements of ideology appear in doctor-patient communication. What patients and doctors say when they meet reinforces their particular ideologic conceptions about the social conditions that they experience. Although ideology has received wide attention in social theory, several previous theoretical contributions are helpful for clarifying ideology in medicine. By presenting these perspectives on ideology, my purpose is to emphasize those theoretical strands that shed light on ideologic processes in medical encounters.

Ideology, work, and the family: perspectives from early Marxist theory. In classic Marxist theory, ideology is an important though inconsistently developed notion. According to the principle of economic determinacy, the events of history emerge chiefly from economic forces and the conflicting relations of social class. From this viewpoint, economic forces affect the ideologies of a specific historical period. Despite the primacy of economic forces, ideology is crucial in sustaining and reproducing the social relations of production, and especially patterns of domination. Marx called attention to the mechanisms by which ideology reinforces capitalist relations of production and the interests of the capitalist class.[4] While ideologies arise in many different areas, including religion, law, aesthetics, and politics, early Marxist analyses did not discuss in depth the ideologic components of medicine.[5]

The Marxist perspective, however, leads to questions about how elements of ideology in medical encounters relate to economic behavior. Ideologic conceptions of work, as they are transmitted in doctor-patient interaction, reflect more general ideologic notions about economic activities in a given society. When they are spoken in medical encounters, these notions reinforce a society's dominant ideologic conceptions about the nature of work and of economic production. For instance, among the many definitions of "health" that have appeared during the twentieth century, modern medicine in practice has emphasized an interpretation of health as the ability to work.[6] There are several ways that this view of health has been reinforced and diffused in the population. The public health policies that large philanthropies and government agencies have initiated in the United States and other countries have consistently stressed the importance of a healthy work force.[7] Images of health conveyed by the mass media also support the symbolism of health as the capacity to do productive work.[8] These images communicate a message that the healthy person is one who produces economically. Moreover, a widely touted standard by which to judge medicine's "cost-effectiveness" involves its contribution to patients' subsequent work productivity.[9]

Doctor-patient interaction, I shall argue, reinforces this same definition of health as the ability to work. In certain encounters with patients, doctors communicate explicitly or subtly a message that work is preferable to idleness. When people become sick, they often stop working, and doctors get involved in this process in several ways. Frequently, doctors certify that a patient is physically disabled and thus unable to work. By the certification of disability, a doctor in effect decides when a patient must return to the job. When judging the seriousness of a patient's complaints, a doctor investigates whether the patient's problems interfere with work. Doctors write letters to employers, insurance companies, and government agencies about patients' work limitations and discuss this correspondence to a greater or lesser degree with the patients themselves. During their routine talk with patients, doctors inevitably convey some attitude about work, usually to encourage patients' continued performance on the job. In these instances and many others, the impact of the doctors' words is to define health as the capacity to work productively.

The family becomes a second focus for ideologic elements in medical encounters, and theorists in the Marxist tradition have emphasized the connections between the family and economic production. For example, Engels claimed that the family, by "propagation of the species," plays a key role in reproducing the labor force. Women's subordinate position in the family, according to Engels, contributes to the family's reproductive role.[10] However, the family's importance goes beyond the physical reproduction of labor. The family also helps reproduce the ideologic framework of the economic system. For instance, patterns of sexuality and child rearing in the family reinforce personality characteristics and attitudes that tend to accept hierarchies of class and authority. By sustaining such patterns, Engels argues, the family becomes an important institution for ideologic reproduction, which helps achieve the population's acquiescence to and participation in current relations of economic production.

Medicine also mediates the family's reproductive role. As noted already, medicine tends to view health as the ability to work. A secondary and related definition is that health is the ability to reproduce labor. Women's activities as homemakers, wives, and mothers are crucial in the family's reproductive activities. Even when women do not work outside the home, they often care for working husbands and for children who later will take part in production and reproduction. Although a greater proportion of women have entered the labor force since World War II, they still face the social expectation that they remain primarily responsible for these reproductive activities. That is, "healthy" women do these things, and doctors predictably aid at least some women in sustaining their reproductive capabilities. For their male clients, doctors also may concern themselves with the stability of family relations. With both men and women, adequate functioning in familial responsibilities thus becomes another criterion in doctors' assessment of health. As discussed later in this chapter, doctors during the twentieth century have joined other expert professionals who increasingly have regulated family life. How the doctor-patient interaction conveys ideologic notions about the family is a question of some interest.

Later theories of ideology. The examples of work and the family lead to a consideration of how certain other theorists—Gramsci, Lukács, Althusser, and Habermas—have treated the question of ideology. A unifying theme among these theoretical positions, all of which are influenced by classical Marxism, is that ideology serves as a subtle mechanism which helps win a population's consent to the ways a society is organized. In addition, these theorists emphasize that ideology helps maintain the economic system and that supporting institutions like the family are key elements in reproducing a society's dominant ideologic patterns. Although the theorists to be considered do not deal specifically with medical encounters, one purpose of reviewing these theories is to apply them to the question of ideology in medicine.

From Gramsci's viewpoint, groups in power use two types of sociopolitical control to maintain and reproduce relations of economic production.[11] First, there is direct coercion; by holding the legal means of violence—in the armed forces, police, prisons, courts, and related institutions—the state protects the established order partly through force and repression. However, Gramsci claims, no regime can hold power for long periods of time strictly by authoritarian rule. Ideologic "hegemony," according to Gramsci, is a second and ultimately more important mechanism of control. Such institutions as the schools, churches, mass media, and family inculcate a system of values, attitudes, beliefs, and morality. This ideologic system supports the established order and the class interests that dominate it. The same ideologic forces achieve consent and mute resistance from disadvantaged groups.

While Gramsci does not consider the ideologic impact of medicine, a similar theoretical perspective would ask to what extent medicine reinforces the dominant ideologic system of a society. When doctors convey ideologic notions about desirable behavior, especially as these notions help shape patients' roles in work and the family, medical encounters contribute to the broader hegemonic impact of ideology. In this sense, medicine exerts ideologic effects that parallel those of such institutions as schools, churches, and the mass media.

Lukács' conceptions of class consciousness and reification also are pertinent to medicine's ideologic impact.[12] Regarding class consciousness, Lukács, like Gramsci, explores how a society's dominant ideologies are conveyed and reinforced. In discussing literature and other forms of cultural expression, Lukács emphasizes the ways that these materials both reflect and strengthen broad ideologic patterns. According to Lukács, such ideologic patterns shape the consciousness of individuals and, cumulatively, of social classes. In this process, the *totality* of social relations in an entire society becomes mystified and blocked from conscious thought. Reification, Lukács argues, involves the transformation of social relations into things or "thing-like" beings that take on their own separate reality in people's consciousness. Shaped by ideology, consciousness focuses on the concrete problems and objects of everyday life, especially economic commodities, rather than on the totality of social relations that lie behind these routine concerns. Through reification, as attention becomes focused on the concrete objects of daily life, the totality of social relations escapes conscious attention.

Reification contributes to the impact of medicine. In medical encounters, technical statements help direct patients' responses to objectified symptoms, signs, and treatments. This reification shifts attention away from the totality of social relations and the social issues that often cause personal troubles. Instead, attention gets paid to problems of individual pathophysiology and personality. By reifying problematic social relations, medicine reduces the potentiality for effectively criticizing those relations. Symptoms, signs, and treatments take on an aura of scientific fact, rather than of subjective manifestations of a troubled social reality. The medical processing of social problems invests them with the symbolism of objects, relatively immune from criticism or change. This same process constricts the level of attention to the disturbed individual, rather than social structures impinging on the individual. For instance, when the organization of work or tension in the family creates personal distress, expression of that distress in a medical encounter tends to reify the social structural roots of the problem. Under these circumstances, it is the objectified symptom or sign that requires treatment—not the institutional sources of individual distress.

Influenced by Gramsci and Lukács, Althusser further analyzes the structures of control in modern societies. Althusser considers the interconnections among repressive and ideologic institutions, as well as their relationships to government.[13] Repressive state apparatuses (RSAs), Althusser argues, include the army, police, prisons, courts, and other institutions that maintain control through violence or repression. Ideologic state apparatuses (ISAs) are institutions that instill dominant ideologies in the population. In Althusser's analysis, ISAs include the family, the legal system, electoral politics, mass media and communication systems, education, and cultural systems. RSAs are not purely repressive, nor are ISAs purely ideologic. Ideologies often legitimate the actions of RSAs. For example, justice and equality are ideologic notions that legitimate the functioning of the courts. Similarly, ISAs may use punishment for discipline, such as physical force or other forms of sanctioning that occur in the family or school system. Althusser argues that ISAs become especially important in reproducing class structure and the relations of economic production. According to Althusser, many social institutions—particularly the educational system—promulgate ideologies that assure the population's acquiescence to and participation in productive work.

Althusser's theoretical position has generated wide debate, the complexities of which are beyond my scope here. In brief, Althusser's interpretation of the state is open to criticism. For instance, he includes essentially all major social institutions within the state apparatus, through these institutions' repressive or ideologic effects. Thus, the state seems to merge into the rest of society. Despite the state's far-reaching impact, the inclusion of such a wide variety of social institutions as parts of the state apparatus becomes misleading. In addition, Althusser has received criticism for his tendency to diminish the possibility of meaningful political action by individuals. From the perspective of Althusser's structuralism, the state overshadows the capacity of individuals to assert themselves politically, and Althusser's critics often have disagreed with this viewpoint.

On the other hand, Althusser's analysis of the wide-ranging repressive and ideologic effects of many institutions in society, though controversial, pertains to medicine as well. In rare instances, medicine exerts directly repressive effects—as when physicians helped implement policies of genocide in Nazi concentration camps. Less obvious instances of medicine's repressive impact include doctors' roles in involuntary mental hospitalization, prison health care, capital punishment (in some cases administering lethal injections or otherwise assisting in executions), involuntary sterilization, and so forth.

Medicine's ideologic impact, however, doubtless becomes much more important than its repressive role. In their encounters with patients, doctors may interpret personal problems and encourage individual behaviors in directions that are consistent with a society's dominant ideologic patterns. From the perspective of Althusser's theory, when medical encounters convey a view of health as the ability to work, they encourage workers' participation in economic production. The doctor-patient interaction also predictably transmits notions about family life that strengthen the family's ideologic impact. In these ways, medicine exerts ideologic effects consistent with those of such institutions as the educational system and the mass media.

Another quite different theoretical approach also pertains to medical ideology. The "critical theory" of Habermas and other analysts of

the "Frankfurt School" provides a link between ideology and science—
and by extension, scientific medicine. Although Habermas' and Althusser's theories both have roots in classical Marxism, these two schools of
thought diverge in fundamental ways. In particular, the Frankfurt School
usually assumes that individuals have the capacity to reflect critically
about society and to take "purposive" political action; as noted above,
Althusser diminishes the potentiality for effective criticism and political
action by individuals. Both approaches, however, emphasize the impact
of ideology. While Althusser focuses on the ideologic effects of various
social institutions in reproducing the relations of production, Habermas
stresses the ideologic components of science.

For Habermas, science is ideology par excellence, precisely because it
claims to be above ideology—that is, objective and value-neutral. Habermas argues that scientific ideology has defined an increasing range of
problems as amenable to technical solutions. In this way, scientific ideology tends to depoliticize these social issues by removing them from
critical scrutiny.[14] According to Habermas, science legitimates current
patterns of domination, including class relations:

> Technocratic consciousness is, on the one hand, "less ideological"
> than all previous ideologies. . . . On the other hand today's domi-
> nant, rather glassy background ideology, which makes a fetish of
> science, is more irresistible and farther-reaching than ideologies of
> the old type. For with the veiling of practical problems it not only
> justifies a *particular class's* interest in domination and represses *an-*
> *other class's* partial need for emancipation, but affects the human
> race's emancipatory interest as such (emphasis in original).[15]

What are the specific processes by which scientific ideology provides
legitimation? One problem in Habermas' account is that it remains on an
abstract level and rarely grounds theoretical claims in empirical reality.
Habermas conveys an impression that scientific ideology creates legitimation through cultural symbols in the mass media, educational system,
and technical organization of the workplace. He also argues that ideology
and domination appear in the face-to-face interaction of individuals.
"Distorted communication," Habermas argues, arises in both the macro-
level realm of politics and the micro-level realm of interpersonal relationships. Domination creates distortion in communication, and undistorted
communication is impossible, according to Habermas, under conditions
of domination. In a major part of his project, Habermas encourages
resistance against domination and aims toward the creation of new, less
distorted forms of communication.[16] Concrete examples of scientific ideology, however, rarely appear in Habermas' work; for this reason, his
account remains abstract and utopian regarding directions of change. On
the other hand, his analysis causes one to look for specific instances of

scientific legitimation and distorted communication in face-to-face inter-action.

These considerations encompass medical encounters, to the extent that doctor-patient interactions convey ideologic messages under the rubric of scientific medicine. From Habermas' perspective, such messages legitimate current patterns in society and further depoliticize these issues by deflecting critical attention from them. In addition, medical interactions show features of distorted communication, fostered for instance by devices of language that reinforce professional domination. In actual encounters between patients and doctors, then, one can ask how and to what extent medical discourse transmits scientific ideology.

PROFESSIONAL SOCIAL CONTROL

Social control refers to mechanisms that achieve people's adherence to norms of appropriate behavior. In medicine, ideology and social control are closely related. When doctors transmit ideologic messages that reinforce current social patterns—at work, in the family, and in other areas of life—they help control behavior in ways that are defined as socially appropriate.

Dealing with problems outside the narrow realm of technical medicine tends to medicalize a wide range of psychological, social, economic, and political problems. Historically, many areas have gradually fallen under medical control. Examples include sexuality and family life, dissatisfaction with work, problems of the life cycle (including birth, adolescence, aging, dying, and death), difficulties in the educational system (learning disabilities, maladjustment, and students' psychological distress), environmental pollution, and many other fields. By participating in these areas, practitioners often believe that they are extending the caring function of the medical role.

On the other hand, medicalization has emerged as the object of a critique that focuses on health professionals' expanding role in social control. As medical management of social problems has increased, the societal roots of personal troubles have become less apparent. That is, by responding in limited ways to some of patients' nontechnical problems, medical practitioners tend to shift the focus of attention from societal issues to the troubles of individuals.[17]

The history of professional social control: Foucault. The intrusion of scientific discourse into many areas of social life has preoccupied Foucault in his work on the history of the professions. Through his studies of what he calls the "human sciences," Foucault has conveyed the connections between knowledge and power.[18] According to Foucault, as such professions as medicine, psychology, law, and social work have developed, they have taken on positions of control in everyday life. By describing the political role of the human sciences, Foucault has clarified how professional social control emerged historically.

While Foucault's early work traces the history of the medical profession's diagnostic and therapeutic ideas, his more recent studies of criminology emphasize how professional control has widened into everyday life.[19] Although modern punishment is more hidden than prior techniques like torture and public execution, Foucault argues, it orients itself to surveillance and professional control over the deviant population. Through new "technologies of power," according to Foucault, the criminologic profession has created what appears to be a humane reform over prior methods of gross corporal punishment. Further, he argues, the administrators of penal institutions have achieved surveillance over those who deviate from society's customary expectations. Most important from Foucault's viewpoint, criminology has become a standard for professional practices throughout society. According to Foucault, similar technologies of surveillance also have emerged to achieve professional power in mental institutions, hospitals and clinics, workplaces, and schools.[20] Foucault's examples show that social control has become more subtle, professionalized, and oriented to surveillance of deviant behavior.

Although Foucault's studies of prisons touch on medicine mainly by analogy, his work on sexuality pertains directly to medical encounters.[21] Foucault's colorful account of modern sexuality begins in the seventeenth century. Until that time, Foucault argues, religious institutions took an interest in sex, mainly through the confessional. When people confessed their sexual activities, priests commented on what liaisons and positions were appropriate and what actions required penance. After the Reformation and Counter-Reformation, according to Foucault, concern gradually shifted from bodily activities to thoughts, fantasies, intentions, and other mental processes related to sexuality. Especially during the nineteenth century, Foucault notes, surveillance and regulation of mental processes pertaining to sex became a preoccupation of science and particularly medicine. Professional practitioners then assumed a measure of control over the activities and psychologic meanings of sex.

In discussing sexuality, Foucault emphasizes professional discourse and links discourse to power. That is, what professionals have said about sexuality has deepened professional power in everyday life.[22] What previously was a concern for the clergy has become a challenge for professionals, who assume various degrees of control over their clients' sexual expression. Medical doctors mediate sex, according to Foucault, but so do psychoanalysts, social workers, educators, bureaucrats in social welfare agencies, and other professionals who lay claim to expert knowledge. The discourse through which professionals communicate their special knowledge, from Foucault's perspective, enhances their ability to intervene in and to control others' behavior.

Where does one find such professional discourse? Foucault of course looks for discourses on sex in the books, articles, and other documents that professionals have written and published. However, for Foucault, unpublished discourse is as important as publications in achieving professional power, if not more so. For this reason, a variety of materials become appropriate sources for study. These materials may include the brochures and files of medical institutions treating sexual disorders, the records of public welfare bureaucracies, therapists' notes, and professional correspondence concerning individuals who are considered deviant. Perhaps most important for the purposes here, one also may look for such discourse, whenever possible, in the face-to-face talk of professionals and their clients. Predictably, for instance, what doctors say to their patients about sex becomes a concrete expression of professional discourse and its power in daily life, probably to a greater extent than what doctors write about sex in textbooks and scientific articles.[23] Although Foucault refers to the usefulness of oral materials, however, he does not use them himself in developing his arguments.

While Foucault documents how professional practitioners of the human sciences have broadened their power in modern society, he develops no systematic theory of professional power and its relation to discourse. In fact, Foucault has maddened critics by his antitheoretical stance. Although Marxist theories, including those discussed earlier, have influenced Foucault, he has distanced himself from Marxism. For instance, while acknowledging the importance of material conditions and ideology, he has refused to identify his own treatment of these themes with a particular theoretical school. Likewise, for Foucault, power derives more from technical knowledge than from the economic resources that Marxists emphasize. The intellectual underpinnings of Foucault's antitheoretical stance emerge from a broader critique of theory, which argues against the primacy of reason and against the ability of a writer to arrive at a conclusive theoretical position. Otherwise, from this view, a theorist could propound a discourse that might potentially be as damaging as the very discourses Foucault criticizes in his own studies.

This theoretical modesty, however, leaves the reader hanging on some key issues. For instance, what is the best way to select and to interpret specific examples of medical discourse? How should discourse be treated if it does not convey the general orientation described? How should variability in discourse be handled? Further, how might these problems of professional power and discourse be improved? Foucault implies that the growth of professional control deserves resistance. But just as he declines to specify his theory or method, he does not spell out how change might occur.[24]

On the unintentionality of medical social control. As noted earlier, social control in medicine is generally an unintended process, dimly if at all perceived by participants in doctor-patient encounters. Health professionals seldom consciously view their activities as contributing to social control. In listening to words of distress from their clients, for instance, doctors usually do not see their responsibility as preserving the current organization of economic production or the stability of the family. Nonetheless, by focusing on individual troubles rather than on social issues, doctor-patient encounters may reinforce the social order as presently constituted. Why do these processes tend to occur without the participants' conscious awareness?

To help explain the unintentionality of medical social control, one may look first to the class origins and position of health professionals. Since the beginning of the twentieth century, the vast majority of doctors have come from upper-middle-class or corporate-class families. In 1920, 12 percent of North American medical students came from working-class families, and this percentage has stayed almost exactly the same until the present.[25] The extremely limited recruitment of doctors from working-class families has persisted despite recent increases in the proportion of women and racial minorities entering the profession. For the small numbers with working-class roots, as for the rest of the profession, the acquired class position of physicians is one of relative privilege. Their predominantly comfortable life-style does not encourage professionals to criticize the social structural roots of their clients' distress, especially the sources of suffering in class structure. Instead, professionals' life experiences predictably lead them to help clients adjust to things as they are.

Professional education and socialization further contribute to the unintentionality of medical social control. A critique of social oppression, needless to say, is seldom part of the medical school curriculum. On the contrary, professionals in training receive many lessons about individual pathophysiology and treatment. Within progressive instructional programs, trainees hear information about emotional disturbances and social problems. But this training consistently emphasizes the importance of psychologic and social knowledge in responding to the needs of the individual patient. Such an approach seeks to help the patient cope with stresses arising in work, the family, and other key institutions. Even in its more progressive and enlightened versions, then, professional education does not foster social criticism or social change as part of the medical mission.

Situational constraints also leave medical social control below the level of consciousness. When a client is in trouble, a professional usually feels that something should be done. Yet the professional also senses the limits of what he or she as an individual can do. For instance, when a patient's symptoms reflect stress at work, a doctor tends to feel that changing the workplace is beyond the responsibility or even the capability of the medical role. With rare exceptions, such as those involving physical abuse, disruption of familial relations is not an appropriate goal of medical intervention. Wanting to help but unable personally to change the social structure, a health professional typically seeks a solution within the existing institutional context. Relaxation techniques, tranquilizers, counseling, family therapy, and related methods all become feasible approaches for the professional who wants to do something. For a patient in crisis, a doctor cannot do everything. What can be done tends to encourage coping and accommodation. Conscious recognition of these choices, or consideration of more critical alternatives, seldom occurs.

These situational constraints contribute to the generally conservative effects of the medical role. On the one hand, medical discourse usually does not attend to institutional causes of suffering. This orientation leads health professionals to overlook social change as a possible therapeutic option. On the other hand, when doctors do consider institutional problems in their encounters with patients, the intervention frequently serves to support the status quo. When a professional encourages mechanisms of coping and adjustment, this communication conveys a subtle political content. By seeking limited modifications in social roles—at work and in the family, for instance—which preserve a particular institution's overall stability, the practitioner exerts a conservative political impact.[26] Despite the best conscious intents, the practitioner thus helps reproduce the same institutional structures that form the roots of personal anguish. This contradiction is one source of pathos in the helping professions.

Medical social control also involves the management of potentially troublesome emotions. Doctors, for instance, regularly deal with patients' anger, anxiety, unhappiness, social isolation, loneliness, depression, and other emotional distress. Often these feelings derive in one way or another from patients' social circumstances, including economic insecurity, racial or sexual discrimination, occupational stress, and difficulties in family life. Such emotions, of course, may become one basis of political outrage and organized resistance. How health professionals manage these sentiments is an interesting question. One of medicine's effects may be the defusing of socially caused distress. Medicine is not the only institution in which such processes occur, nor do these phenomena necessarily occupy a major part of medical encounters. Still, it is worth asking how such largely unintentional, micro-level processes take place in practice.

THE LANGUAGE OF MEDICAL ENCOUNTERS

In adapting prior theories to medical encounters, I also want to point ahead to the next chapter, in which I present a new theory of medical discourse. Ideology and social control are essential features of that the-

ory, but so is the nature of language. Before spelling out the theory, I need
to look more closely at how language is used in medical encounters, as
revealed by studies in the fields of sociolinguistics, conversation analysis,
and discourse analysis.[27]

First, differences in language use among social classes pattern the
ways that professionals and clients either deal with, or exclude from
verbal consideration, the social roots of personal troubles.[28] Within the
medical encounter, the linguistic performance of working-class patients
may not lend itself to developing verbally such linkages between individual distress and social issues. Because of class-based sociolinguistic differences, working-class patients tend to take little verbal initiative in questioning and directing doctors' attention to matters of concern, including
sources of suffering in the social context. Working-class patients are also
less likely than middle-class clients to express verbal disagreement with
physicians who hold a higher class position. From this perspective, one
expects that the patterning of ideology and social control in medical
encounters varies, depending partly on the class positions of the participants.

Beyond such class differences, the language of medical encounters
contains common structural features. For instance, in an analysis of
doctor-patient conversations, West has found typical "troubles" that arise
in encounters.[29] When patients express concerns about events in their
lives that are not amenable to doctors' technical intervention, West argues, questions and interruptions are mechanisms by which doctors
steer patients' concerns back to a technical track. As West notes, other
studies also have observed that doctors interrupt patients frequently and
initiate more questions than patients do. In West's tape-recorded sample
of medical interactions, male doctors tended to interrupt patients more
often than did female doctors. West interprets interruptions and frequent
questioning as gestures of dominance, by which doctors control the flow
of conversation. She also postulates a connection between social power
and sexual differences in language use, both generally in conversations
and more specifically in professional-client encounters.

By questioning, by interrupting, and by otherwise shifting the direction of conversation from nontechnical problems to technical ones, doctors *exclude* certain topics from talk and *include* others. Of particular
interest here are the verbal techniques that divert attention from sources
of personal distress in the social context. Such techniques cut off the
possibility of considering the context critically, let alone changing it.
How medical encounters convey ideologic messages, and how they
invoke social control, sometimes involves doctors' explicit pronouncements about what patients should or should not do. It is also likely that
ideology and social control emerge from what doctors and patients exclude from their talk, and how it comes to be excluded.

In another study of medical encounters, Mishler demonstrates how medical discourse cuts off contextual issues and redirects the focus to technical concerns.[30] Mishler presents transcripts from my own recordings of doctor-patient communication and describes two "voices" that compete with each other. The "voice of medicine" involves the technical topics (of physiology, pathology, pharmacology, and so forth) that concern doctors in their professional work. Alternatively, the "voice of the lifeworld" comprises the everyday, largely nontechnical problems that patients carry with them into the medical encounter. According to Mishler's analysis of transcripts, patients often try to raise contextual issues through the voice of the lifeworld. Doctors, however, are ill-equipped to deal with such issues and therefore repeatedly return to the voice of medicine. For instance, patients raise personal troubles that do not pertain to technical problems. Or, these personal troubles, although related to technical problems, do not seem amenable to technical solutions. Or, the raising of personal troubles leads to discomfort for the professional, the client, or both. Under these circumstances, doctors typically introject questions, interrupt, or otherwise change the topic, to return to the voice of medicine.

Although Mishler's approach conveys how medical language encourages the saying of some things and the leaving unsaid of others, the "lifeworld" remains rather general. Mishler implies that patients' concerns about contextual issues in the lifeworld are very important to them and that cutting off these concerns is undesirable. When the voice of medicine gains sway, however, this achievement has much to do with ideology and social control. In diverting critical attention away from the lifeworld, doctors subtly reinforce the ideas that pattern the lifeworld and help win acquiescence to those features of the lifeworld that patients find most disconcerting. In short, a rereading of Mishler's materials might emphasize that the voice of medicine not only tends to suppress the voice of the lifeworld but also reinforces the lifeworld's orderliness in its present form.

What is left unsaid or hidden in medical encounters has fascinated other researchers, who have interpreted rich textual materials using little or no contextual theory. For instance, Katz provides an extensive account of the "silent world" of the doctor-patient relationship.[31] He shows how medical language overlooks or downplays some important features of doctors' and patients' experiences. Thus, Katz argues, doctors tend to gloss over their patients' concerns, and patients tend to leave these concerns unsaid. In Katz's account, doctors and patients tend to remain silent about many topics, especially those that would require patients' informed consent in such spheres as cancer treatment and intensive care. Similarly, Cassell gives a thorough interpretation of confusions, misunderstandings, insensitivities, and communication lapses in transcripts of doctor-patient interactions. He reiterates a viewpoint frequently expressed—that doctors in training should learn better communication skills to avoid such gaffes in practice.[32] Commenting on the unsaid socioemotional content of medical encounters, Cassell urges that health practitioners pay more attention to what is excluded from conversation, as well as the reasons why.

These accounts of the unsaid in medical language—based in the fields of sociolinguistics, conversation analysis, and discourse analysis—do not emphasize enough the pertinence of the unsaid for the context of professional encounters. In chapter 4, I raise other methodologic problems with work in these fields. Meanwhile, it is enough to say that doctors do not simply overlook or downplay or suppress patients' contextual concerns. The exclusion of social context from critical attention is a fundamental feature of medical language, a feature that is linked with ideology and social control. Inattention to social issues, especially when these issues lie behind patients' personal troubles, can never be just a matter of professional inadequacy, or the inadequacy of professional training. Instead, this *lack* is a basic part of what medicine *is* in our society.

This chapter has asked, why look at medical encounters from a theoretical point of view? I have argued that the personal troubles which patients bring to doctors often have roots in social issues beyond medicine. Further, I have claimed that the micro-level processing in medical discourse of these macro-level issues is a phenomenon of some importance. Moving toward a critical theory of medical discourse in the next chapter, I have examined previous theoretical works that prove helpful in thinking about medical encounters. These prior theories have led to further claims: that at least some medical encounters convey ideologic messages supportive of the current social order; that these encounters yield repercussions for social control; and that medical language tends to exclude a critical appraisal of the social context. All such effects are usually subtle, often hidden, and generally unconscious phenomena that arise in communication between people whose intentions are beyond reproach.

In the next chapter, I ask if spoken medical discourse can be read and analyzed as a text. In answering yes, I will rely on some developments in critical theory that offer a useful framework for understanding professional encounters.

CHAPTER 3

A CRITICAL THEORY OF MEDICAL DISCOURSE

Before asking if medical discourse can be read as a text, I want to ask another question, which will both begin and end this chapter: Does medical discourse have a typical structure? First, I summarize the medical encounter's structure as traditionally seen by health professionals. Then I move behind this traditional view to search out a deeper structure that may have little to do with professionals' conscious thoughts about what they are saying and doing.[1]

THE TRADITIONAL FORMAT OF THE MEDICAL ENCOUNTER

The traditional format of the medical encounter is as follows:

Chief complaint (CC) → present illness (PI) → past history (PH) → family history (FH) → social history (SH) → systems review (SR) → physical examination (PE) → other investigations (OI) → diagnosis (Dx) → plan (P).

During a typical encounter, the doctor tries to cover some or all of these components in his or her spoken interaction with and examination of the patient. In addition, the doctor provides a written version of the encounter, in the medical record. There, the doctor usually labels each component of the encounter with the same abbreviations that I use here. This traditional format appears in most textbooks that provide instruction on clinical methods for trainees and practitioners of medicine. Research on doctor-patient communication also has confirmed that medical practitioners actually do use the traditional structure as an organizing framework for their encounters with patients.[2]

To define and to comment on each of these elements, I will focus first on the components of the medical history (Hx), which comprises CC, PI, PH, FH, SH, and SR in the above scheme. In the chief complaint (CC), the physician elicits what is troubling the patient, in the briefest possible terms. The physician leads into the CC usually with an opening question like: "Hello, what brings you in today?" or "Well, what's bothering you today?" or "How can I help you?" To these or similar questions, the patient might answer, "Headaches," or "My back hurts," or "I've got pain in my chest," or "I can't sleep," or "I want a check-up," and so forth. In asking for the CC, the physician seeks to bring out the patient's foremost concern.

Through the present illness (PI), the patient elaborates on the CC. He or she tells the doctor when the problem began, what the specific characteristics of the symptoms are, which medications or other measures relieve the symptoms, what prior medical attention he or she has received for the problem, and similar details that may contribute to the doctor's attempts to reach a diagnosis. Eliciting the CC and PI purportedly is the greatest skill that doctors develop in taking a medical history; some commentators argue that this is the most important skill in medicine. Doctors in training presumably learn a comfortable and effective balance between open-ended listening to the patient's story and more directive questioning that clarifies the patient's problem in terms of medical diagnoses.

Interruptions by doctors commonly begin to occur during the PI. Such interruptions are basically attempts to curtail storytelling by patients, for the following reasons (among others): the story may not contribute to the doctor's cognitive process of reaching a diagnosis; the patient's version of the story may be confusing or inconsistent; telling the story may take more time than is perceived to be available; or parts of the story may create feelings that are uncomfortable for the doctor, the patient, or both. The circumstances under which the doctor interrupts the patient's story to focus the PI—that is, what is interrupted, when it is interrupted, what reason is given for the interruption, and so forth—are important, especially to the extent that they cut off concerns about the social context of the medical encounter. Predictably, the PI is a critical juncture, during which certain elements, though they may be quite important in the patient's experience, come to be excluded from discourse, while other elements are included.

What is the relationship between the spoken PI and the version that the doctor writes in the medical record?[3] Although writing a comprehensible PI may involve skillful effort by a doctor, its orderliness invariably gives a false sense of what happens during the spoken PI. For example, the doctor never writes, "I interrupted the patient at this point," or "I thought the patient's comments about his family here weren't pertinent to his pain, so I asked him about what medications he was taking," or "I was in a hurry to get my daughter from child care so I cut off the patient at this point," and so forth. Instead, the written PI represents the doctor's interpretation of a disorderly series of spoken exchanges. The orderliness of the written version belies what actually gets said during the PI, which is my chief focus here. This is not to say that the written PI is uninteresting, and others have documented the substantial differences in content between the spoken and written versions.[4] However, I am mainly concerned with the spoken PI in all its disorderliness.

While the CC and PI are almost always present in medical encounters (assuming the patient is awake and conversant), other components may appear or not, depending on time, the doctor's desire to complete a comprehensive evaluation, such financial issues as the patient's insurance and how extensive an evaluation it permits, and other situational constraints. A doctor may choose to defer some or all of the remaining components to future visits, or may not cover them at all, although there is usually some attempt initially to develop a diagnosis and plan.

In the past history (PH), the doctor gathers information about past medical events in the patient's life that are not directly pertinent to the PI. This information typically includes prior hospitalizations and surgery, other major illnesses, medications, allergies, immunizations, smoking and drinking habits, and use of recreational substances.

The family history (FH) includes data about illnesses and deaths in the patient's immediate family: mother, father, sisters, brothers, spouse, and children. Additionally, in this section many doctors routinely elicit information about family occurrences of cancer, heart disease, hypertension, diabetes mellitus, and other common problems that may carry an increased risk in certain families.

Although one might expect the social history (SH) to be important for a contextual analysis of medical encounters, it is usually a perfunctory listing of demographic data. For instance, the doctor typically asks about birthplace, occupation, educational attainment, living situation, and insurance status. The contextual concerns that pertain to a patient's distress usually appear, subject to interruption and curtailment, during the PI, rather than the SH. In the SH itself, the doctor traditionally tends not to pursue in much depth how the patient's social circumstances might relate to the difficulties for which he or she is seeking medical attention.

Presumably, the purpose of the systems review (SR) is to elicit any additional information about the patient that might be left out or missed by other parts of the history. The SR is sometimes very brief and sometimes quite lengthy; scuttlebutt among medical practitioners has it that the SR's length is inversely related to clinical experience. The expectation, however, is that the doctor will ask the patient whether he or she has experienced symptoms in each of the following organ systems: skin, lymph nodes, head, eyes, ears, nose, throat, neck, respiratory system, cardiovascular system, gastrointestinal system, genitourinary system, reproductive system, neurologic system, endocrine system, and musculoskeletal system. For instance, under the gastrointestinal system, the doctor would question about symptoms or prior conditions of the esophagus (principally swallowing), stomach (heartburn, ulcers, cancer, and so forth), duodenum, small intestine, large intestine (irregularity in bowel habits, bleeding, infections), rectum (hemorrhoids, fissures, bleeding), liver (jaundice, hepatitis, toxic exposures), and pancreas. In other words, the SR can be quite exhaustive, even more so if the patient happens to be a "yea-sayer." Then, doctor and patient enter potentially endless labyrinths of questions and answers, leading to frustrating excursions through a welter of symptoms and diseases that have little to do with the current purposes of the medical encounter. Gradual recognition of these pitfalls during a medical career accounts for the exhaustive efforts that medical students devote to the SR, while their supervising physicians often truncate the SR to a very brief series of questions, for which they do not expect to hear *yes* as an answer.

The physical examination (PE) involves the laying on of hands, whose impact in medicine has been so highly touted. Without intimate touch, medical interaction would not differ nearly so much from other types of commonplace interactions. Often doctors wait until completing the medical history before they begin the PE, although many experienced practitioners continue to ask questions about the history during the PE and even after it is completed. If time is available, a doctor will examine the body's entire external surface during the PE, as well as within its orifices. When time is not available, or if the doctor is not inclined toward comprehensiveness, he or she does a more focused PE, concentrating on those parts of the body that might be related to the CC and PI.

After the PE, the doctor sometimes initiates one or more other investigations (OI)—laboratory tests, x-rays, electrocardiograms, and so forth—whose purported aim is to clarify the diagnosis or to gather data that may be useful for treatment or prevention. OIs also seem to communicate something. Specifically, they may convey an impression of thoroughness and concern. A scientifically oriented intervention may be reassuring because of the technical knowledge it presumably reflects. Further, when an OI leads to a negative finding, it doubtless produces a feeling of relief and well-being. In fact, one research study has shown that normal results lead to improvement in symptoms, even when OIs are not ordered for a specific clinical reason from a doctor's point of view.[5] Thus, a doctor's act of recommending an OI may have several meanings in a medical encounter, aside from the specific results that are obtained.

With the data gleaned from the various components of the medical history, the PE, and the results of OIs, the doctor reaches a diagnosis (Dx), which may be provisional or confirmed. The cognitive operations involved in making a diagnosis undoubtedly are complex, and they are poorly understood. Essentially, the doctor takes the patients' comments in the medical history, the observations made during the PE, and data from OIs, and shapes this information into one or more diagnostic categories.

The drive to reach a diagnosis is extremely strong. Practitioners and doctors in training view facility of diagnostic categorization as one of the most important professional skills in medicine. The "differential diagnosis" involves a list of all possible categories into which a patient's physical problems might fall. Most practitioners would acknowledge that the tendencies to interrupt, cut off, or otherwise redirect the patient's story during the PI derive at least partly from the drive to make a diagnosis. That is, a doctor wants to hear those words that are consistent with previously defined diagnostic categories. Parts of patients' stories that do not fit neatly into these categories function as unwanted strangers in medical discourse and tend to be shown to the door.[6]

Diagnostic reasoning tends to be limited and exclusionary. True, doctors and doctors-in-training must learn to deal with an awesome number of diagnostic categories and subcategories. On the other hand, it would be presumptuous to assume that this set of diagnoses corresponds to more than a tiny fraction of human experience. In large part, the cognitive process of reaching a diagnosis involves excluding a substantial part of a patient's experience that—no matter how relevant to the patient—is not relevant to the diagnosis. Features of patients' social context may be very troubling to patients and may affect their physical conditions in fairly direct ways. These contextual issues, however, are almost always difficult to define with precision, are loaded with ambiguity, and are not completely consistent with the technical categories of differential diagnosis. The exclusionary drive, so much a part of reaching a medically proper diagnosis, profoundly affects what is said during medical encounters. Contextual concerns that do not lend themselves to the technical lexicon of diagnostic possibilities tend to gravitate toward the margins of medical talk.

The medical plan (P) constitutes the interventions that the doctor suggests, usually toward the end of an encounter. Traditional teaching about the medical plan holds that it contains two components. First, there is a diagnostic plan, which involves the OIs that the doctor wishes to obtain after the present encounter ends. Second, in the therapeutic plan the doctor recommends the medication, surgery, diet, rest, exercise, counseling, relaxation, change in attitude, and so forth that he or she believes the patient's diagnosis warrants. A substantial part of medical education involves learning and "keeping up" with current vogues of preferred diagnostic and therapeutic plans.

Just as it affects diagnostic reasoning, the exclusionary drive also shapes the plan that is formulated. Among the infinitely varied possibilities for human action, the limited range of medical diagnoses encourages relatively few options. Usually, these options involve OIs that create more technical data, or treatments that use medication, surgery, or similar technical intervention. Alternatively, a doctor may suggest nonintervention, which includes reassurance that a problem is not serious enough to require technical action, or a schedule of follow-up to be sure that the problem does not become worse. Sometimes, a doctor recommends maneuvers like dietary improvement, changes in habits like smoking and alcohol consumption, counseling, psychotherapy, or behavioral change. In such situations, the problems under consideration often have roots in the social context of the encounter.

Partly because the medical diagnosis rarely provides a technical name for such contextual problems, the plan does not generally call for a contextual intervention. Instead, the medical plan tends to accept the social context as a given. Even the limited behavioral changes that doctors may encourage generally aim at a patient's less troublesome reconciliation with his or her context, rather than change in the context itself. The range of plan that is perceived as possible is usually quite restricted.

Where does giving information to the patient fit in the traditional format of the medical encounter? Remarkably, as taught to generations of doctors in training, this format does not include a specific niche for providing information. It is probably for this reason that information giving in medicine has often been a catch-as-catch-can phenomenon. Similarly, the lack of a specific place to give information in the format of the encounter doubtless has contributed to the deficiencies and dissatisfactions that have arisen in this arena.[7] Suffice it to say, the traditional format does not guide the doctor in communicating information about contextual issues.

As I conclude this overview of the medical encounter, the puzzling history of the encounter's format deserves a brief comment. How this format emerged historically is currently a mystery.[8] The preferred and widely taught sequencing of CC → PI → PH → FH → SH → SR → PE → OI → Dx → P probably goes back to late-nineteenth-century Europe. Most of these components appeared in textbooks of clinical medicine published in Germany during that period. Although Foucault and others who have studied the history of medicine in Europe do not deal with the format of the encounter, a similar format presumably arose in France and Britain as well. As with most of the other features of laboratory-based "scientific" medicine, North Americans probably brought the medical encounter's format to the Eastern seaboard of the United States in the late-nineteenth or early-twentieth century. To what extent similarities existed between this format and those used earlier in North America is unknown. Likewise mysterious at this time are the formats of medical encounters in most premodern societies. For instance, although much anthropologic data are available on "ethnomedical" beliefs, little is known about how encounters between so-called primitive healers and their clients are organized. What is known indicates that some kind of history taking, physical examination, diagnostic categorization, and medical plan appears in most if not all ethnomedical encounters.[9]

While elaborating the history and prehistory of the medical encounter comprises a worthy enterprise, beyond my scope here, there is little doubt that the traditional format now is commonplace in many or most human societies. That this particular format should have arisen is remarkable partly because its effectiveness in improving medical conditions remains unproven. Like many other aspects of modern medicine, the beneficial impact of the format on the morbidity and mortality of large populations, as well as on individual patients, is difficult or impossible to demonstrate.[10] This is not to deny that modern medicine has accomplished great things. Many of the medical encounter's most time-consuming and thus costly components (such as the FH, SR, and much of the PE), however, have never been put to the test of cost-effectiveness. If effectiveness has not been proven, why has the medical encounter's traditional format received such wide and unquestioning acceptance that it is now essentially a sacred cow?

My purpose in the remainder of this chapter is to uncover a deeper structure within the medical encounter. The traditional format conveys a fairly accurate sense of the encounter's technical structure and also defines the concept that doctors generally hold about what needs to be accomplished during one or more visits. I will argue, however, that the traditional format masks another, underlying structure within the medical encounter. Moreover, the appeal of the traditional format may derive at least in part from its tendency to exclude or to marginalize contextual difficulties. In looking for a deeper structure, I will consider how broad social issues arise in medical discourse and how the participants either deal with these concerns, or do not.

APPROACHES TO MEDICAL DISCOURSE FROM STRUCTURALISM

Structuralist theories, though now considered by some to be relics of a bygone heyday, can help in any search for deep structures that lie within the more obvious meanings of discourse. While I will adapt a structural approach to help explain how medical discourse deals with social issues, I also want at the outset to clarify two points about my use of structuralism.

First, I am arguing that an underlying structure in medical discourse manifests itself in a substantial number of doctor-patient encounters at a specific place and time in history: the United States and probably certain other advanced capitalist countries during the late twentieth century. I am not arguing, as some structuralists might, that a similar structure arises as a universal feature of medical discourse at all times and places. In other social contexts, different structures of medical discourse predictably become apparent, and the current structure might well change in the future. Because I view the structure of medical discourse as a historically specific pattern, I want to avoid a quest for universal, invariant, or essential structures—a quest for which structuralism has received wide criticism. By acknowledging the possibility of, and in fact hoping for, change in the structure that I describe, I accept the common post-structuralist argument that no deep structure continues to exist (or to remain, as it were, "ontologically grounded") in all historical circumstances. On the other hand, I try to show how a characteristic structure does emerge in the medical discourse that confronts many of us during the current period of history.

Second, the structure of medical discourse does not emerge in the abstractions of language alone, but rather within the concrete interactions of individuals who deal with specific material conditions in the here and now. From this view, medical discourse does not occur as an isolated phenomenon of language, as it might be seen by at least some traditional structuralists, but rather within a social context. As a micro-level process, doctor-patient communication reflects macro-level patterns in a given society and helps reproduce those patterns. Other research on medical discourse (for instance, in the fields of sociolinguistics, discourse analysis, and conversation analysis) has looked for structures in interpersonal speech, and the links between micro-level speech and macro-level patterns of society often have remained ambiguous. Further, in seeking these structures, such studies generally have not tried to adapt structuralist theories to doctor-patient communication.[11] By applying some features of structuralism to medical discourse, I try to base my arguments on concrete instances of interpersonal interaction, involving patients and doctors who face the material conditions of everyday life.

Among the rich and controversial contributions of structuralism, the ones that I want to emphasize involve a search for underlying structure beneath the diverse surface details of interpersonal discourse. In structuralist thought, this quest for underlying structure began with linguistic research concerning the nature of language itself but later extended to studies of literature and eventually to nonliterary discourse. As background for my own later attempt to locate a structure that links medical discourse with its social context, certain structuralist accounts of language, literature, and nonliterary elements of culture become pertinent.

Structural linguistics treats language as a system of signs in structural relationship with each other. From this viewpoint, a sign contains two components: a signifier, which is its sound or graphic equivalent in writing, and a signified, which is its meaning in structural relation to other signs. Saussure, the founder of structural linguistics, argued that *langue*, the underlying structure of signs that makes speech possible, is much more important for an understanding of language than is *parole*, which consists of actual speech.[12] From a Saussurian perspective, medical discourse involves a system of signs whose surface meanings prove less important than their structural relationships with one another. For instance, it is revealing to look behind such signs as the CC, PI, and other surface features of the medical encounter, to locate an underlying structure that goes beyond the words exchanged by a particular doctor and a particular patient.

A similar search for structure emerges in literary criticism influenced by structuralism. The structural analysis of literature seeks constancy of structure amid a great diversity of texts. Among structuralist critics like Jakobson, for instance, the surface meanings of particular poems, stories, novels, and folktales hold interest—no matter how intriguing in their separateness—mostly insofar as they manifest common structural elements. Further, these underlying structures are usually unconscious, intuitive, or "subliminal."[13] Thus, a poet or artist rarely recognizes on a conscious level the structure that a creative product manifests. From this viewpoint, a writer or artist expresses these structures through a creative process whose rules, though socially learned, usually remain below the level of conscious intentionality.

Seen in this theoretical perspective, the oral elements of medical encounters reveal common structural elements within a diversity of surface meanings. That is, while doctors and patients converse about many topics and express a wide spectrum of concerns, a structuralist critic would see a smaller number of structures that cut across many superficial differences in encounters. Further, from Jakobson's viewpoint, participants in medical encounters most likely would not perceive these structures consciously. Instead, commonalities of structure would emerge for the most part unintentionally in discourse, without doctors' or patients' conscious awareness.

Beyond linguistics and literary criticism, structuralist analysis has extended to nonliterary elements of culture; this line of work, I will argue, also pertains to medical discourse. In anthropology, for example, Lévi-Strauss looks at the structural relationships among elements of culture, including language, magic, religion, art, kinship, and myth.[14] By grouping these elements into structural units, he uncovers commonalities that appear within varying types of cultural expression. In his reading of myth, Lévi-Strauss uses a two-dimensional scheme of categorizing binary oppositions. The surface elements of the myths appear on the horizontal axis; the structural "features" then emerge through interpretive grouping on the vertical axis. He applies this approach to the Oedipus myth, the Zuni origin and emergence myths (which themselves strikingly resemble the Oedipus myth), the Ash-Boy and Cinderella tales, and eventually other forms of cultural expression, such as science, art, dress, and food preferences.[15] By recognizing both the similarities and differences among the versions, and by allowing some "simplifications," Lévi-Strauss claims that the reader then can clarify a unifying structure despite wide surface variations.

While medical discourse is not exactly mythic, or even literary, it does comprise a series of surface elements whose underlying structure might become apparent through a similar kind of reading. Lévi-Strauss himself confronts medical discourse as he interprets a South American song that a shaman sings to facilitate a difficult childbirth.[16] The song's therapeutic impact, to which Lévi-Strauss refers as "the effectiveness of symbols," arises from the verbalization and bringing to consciousness of previously unconscious conflicts and resistances. In this sense, he claims, the shamanistic cure compares favorably with psychoanalytic technique. Although Lévi-Strauss' structural analysis of ethnomedical discourse explores a confluence between primitive and psychoanalytic "myth," he does not try to navigate the more humdrum texts of modern medicine.

That is the next destination. To get there, I need to look more closely at the flow of medical talk. While a structuralist compass might help to see what is present in medical discourse, other theoretical scopes are useful to discover what is absent and why what is absent might have import.

APPROACHES TO MEDICAL DISCOURSE FROM POST-STRUCTURALISM, DECONSTRUCTION, AND MARXIST LITERARY THEORY

Can medical discourse be read as a text?

Reading nonliterary texts. I will contend that both structuralist techniques and techniques of "deconstruction"—perhaps the hallmark of the post-structuralist period—can help in understanding medical discourse. As noted already, such an approach takes into account the much discussed weaknesses of structuralism by looking for underlying structures as historically specific parts of current medical discourse, rather than as universal or invariant structures. The approach also addresses weaknesses in the fields of sociolinguistics, conversation analysis, and discourse analysis, by emphasizing elements of social context and how they come to be excluded or marginalized.

Literary theory of the past two decades has effaced the boundary between literature and nonliterary discourse as targets for critical interpretation. That the tools of literary criticism can and should be brought to nonliterary texts has become a frequent call among critical theorists.[17] These
efforts begin to move beyond literature in the traditional sense as a focus
of critical theory. Influenced by deconstruction and post-structuralist
thought, some Marxist literary critics also have argued that nonliterary
texts are appropriate for critical reading. From this view, television programs, popular romances, films, advertisements, and public policy statements in such areas as law, housing, and health care all merit attention, especially as they reinforce current patterns of political-economic
power.[18] Unfortunately, such calls for critical work on nonliterary texts—
like those of medical encounters—to illuminate social problems often
appear toward the end of critical studies of literary texts, with little
indication of how such efforts might proceed.

In the pages that follow, then, I will use an expansive definition of *text*.
Specifically, a text is a written or spoken unit of language that is available
for appraisal by one or more observers. This definition assumes that a
critical analysis of nonliterary, spoken texts is both acceptable and desirable. The texts to be considered are those of spoken medical discourse in
actual encounters between patients and doctors.

Margin, context, and ideology. Deconstruction, among its goals, tries
to clarify what is marginal, absent, or excluded from a text. Although
deconstruction has mainly studied the margins of philosophy and literature, this approach can help bring into focus what does and does not
happen in the spoken discourse of medical encounters.

In emphasizing what is strategically excluded or marginalized within a
text, deconstruction holds that the absence or de-emphasis of one or
more elements is key in trying to interpret a text critically. According to
Derrida, for instance, such elements often appear at the margin of a text,
within passages that superficially seem tangential, extraneous, unessen-
tial, or otherwise unimportant. Yet these same elements, Derrida argues,
tend to break down the explicit principles by which the text is organized.
Studying the margin then becomes a way, perhaps the best way, to study
a text.[19] Where is the appropriate margin to study for a given text?
Derrida refers to elements of history, politics, economy, sexuality, and so
forth, as constituents of a text's margin. In short, a critical reading of a
text may find many marginal elements, and these elements are likely to
reflect the text's social context. Derrida's readings through a wide range
of philosophical, literary, and anthropologic texts have shed light on contextual concerns that appear at the margins, expressed by de-emphasis,
absence, or exclusion.

A text, then, tends to break down at its margins, facing tensions,
incompatibilities, and contradictions between itself and its social context.

While Derrida—ever mindful that his own texts are subject to decon-struction—is reluctant for theoretical reasons to voice calls to action, Marxist critics influenced by him have argued that the search for ele-ments of social context in the margins should be an essential task for critical theory. Jameson, for instance, has suggested that criticism should elucidate the social contradictions that are absent causes underlying a given text.[20] This search involves a close reading of the inconsistencies, the breaks in logic, the interruptions, the overlooked, the ignored, and the otherwise absent though pertinent components that a text either expresses or might express. Accordingly, criticism finds its most fertile ground at the margin between text and social context. This productive space presumably exists no less in nonliterary, spoken discourse than it does in more traditional literary or philosophic texts.

Ideology predictably appears at the margins of discourse, including nonliterary discourse like that of medicine. How and to what extent ideologic notions are transmitted in medicine, as noted in the last chap-ter, is not entirely clear. It is likely, however, that ideologic notions about work, the family, and other parts of the social context arise subtly, if they are voiced at all. Further, ideology may manifest itself through lack of explicit discussion of alternatives to the present, by a de-emphasis of contextual problems, or by the absence of critical attention to such prob-lems.

The apparent absence of explicit ideologic statements in discourse becomes an important mechanism by which ideology is reproduced. Eagleton, a Marxist critic influenced by deconstruction, gives a forceful statement of this point, as applied to literary texts: "Ideology, rather, so produces and constructs the real as to cast the shadow of its absence over the perception of its presence. . . . These absences—the '*not-said*' of the work—are precisely what bind it to its ideological problematic: ideology is present in the text in the form of its eloquent silences."[21] Eagleton applies this perspective to interpret the underlying ideologies of literary texts by examining what alternatives remain unsaid. Further, he argues that the illumination of textual absence is one of literary criticism's most challenging tasks. There is ample reason to extend this perspective to nonliterary texts as well. In doing so, it is reasonable to expect—for instance, in medical discourse—that ideology presents itself explicitly at certain times, but more often through key themes that are unspoken or referred to in a marginal way.

Understanding the ideologic components of discourse, however, de-pends on seeing the relationships between discourse and its social con-text; as Bakhtin, Jameson, and other Marxist literary critics have argued, social class is a key contextual element that shapes the ideologic content of discourse.[22] To state what probably is already obvious: relationships of social class are crucial parts of the context in which discourse arises and in which ideology is transmitted. From this contextual viewpoint, a dominant ideology conveyed through discourse tends to legitimate the position of whatever class holds power during a given historical period. Discourse, according to Jameson, often is the scene of a subtle struggle between this dominant ideology and an oppositional ideology that "will, often in covert and disguised strategies, seek to contest and to undermine the dominant 'value system.' "[23]

In the nonliterary discourse of face-to-face speech, social class also becomes a critical contextual element that shapes the transmission of ideology. To the extent that doctors and patients occupy different class positions, this class difference patterns the ideologic content of their medical discourse. Predictably, doctors sometimes voice explicit ideologic messages that legitimate the current class structure of society; or the transmission of ideology occurs more subtly, conveyed by the absence of criticism about class structure and its various injuries. In medical encounters, marginalization constrains an oppositional voice, perhaps that of a patient in distress, through interruption, truncation, or de-emphasis. This way of looking at medical discourse provides a slightly different theoretical prism for seeing the same problems uncovered (as discussed in the last chapter) by sociolinguists who observe a "diffidence" of working-class patients in medical encounters, or who note contention between the "voice of medicine" and the "voice of the life-world."[24] Such observations confirm that social class relations, as an element of context, pattern ideology within discourse.

But social class is not the only contextual element that affects discourse; other crucial elements include gender, age, and race.[25] All these contextual elements can become the basis of dominance and subordination, and they are closely linked to social class. Ideologies of gender pertain in large part to the roles that men and women occupy in the family and at work. Through ideologies of gender, expectations about what men and women appropriately should and should not do enter everyday language. Arising in the context of discourse, these ideologies profoundly affect what is or can be said, what appears at the center of discourse, and what slips in at the margins. Similarly, as people age, they encounter a changing set of expectations and demands, which vary a great deal among societies. In the United States, for instance, ideologies of aging can convey the image of a trash heap, where elderly people move when their productivity, or reproductivity, is used up. Other societies tend to be more lenient, or even respectful, in ideologies of aging. Ideologies of race have entered discourse, whenever societies have encountered the contrast between majority and minority groups. Expressions of racial ideologies have ranged from the master-slave vernacular to the only slightly more subtle versions of modernity.

Why highlight these contextual elements here? Class, gender, age, and race are some of the contextual elements that pattern ideologic language in face-to-face discourse, like that of medicine. It is not enough to acknowledge that ideology may be reproduced in medical discourse, as I have done in the previous chapter. The important question is how this happens. That is, in concrete examples of discourse, the critical reader needs to seek specific places where ideologic reproduction occurs and where context impinges on discourse. From structuralism, one expects that these places may become apparent as part of an underlying structure that is not obvious or consciously appreciated in surface meanings. From post-structuralism and deconstruction, one expects that such a structure is a historically specific one, contingent on a certain social context and changeable in other contexts, and also that ideology and context make themselves felt, at least partly, in the margins of discourse—in what is left unsaid, interrupted, cut off, or de-emphasized.

Unintentionality and consent. As noted already, ideologic reproduction and social control in medicine are subtle processes, which rarely reach consciousness, but their unintentionality goes beyond the level of individuals engaged in discourse. Jameson argues that a political unconscious, embedded in language, patterns the discourse of everyday life.[26] The political unconscious, according to Jameson, shapes discourse particularly through "strategies of containment," which express only a narrow range of possibilities for action, while repressing others. Specifically, these strategies within discourse repress the possibility of alternatives, such as collective action, that would fundamentally change present social organization. By leaving alternatives unsaid, Jameson claims, strategies of containment also help make these alternatives unthinkable. That is, while ideology is conveyed by an absence of criticism, possibilities for change become drastically constricted, to the extent that they remain unexpressed in discourse. When alternatives are left unsaid and thus marginalized, in Jameson's view, the most profound historical, social, and political impulses can be subtly "managed."

Similarly, social control in medicine usually remains a subtle process, based in the structure and margins of discourse. While Foucault and other writers who have analyzed social control in medicine portray it as rather straightforward and obvious, the language of control as actually enunciated is much more likely indirect. That is, social control predictably achieves its impact through the absence of key alternatives and through marginalization of certain concerns, rather than through specific controlling statements. Such subtle mechanisms in discourse then help achieve consent to current ways of organizing society.

On the other hand, the participants in medical discourse also obtain gratifications that can overshadow in consciousness whatever ideologic reproduction and social control occur. All that doctors have to offer contributes to the gratification that patients experience in medical encounters. These offerings include technical intervention, advice, emotional support expressed through words or nonverbally through the laying on of hands, and so forth. Further, doctors gain innumerable sources of gratification from interacting with patients. Among other things, these rewards include experience of technical mastery, money, prestige, gratitude, and the pleasing though complex sensations of helping those in need. It would be a great mistake to underestimate such gratifications, since they comprise so much of the conscious experience of medical encounters. Yet these undeniable gratifications of medical discourse also tend to obscure its less pleasurable and much less obvious characteristics.[27]

That medical discourse becomes consciously gratifying to its participants while it helps achieve consent through ideologic language should come as no surprise, since much of modern culture operates in similar ways. During recent decades, such dubious cultural achievements have disconcerted many commentators, who have noted the ideologic and controlling effects of the mass media, art, film, music, literature, and science. Meanwhile, all these cultural forms have generated enormous popular enthusiasm.[28] Similarly, professional-client discourse provides keenly felt gratifications, which mask elements of ideology and social control that are present on a deeper level.

The subtle yet powerful ways that the political unconscious operates in discourse lead to what seems a discouraging view. If problems of context present themselves marginally or through absence, and if the participants in discourse are mainly unaware of elements that reproduce ideology and achieve social control, the potentialities of language become rather drab and unappealing. Even the task of bringing these matters to awareness takes on an aura of futility. As Eagleton has written, such a perspective leaves us "in the grip of ideology, conforming to social reality as 'natural' rather than critically questioning how it, and ourselves, came to be constructed, and so could possibly be transformed."[29] For instance, is the clarification of ideologic reproduction and social control in actually spoken medical texts worthwhile? Are such problems and processes pervasive enough that they cannot be modified or improved upon?

Critical theorists vary widely in their opinion of their work's social import. Practically oriented theorists—usually influenced by characteristically Marxist concerns—do hope to help bring about change in society, especially to the extent that current forms of social organization cause or maintain human suffering. This approach to politically engaged criticism links the analysis of discourse to collective political action. From this viewpoint, the critical theorist's "praxis"—his or her attempt to unite theory with action—aims toward basic change in the contradictory social context in which discourse occurs.[30] A critic therefore points out troubles in the relation between discourse and social context, but one underlying goal of this analytic effort usually involves making a contribution to change in the context itself. How to translate analysis into social change, of course, is never a straightforward matter. But it is a goal that moves beyond the pessimism of the critic and a goal to which I return later.

A CRITICAL THEORY OF MEDICAL DISCOURSE

In the past two chapters and the prior sections of this one, I have tried to build some new theoretical channels from several sources. Setting out in the first chapter from the actually spoken discourse of doctors and patients, I examined the medical mediation of work, family life, sexuality, "deviant" activities, and emotional problems. In the second chapter I explored the connections between "micro-level" personal troubles in medicine and "macro-level" social issues; I also considered medical discourse in light of prior theoretical interpretations of ideology, professional social control, and the language of the medical encounter. Earlier in this chapter, I presented the traditional and technical view of the medical encounter and asked whether a deeper structure might be present beneath the surface meanings of medical discourse. In trying to answer this question, I drew selectively from structuralism, post-structuralism, deconstruction, and Marxist literary theory.

Now let me return to the three summaries of actual doctor-patient encounters that introduced the first chapter. After reiterating the summaries for convenience, I try to reorganize the elements of discourse so that some underlying structures become apparent. As heuristic tools, I also present a series of schematic figures that give visual pictures of the structures I am proposing. At this point, the structural analysis of these particular materials is quite preliminary (later chapters present more detailed analyses of the encounters and their transcripts). After reviewing the three encounters, I present a general structural view of medical discourse.

> A man comes to his doctor several months after a heart attack. He is depressed. His period of disability payments will expire soon, and his union is about to go on strike. His doctor tells him that he is physically able to return to work as a radial drill operator and that working will be good for his mental health. The doctor also prescribes an antidepressant and a tranquilizer.

Figure 3.1 shows some structural elements of discourse in this encounter. Seen in this way, the contextual issue of uncertain employment presents itself first (A). Depression is a personal trouble that the patient experiences in anticipation of a return to uncertain employment (B).

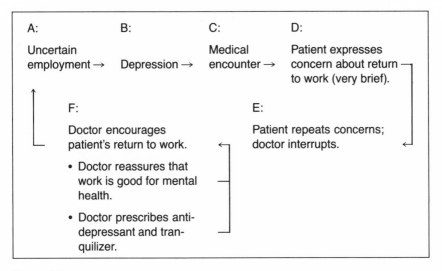

Figure 3.1
Structural elements of a medical encounter with a man anticipating return to work after a heart attack

Coming to the medical encounter (C), the patient tentatively and briefly expresses concern about his impending return to work when his union intends to go on strike (D). He repeats this concern at several points, but the doctor de-emphasizes it (E). Rather than pursuing the contextual problem, the doctor reassures the patient that work is good for his mental health; further, the doctor prescribes both an antidepressant medication and a tranquilizer (F). After the encounter, one assumes, the patient continues to prepare himself for a return to work.

> A woman visits her doctor because of irregularities in her heart rhythm. She complains that palpitations and shortness of breath are interfering with her ability to do housework. The doctor checks an electrocardiogram while she exercises, changes her cardiac medications, and congratulates her in her efforts to maintain a tidy household.

Structural elements of this encounter appear in figure 3.2.

Here the contextual issue involves expectations about women's social role in the family (A). Housework, as many have noted, is an important activity in economic "reproduction," which traditionally is the responsibility of women. Because this patient's cardiac symptoms interfere with her housework, she experiences emotional distress (B). When she sees her doctor (C), the patient mentions this concern (D). Rather than exploring her concern in depth, the doctor does an electrocardiogram while the patient exercises (E). Based on the results, the doctor changes the pa-

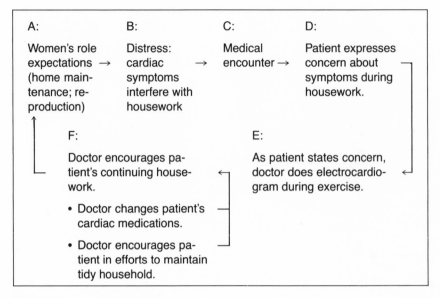

Figure 3.2
Structural elements of a medical encounter with a woman whose cardiac symptoms interfere with her housework

tient's cardiac medications. He also encourages her efforts in at least trying to maintain a tidy household (F). The patient thus returns to her personal challenge of doing housework in the face of serious heart disease.

> A man goes to his doctor for a premarital blood test. The doctor questions him closely about his drinking problem, his smoking, his job as a netmaker for fishermen, his family, and his plans for married life. Then the doctor encourages attendance at Alcoholics Anonymous and orders tests of liver function, in addition to the premarital blood test that the patient requested.

Figure 3.3 gives some structural elements of this encounter.

This patient faces a contextual issue that derives from the patterning of role expectations that affect men (A). Like most men, this patient finds that he must hold a job steadily to support himself and his family—to use a convenient term, he must earn the "means of subsistence." Further, as he approaches marriage, he also encounters an expectation that he stably perform as "head" of a family. Such expectations about work and the family, however, are not simple ones, since the patient is a habitual, heavy drinker. The patient therefore experiences a personal trouble that pertains to actual or potential conflicts deriving from alcohol use (B). During the medical encounter (C), the doctor takes the lead in expressing

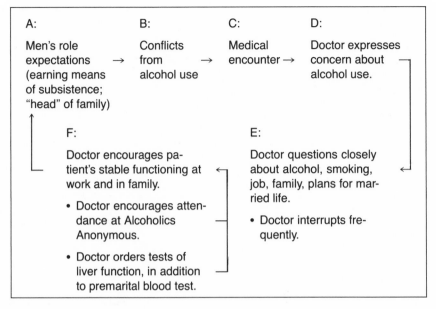

Figure 3.3
Structural elements of a medical encounter with a man whose alcohol problem potentially interferes with work and family relations

concern about alcohol use (D). The doctor questions the patient closely about alcohol, as well as his heavy smoking, job, family, and plans for married life. In pursuing these questions, the doctor interrupts the patient frequently (E). Beyond voicing strong encouragement that the patient attend Alcoholics Anonymous, the doctor also orders tests of liver function. In this discourse, the doctor encourages the patient's stable functioning at work and in the family (F).

In the paragraphs that follow, reasoning from the above three encounters and from others that appear in later chapters, I map some islands around which medical discourse seems to flow (figure 3.4). I interpret these islands as underlying structures of medical discourse, rarely discerned consciously by the doctors and patients who travel there.

A. *Social issue as context:* The economic, social, and political context of society contains many difficult conditions. These "social issues" often lie behind and help create some of the "personal troubles" that clients experience in their everyday lives. (In the three encounters above, the pertinent social issues are uncertain employment, women's role expectations, and men's role expectations.)

B. *Personal trouble:* Clients tend to experience these troubles privately, as individual problems. They are unlikely to recognize consciously the social issues that lie behind their personal troubles. (In the same three

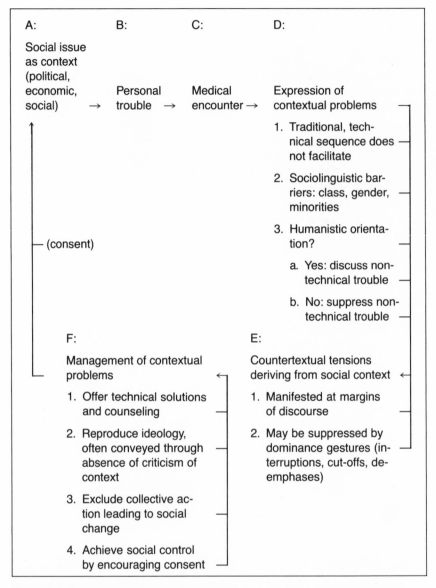

Figure 3.4
The micropolitical structure of medical discourse

encounters, personal troubles include depression, distress that cardiac symptoms interfere with housework, and conflicts from alcohol
use.)
C. *Medical encounter:* Clients come to medical professionals with complaints that very often (though not always) have economic, social,

and political roots. The contextual sources of personal troubles include class structure and the organization of work; family life, gender roles, and sexuality; aging and the social role of the elderly; the patterning of leisure and "substance use"; and limited resources for dealing with emotional distress.

D. *Expression of contextual problems in medical discourse:* The traditional and technical sequence of the medical encounter does not facilitate the expression of contextual concerns. Further, the relations between language and social structure predictably make the expression of contextual concerns more difficult for working-class people, women, and racial minorities. Certain "humanistic" or "progressive" doctors encourage patients to talk about the nontechnical components of problems that pertain to their "lifeworlds." These patients can express concerns and vent emotions about such personal troubles. Less humanistic or progressive doctors tend to discourage patients from expressing such concerns or to ignore them when expressed.

E. *Countertextual tensions deriving from social context:* However, contextual problems create tensions in medical discourse. Periodically, such tensions that derive from troubling social issues erupt into the discourse, or appear at its margins, and create a countertextual reality that cannot be resolved in the framework of a medical encounter. Doctors tend to suppress such tensions by dominance gestures like interruptions, cut-offs, and de-emphases, that get the discourse back on a technical track. The inherent hierarchy and asymmetry of the doctor-patient relationship reinforce this pattern of dominance in discourse.

F. *Management of contextual problems:* Whether such tensions are expressed or suppressed, the language of medicine leaves few options for action. Limited options for action apply to both "humanistic" encounters, when doctors encourage patients to talk about nontechnical components of their personal troubles, and to less humanistic encounters, where such concerns are discouraged. Generally, doctors respond with technical solutions and counsel patients how best to adjust to their previous roles. The language of medical science can convey ideologic content, especially when it converts social problems into technical ones. Ideologic language also arises at the margins of medical discourse or achieves its impact through absence. That is, by a lack of criticism directed against sources of distress in the social context, medical discourse ideologically reinforces the status quo. The discourse of medicine thus tends to exclude basic social change as a meaningful alternative. In accepting the present context as given, and in remaining silent about collective political action, medical discourse encourages consent by rendering social change "unthinkable." This latter accomplishment of medicine may be its main contribution to social control.

In later chapters I will show how this structure helps us understand what is happening as doctors and patients deal with problems of work; the family and gender roles; aging; sexuality, leisure, substance use, and other "vices"; and troublesome emotions. In addition, medical discourse in which this structure is not apparent will become a matter of particular interest.

To whatever extent this theory is persuasive, other questions immediately suggest themselves: Can the structure of medical discourse be reformed? Can medical discourse include a criticism of the sources of personal distress in the social context of the professional encounter? A reformed medical discourse would encompass self-criticism of its own micropolitical structure and would no longer encourage consent to contextual sources of personal troubles. By suggesting collective action as a meaningful option, medical professionals perhaps might begin to overcome the hurtful effects that its exclusion exerts. Can this be done without further medicalizing social problems? If so, critical discourse in medicine also would recognize the limits of medicine's role and the importance of building links to other forms of praxis that seek to change the social context of medical encounters. Moving beyond the current structure of medical discourse is one goal of my attempt to analyze it, and this concern is a focus of the final chapter of this book.

Meanwhile, before trying to interpret some actual medical texts and to discern their structure, I need to ask: What is the best way to write them down and then to read them? In short, the question of method.

CHAPTER 4

ON METHOD

Deciding how best to write down medical texts and then to read them should take into account generations of debate about ways to interpret texts. Within philosophy and literary criticism, this debate comprises the field of hermeneutics. However, since hermeneutic principles usually focus on literary texts, or texts that at least have reached printed and published form, the interpretation of nonliterary materials presents special problems. Research on spoken discourse in the social sciences offers assistance, though less than one might expect.

Partly due to weaknesses in prior methods of studying nonliterary discourse, like that of medicine, I want to propose a new methodologic approach, influenced by techniques of literary criticism. With the theoretical perspective developed in the previous chapters, my goal is to work out a method that, first and foremost, helps explain the interrelationships between "micro-level" processes in professional encounters and "macro-level" social issues.[1] From this standpoint, the interpretation of medical discourse places the encounter between patient and doctor within a broader social context. As noted earlier, patients present to their doctors a variety of personal troubles, many of which have roots in social issues beyond the individual level. These issues often have impact on physical disorders, and words exchanged in the medical encounter frequently focus on the patient's roles in work, the family, and other areas of social life. Ideology and social control figure in the medical processing of such problems, as part of an underlying structure of discourse that initially may not be apparent. The interpretive method that emerges therefore focuses on how the structure of medical discourse does or does not deal with contextual concerns.

The new method that I describe involves certain compromises. I say compromises because I doubt that one can reach total solutions to the methodologic questions raised by interpretive practice.[2] While I hope that my interpretations prove convincing, I also aim to make these non-literary materials accessible for review and alternative interpretations by skeptics. For now, I want to describe a bit more fully the methodologic challenge posed by medical discourse. To begin, I criticize both quantitative and qualitative methods that I and others have used previously to study such materials. After that, I sketch out some criteria of an appropriate method—one which is oriented to the hermeneutic approaches of structuralism and post-structuralism, as outlined in the last chapter. I also explain how these criteria have affected what appears in the later chapters, in which I seek to write down and to read critically a series of texts from actually spoken medical discourse.[3] While such compromises do not completely solve the problems of method, at least they are methodical.

A CRITIQUE OF QUANTITATIVE METHODS APPLIED TO MEDICAL DISCOURSE

Developing a suitable method for studying medical discourse has challenged scores of investigators drawn by the fascination of what goes on in encounters between health professionals and clients. Until the mid-1970s, the clinical literature contained many prescriptions for communication that was "good," "effective," "compassionate," and so forth, but these claims were derived from remarkably little research.[4] During the past decade, studies of doctor-patient communication have multiplied. Influenced by quantitative methods in the social sciences, such studies have developed various schemes for analyzing statistically both verbal and nonverbal behaviors. From this research, much descriptive information about the nature of doctor-patient communication has emerged.

Yet something is missing from nearly all these quantitatively oriented studies. Specifically, such methods tend to treat discourse as self-contained and separated from the social context in which encounters between professionals and clients actually occur. That is, counting categories of communication and analyzing them statistically shed little light on how patients and clients deal with contextual issues when they arise. Further, quantitative descriptions of medical communication generally do not help in the search for a deeper structure that may lie beneath the surface meanings of language.

In any critique of methods, the best place to start probably is at home.

Beginning in the mid-1970s, I coordinated a largely quantitative study of doctor-patient communication. This study focused on the giving and withholding of information in a large random sample of medical encounters. The research attracted substantial funding from governmental and philanthropic agencies, required a sizable research staff working in three states for nearly a decade, and led to a series of influential publications that reported the findings. Whereas very few such studies had appeared before our research, other investigators have subsequently reported similar studies of verbal and nonverbal behavior in doctor-patient communication.[5] These approaches differ somewhat in their specific details, but they use techniques that resemble those my coworkers and I adopted. For this reason, I undertake a self-criticism, applied to my own quantitative research. The same limitations, however, also apply to the ever-expanding number of quantitative research projects in this field, some of which, for better or worse, our own work has influenced.

Quantification alone does not deal with the complexities of discourse. To understand such complexities adequately requires an in-depth interpretive analysis. This is not to say that well-thought-out quantitative methods cannot convey complexities of discourse at all. As our own research group and as other researchers have found, quantification can convey certain realities of medical or other interpersonal talk. However, the taxonomic pigeonholing required by the coding of quantitative variables inevitably constrains the critical interpretation of texts.

For instance, the categories of communication by which we and others have measured doctor-patient communication quantitatively require that we overlook or downplay many of the subtleties of medical talk, which cannot be categorized in a straightforward way.[6] In the achievement of statistical reliability among different observers, who apply the coding scheme to interactions, nuances of discourse—especially the impact of interruptions, cut-offs, pauses, and so forth, on the meaning of the words exchanged—become a peripheral concern. The quest for reliability, a euphemism that quantitative methodology applies to what is actually a distrust of idiosyncratic observation, drastically reduces the interpretive discretion of an individual observer. Demands of quantification lead to the exclusion of meanings in discourse that do not readily fit into whatever taxonomic coding scheme has been adopted. Since this exclusion leads to substantial interpretive sacrifices, one wonders if the advantages of quantitative methods really justify such losses.

Quantitative methods usually are not helpful in analyzing the context of discourse. In particular, they do not help very much in understanding the social, political, economic, and historical context in which micro-level encounters occur. For our study of doctor-patient communication, we actually developed some coding categories that allow us to count contextual elements of discourse. That is, we can look for verbal allusions to work, family life, sex roles, aging, substance use, and so forth, within encounters, can tally them, and can use these numbers as "variables," to analyze statistically with our other measures. Contextual concerns, however, typically appear in several different categories of interaction, such as history taking, general reassurance, and miscellaneous comments. Because of this overlap, the category of contextual concerns cannot be mutually exclusive from the other categories.

Even more important, in pretesting this approach, we found that the statistics usually pale in comparison to the richness of the original discourse, where contextual issues are expressed and discussed, and/or interrupted and cut off. Quantification of context inevitably loses the flavor of what actually occurs in the spoken discourse. The weakness of quantitative methods in representing the contextual components of discourse adequately, at least in our hands and those of others we know, seems at this point an intractable limitation.

These methods do not clarify the underlying themes and structures of discourse. Quantitative techniques applied to discourse produce statistical counts of categories. The numerical processing of such counts can comprise a simple-minded statistical distribution of categories, or this numerical work can become quite sophisticated, leading to statistically driven, multivariate "models" of communicative behavior.[7] Some quantitatively oriented researchers argue that deeper structures, not apparent on the surface, can indeed emerge from such statistical approaches. From this viewpoint, quantitative "content analysis" sometimes seeks to uncover textual themes through statistical modeling from the numerical distribution of counted categories.[8] Computers presumably can assist in combining such statistical distributions to discover mathematically the underlying themes within discourse. Ironically, in his classic exposition of the structural method in anthropology, Lévi-Strauss himself expressed guarded optimism about the eventual contribution of quantitative, computerized techniques to the structural study of myth and other elements of culture.[9]

In general, such optimism has proven unwarranted. (Lévi-Strauss, for instance, did not pursue the quantitative direction seriously after he saw its limitations.) While quantitative approaches sometimes do provide data about texts that assist in the analysis of underlying structure, they have not yet replaced the nonmechanical interpretation of texts by live readers. This conclusion, so disappointing to so many, applies especially to spoken discourse, in which nuances and disjointedness remain least amenable to quantification yet provide the most important clues to deeper structure.

Quantitative methods are costly and tedious to use; they yield summary statistics that increase knowledge little in consideration of the time and expense required. Beyond the interpretive sacrifices mentioned earlier, quantitative methods also entail more palpable costs. For quantitative work with discourse like that described earlier, consider: Sampling and data collection can easily consume several years and require salary support for multiple research assistants. One cannot cut these costs simply by reducing the number of encounters studied; the reason is that achieving a large sample size is necessary if multivariate statistical techniques are performed according to current methodologic standards. Transcript preparation (which also, by the way, is essential in nonquantitative research) demands the hiring and training of expert transcriptionists who must work approximately six hours to transcribe one hour of spoken speech. To avoid idiosyncratic interpretation, research assistants must spend months in reliability checks of coding techniques. Then they and their leaders pass more months, at a rate of about three hours per hour of recorded conversation, in the coding of actual materials. Later, the researchers must convert the coded data to a computerized format, review statistical outputs of the data, prepare reports according to current quantitative standards, and so on.

Especially because few researchers emphasize these details in public, it is easy to underestimate the vicissitudes of obtaining funds, space, and time to administer and to conduct such activities. To ask a question common in quantitative circles, are the benefits worth the costs? Asking this question does not imply that nonquantitative methods are without costs. But when quantitative methods sacrifice so many important elements of substance, the costs of these techniques should make the buyer beware.

A CRITIQUE OF QUALITATIVE METHODS APPLIED TO MEDICAL DISCOURSE

Generations of philosophers, literary critics, and social scientists have used nonquantitative techniques to study discourse. Regarding medical discourse, this brand of scholarship has led to some of the most profound, or at least troubling, conclusions about what goes on in medicine. Such qualitative observations have focused especially on ideology, social control, and the nuances of communication in medical encounters.

Before reviewing qualitative methods critically, I should say a few more words about what I mean by *qualitative*. The quantitative toolbox of modern science carries a forceful symbolism. This symbolism includes a subtle dichotomy between the quantitative and the qualitative, with an explicit or implicit devaluation of qualitatively derived knowledge. Thus, the application of numbers to concepts entails a mystique that conveys a sense of rigor and superiority. In the common parlance of science generally and social science specifically, qualitative research reeks of personalism, bias, subjectivity, weakness, and similar unworthy attributes. From this perspective, qualitative inquiry is not simply "nonquantitative"; the quality of qualitative work is also somehow inferior. This judgment often applies, even if the subject matter of inquiry remains intractable to quantification, or if quantitative methods prove less than fully adequate (for example, in the study of medical discourse). As a veteran of quantification, I do not appreciate such derogatory imagery. By qualitative methods, then, I mean simply those techniques that depend on nonquantitative interpretation of data. As used here, *qualitative* is not a pejorative term, and it even implies a measure of esteem.[10]

Again, let me offer a critique of qualitative methods mainly by casting stones at my own house. Periodically, through the decade that our quantitative study of doctor-patient communication consumed, I could not resist the temptation to talk qualitatively about our findings. For instance, observations of medical encounters in my family and during medical training led to my theoretical concerns about power and the withholding of information in the doctor-patient relationship. Qualitative interpretations of these observations generated the working hypotheses that I later tried to test in our quantitative research project. Eventually, I published theoretical accounts of power and information control, based on these qualitative interpretations. This theoretical work conceptualized the medical encounter as a "micropolitical" situation, in which the control of information reinforces power relations that parallel those in the broader society, especially those related to social class, gender, race, and age.[11]

Later, our group extended the theoretical work to consider the problems of ideology and social control. This theory linked "professional-client interaction with ideology and consciousness, social institutions, social relationships of daily life, and the material conditions and class relationships of the workplace and economic system."[12] Arguing in behalf of this theory, I presented a qualitative analysis of excerpts from transcripts that we had prepared from the sampled medical encounters.

What follows represents a self-critical effort to appraise qualitative methods as applied to medical discourse. As in the case of quantitative methods, the self-criticism unfortunately also applies to much of the similar work in this field.[13] The intention again is to move beyond these difficulties, to work out later some more useful compromises.

The selection of discourse for qualitative analysis is not straightforward. Theory that is "grounded" in empirical observations does not develop easily from unsystematic accounts of a few cases.[14] For instance, in selecting passages that conveyed ideology and social control in medicine, our own research group initially picked out a small number of transcripts that appeared both "typical" in content and "juicy" in the interest that they would provoke in readers. In our publications, these largely implicit criteria of typicality and juiciness guided our selection of the transcripts and passages within transcripts that we chose to report. When one selectively samples the materials for study according to his or her own concerns, however, it is hard to know whether the conclusions shed light on general tendencies in discourse, or whether they reflect the theoretical ax that a given observer wishes to grind.

This routine objection, referring to what is commonly known as "bias" in selection, applies to several kinds of qualitative research. Selectivity that leads to consideration of some doctor-patient encounters but not others, or some passages within encounters but not others, may determine whether or not an observer finds a problem worthy of criticism. For instance, nonquantitative studies of doctor-patient communication in the fields of sociolinguistics, conversation analysis, and discourse analysis generally have paid little attention to this problem of selection bias. In such studies, researchers generally have selected medical encounters based on convenience, rather than systematic sampling. Further, the selection of excerpts within encounters for analysis usually has depended on the theoretical concerns of the investigators; passages in encounters that might prove less consistent with a particular interpretation seldom become available in the published reports of such research.[15] This caution about selectivity also applies to such endeavors as the search for messages of ideology and social control, which predictably may occur in some medical encounters but much less in others.

The quality of qualitative interpretation is difficult to evaluate. In our initial qualitative analyses of transcripts, for example, the research group developed four categories of interest: relations of production, class relations, the role of science under capitalism, and medical control of everyday life. Having found typical and juicy examples of each, I then wrote up each category briefly, juxtaposed to a short illustrative excerpt from a sampled transcript.[16] However, it is usually unclear how valid, reliable, and representative such interpretations actually are. These concerns pertain, in turn, to how well a qualitative measurement technique conveys the empirical reality of a concept under study, how consistently one or more observers apply a technique to the data, and how the interpreter emphasizes certain elements of observations rather than others.[17] Because of these concerns, success in interpretation becomes an elusive goal. A reader of qualitative interpretation may form a subjective opinion about whether an interpreter's analysis represents the original materials in a convincing way. What criteria one should apply in reaching this opinion, however, may not get stated explicitly.

Problems of interpretive practice arise even when qualitative researchers use sophisticated techniques to avoid such difficulties. For instance, in trying to present accurate transcripts and analyses of spoken language, some investigators in sociolinguistics and conversation analysis have argued for the importance of putting aside their own analytic assumptions by letting the speakers' words speak for themselves. These researchers have attempted not to interpret speakers' meaning or intention from a particular theoretical viewpoint, but rather to deduce regular patterns of speech from a close reading of transcribed conversations. Examples of this approach, as applied to medicine, include some very revealing studies of turn taking, interruption, and nonverbal behavior in doctor-patient encounters. Yet, despite claims of interpretive neutrality, such research often contains subtle assumptions that, for instance, treat the physician as the central figure in the interview, or that focus on predetermined issues like gender differences in interruptions and other conversational behavior. Even more important, by emphasizing fragments of talk, conversation analysis of medical encounters tends to strip away the social context of discourse, thereby shifting attention away from the crucial ways that contextual issues pattern the meaning of words exchanged by patients and doctors.[18]

There are many schools of thought about whether and to what degree standards of qualitative interpretation should be agreed upon at all. Qualitative methodologists in the social sciences tend to be optimistic that standards of validity, reliability, and representativeness can be developed and accepted; critical theorists in the humanities usually put these concerns on a back burner, since they doubt that interpretation can or should be removed from the subjectivity by which an individual appraises a particular text.[19] Such diverse views do not provide clear guidelines on the best way to interpret spoken discourse like that observed in medicine.

How to present medical discourse as a text also is not a clear-cut decision. To evaluate a piece of literary criticism, for instance, a reader often knows the text on which the criticism is based, or almost always can gain access to the text through a library or bookstore. By reviewing the text and comparing it to the interpretation, a reader can decide how convincing the interpretation seems to be. A reader of nonliterary, and especially spoken, texts has no such luck. In most cases, such texts are previously unknown to the reader. Further, the texts are not even written down, let alone sold in bookstores or loaned from libraries. Therefore, if a reader is to evaluate an interpretation of a nonliterary text, the interpreter must create some device to make the text accessible, along with the interpretation. Some questions immediately arise:

■ How should the account of interpersonal talk be prepared? Should the discourse simply be summarized, or should a transcript be presented? A summary might be easier to read, but it would require great editorial discretion. That is, the researcher would need to summarize the discourse in a way that accurately conveys what has happened, rather than simply what the researcher's theoretical bent has led him or her to see and hear (again, the issue of the "biased" theoretical ax, slicing qualitative observations).

Qualitative studies of social control in medicine and psychiatry, including my own, usually have provided historical or anecdotal summaries of medical encounters. Whatever success that such approaches enjoy has depended on the interpreter's skill at argument and the reader's suspending judgment about the accuracy of the summaries.[20] Making a transcript available might facilitate the reader's evaluating a particular interpretation; at least the reader could judge how well an interpretation stands up to the original text. Reviewing a text to appraise an interpretation then would resemble the process by which critics traditionally judge a piece of literary criticism.

■ If a transcript appears, should it be prepared so it can be read easily (as in the smoothly flowing conversations of novels), or should it accurately convey the nuances of talk that are much more difficult to read (examples include interruptions, speech enunciated by more than one person at the same time, pauses, mumbling, tone and volume of speech, stuttering, and so forth)? In my earlier attempts to quote from transcripts of medical encounters, I edited the chosen passages to make them easier to read.[21] However, nuances of discourse, particularly "marginal" components like interruptions, changes of direction, and excluded topics, comprise some of the most important elements that deserve interpretation. This point has been made both by researchers in sociolinguistics and conversation analysis, who have developed standard conventions for transcribing conversations, and by critical theorists, who have analyzed marginal elements in literary texts while calling for a similar approach to nonliterary discourse.[22]

■ Whether the transcript includes or intentionally excludes such subtleties, who should do the transcribing, and how can the quality of transcription be assured? In my early efforts to depict elements of ideology and social control in medical discourse, I personally listened to tape recordings and transcribed selected passages. Since one's own theory may distort what one hears and writes down, however, considerations of "bias" again might dictate that someone other than the interpreter do the transcribing. Constraints of time and workload lead to the same conclusion. In that case, training and accuracy checks become necessary, all the more so because professional transcriptionists usually try to edit recordings so that marginal elements (pauses, mumbling, interruptions, simultaneous speech, and so forth) do not appear in the polished transcript. What rules one should adopt for transcription, how transcriptionists should be trained, and which procedures are needed to assess the quality of transcription—all these questions deserve explicit answers.[23]

■ How should the transcript appear in relation to the interpretation? I have wrestled with several options in my own previous attempts to interpret medical discourse. First, the entire transcript of speech might be printed verbatim, before the interpretation begins.[24] Although this technique allows the reader to approach the material with as fresh a viewpoint as possible, the full transcript can become quite tedious to read in its entirety. Alternatively, the interpreter might choose specific excerpts from a transcript and present them verbatim at strategic points within the interpretation.[25] For evaluating an interpretation of spoken discourse, however, the reader remains at a disadvantage in appraising selected quotations, if the entire text is not available. A third option involves printing the entire transcript alongside the interpretation, on adjoining pages.[26] Although this alternative implicitly lets the reader decide how much of the transcript requires reading to evaluate the interpretation, the positioning of transcript and interpretation on opposing pages can lead to disjointed and distracting reading, especially since this format requires the reader to flip back and forth to find those parts of the text to which the interpretation alludes at a given moment.

A mixed approach to transcript presentation includes elements of these various options. Thus, for instance, the interpreter might summarize the transcript before the interpretation begins, might offer quotations from or allusions to the transcript to substantiate certain interpretive points, and then might append the entire verbatim transcript at the end or otherwise make it available for interested readers. The mixed option permits discretion for the reader, who may selectively choose to evaluate an interpretation, or parts of it, against the original transcript. In this approach, the reader also need not experience the tedium of wading through the whole transcript at the beginning, or the distraction of seeing it on opposing pages. While the mixed approach improves on some of the difficulties that arise in the other options, it also requires more space and thus becomes expensive to print.

In summary, the question of how to present medical discourse requires decisions about summarizing the material or reproducing it verbatim, transcribing superficially or according to detailed rules, training transcriptionists and performing accuracy checks, and organizing transcripts on the printed page to help the reader but not to burden him or her with the tedium of wading through too much unedited discourse that is uninteresting or irrelevant to the theoretical issues at hand. While calling for the application of their techniques to spoken texts, literary critics have offered few clues about how best to present such materials. Researchers in sociolinguistics, conversation analysis, and discourse analysis have experimented with various options for presenting spoken discourse, but no single alternative has emerged as clearly the best.

CRITERIA OF AN APPROPRIATE METHOD

Several criteria offer reasonable compromises in dealing with the problems of both quantitative and qualitative methods as applied to medical discourse. Again, I say compromises because I do not feel that these criteria in any sense provide the final methodologic word on these problems. The difficulties of selecting, interpreting, and presenting spoken texts remain substantial, and I do not pretend to have resolved them fully. Still, such criteria may stake out the territory for the textual analyses that later chapters offer. Before listing the criteria themselves, I want to mention some considerations that led to choosing them rather than others.

First, as indicated in the previous chapter, the methodologic techniques of textual analysis in structuralism and post-structuralism have much to offer for the interpretation of spoken discourse like that in medicine. In particular, these techniques help focus on the relations between text and social context, for instance, when the discourse of medical practitioners and patients deals with contextual issues. Such perspectives lead one to look for a deeper structure lying beneath the surface details of conversation and to examine carefully elements of discourse that may be marginal, de-emphasized, interrupted, cut off, or absent. Clearly, the history of hermeneutic debate offers a galaxy of alternative methods to interpret texts. Among these options, however, techniques from structuralism and post-structuralism provide useful ways to grapple with the nonliterary texts of medical discourse.

On the other hand, methods from the social sciences, and especially the field of sociolinguistics, help respond to some common quibbles and sources of distrust that inevitably arise in this line of work. Critical theorists in structuralism and post-structuralism frequently convey an implicit optimism that convincing interpretation can emerge from the gifted reader's careful (though ultimately subjective) selection and reading of a given text. Distrust of idiosyncratic interpretation, however, has led social scientists to emphasize such issues as validity, reliability, and representativeness in qualitative research. Without being taken so seriously that they stifle imaginative readings, these concerns do deserve a place in the compromises reached about appropriate methodology. That prior studies have at least tried to work out suitable methods for selecting, transcribing, and analyzing conversation may contribute to methodologic decisions about how to cope with discourse in medicine.

In adapting methods from the social sciences, however, one also perceives some danger. Although they are nonliterary, spoken texts like those of medicine nonetheless tell a story. "Narrative" is the term by which literary criticism refers to story telling in literature or oral tradition. The discourse that arises in medical encounters often involves a patient's telling a story, which a doctor may elicit by questions like: "How can I help you?" "What brought you here today?" or "What's bothering you?" Such questions introduce the procedures commonly known as history taking in medicine. In response, a patient may try to offer a lengthy and rambling narrative about what is wrong and how that came to pass. Contextual concerns may arise within the patient's narrative. Through questions, interruptions, de-emphases, cut-offs, and other mechanisms of speech, a doctor may direct the patient's narrative in ways that make it more consistent with a medical model. As noted in the last chapter, the drive to include elements of experience consistent with diagnostic categories, while excluding or de-emphasizing other elements, has become a characteristic feature of physicians' professional work in history taking.

Within the doctor-patient encounter, then, a narrative voice confronts a voice accustomed to the abstractions and categories of medical science. The diagnostic drive may jam patients' narratives about experience into convenient diagnostic compartments, but only by sacrificing elements of storytelling. While observers of medicine have described this clash of voices in different ways,[27] for both doctors and patients the incompatibilities between narrative discourse and scientifically oriented discourse in medical encounters doubtless have caused much heartbreak.

If the differences between narrative and scientific language affect what is said in medical encounters, these differences also impose certain methodologic limits on the study of medical discourse. That is, the language of science constrains the reading and interpretation of texts that remain, on many levels, narratives. The social scientist, for instance, applies a series of categories to recorded medical encounters. Pigeonholing medical discourse into analytic categories, however, converts stories into data. Much of the discomfort about what is lost in quantitative research on medical encounters, as discussed earlier, derives from this incompatibility between the richness of narrative and the poverty of analytic categories required by quantification. The quest for sensitive and sophisticated categorization schemes does not acknowledge a troubling realization: Elements of narrative in spoken discourse remain intractable to the customary techniques of categorization in science. Interpretation of narrative elements in discourse requires a method that is quite different from scientific categorization—an interpretive method that is probably more akin to those customarily used in the critical reading of literature. In short, while techniques from the social sciences deal with such problems as validity, reliability, and representativeness, they ought not sacrifice the richness of the stories told.

The criteria of an appropriate method thus ought to be rather eclectic. Certain approaches from the social sciences respond to the distrust of idiosyncratic interpretation that inevitably arises when one tries to read texts of spoken discourse like that in medicine. In particular, the method chosen can introduce a series of checks and balances, by which a researcher's zeal to interpret materials in a certain way is countered by others' opinions. One way to achieve this goal is through a group process, in which several readers come to some agreement on how to interpret a given text, without being dominated by one interpreter's point of view. Further, because of the profound limits of social scientific categorization in interpreting components of narrative within medical discourse, an appropriate method would include techniques more commonly used in literary criticism. The method also would benefit from the emphases on underlying structure and marginal elements of discourse that characterize structuralist and post-structuralist interpretation.

Such eclecticism in method does not exactly espouse a philosophy of science that advocates the methodologic anarchism of "anything goes."[28] This approach does, however, permit a freer play of interpretation, especially concerning narrative elements of discourse, than is possible within the categorization schemes of the social sciences. It also allows the reader to evaluate an interpretation, with reference to the original text. The eclecticism, in sum, is a controlled one that seeks to honor both the discourse as spoken and the traditional quibbles about idiosyncratic interpretation.

Here then are some criteria, compromises though they may be, for methodically studying medical discourse:

a) *The discourse under study should be selected through some kind of sampling procedure, preferably a randomized procedure, to increase the degree to which it is "representative" of discourse in similar settings and under similar conditions.* Systematic sampling reduces the probability that the researcher's theoretical leanings will affect the selection of discourse to be interpreted. Rather, the sampling procedure requires that the researcher consider a range of texts, some of which may become startling examples that confirm the investigator's theoretical expectations, but many of which may not.

b) *The sampled discourse should be recorded so that the primary recordings can be heard by other observers if interested.* The availability of primary audio or video recordings provides a mechanism by which skeptics can evaluate all later steps in analyzing discourse. Video recordings are often preferable, because they can assist in the analysis of nonverbal components of communication. If doubt arises about the quality of transcription or interpretation, for instance, a skeptic can listen to or look at the original recordings. The recordings permit replication or nonreplication of findings by other investigators. Further, different researchers can exploit the recordings to study discourse in their own ways.

c) *Standardized rules of transcription should be applied to the recorded discourse in producing texts for subsequent analysis.* For instance, sociolinguistic procedures that take into account such features of discourse as interruptions, pauses, questions, simultaneous speech, changes in tone of voice, and so forth, provide a useful standard for transcript preparation. To make such transcripts easier to read, however, these sociolinguistic conventions may need to be simplified to some extent.

d) *The reliability of transcription should be assessed by multiple observers.* Whatever transcription procedure is adopted, it should be applied consistently. Checking for consistency becomes especially important if the same person does the theorizing, transcribing, and interpretation, since "bias" is then more likely to show its ugly face. If one or more transcriptionists prepare the transcripts, training procedures and accuracy checks should assure the product's quality.

e) *Procedures for interpreting the prepared texts should be decided in advance. The validity of these procedures should be assessed in relation to theory. The interpretive procedures should address both the content and structure of texts.* Spelling out interpretive procedures in advance stays a step short of the methodologic anarchism of "anything goes." This criterion provides a framework, but also a degree of latitude, within which one or more readers can interpret the sampled texts. The procedures selected may turn out to be rather loose, as dictated largely by common sense[29]—for instance, identifying passages that reflect theoretical problems such as ideology and social control; or noting excerpts that concern contextual issues like work, the family, aging, sexuality, and so forth; or focusing on the absence, exclusion, interruption, or de-emphasis of such contextual elements. By agreeing upon interpretive procedures beforehand, however, one at least tips one's hat to the distrust of idiosyncratic interpretation so prevalent in scientific circles.

f) *The reliability of applying these interpretive procedures should be assessed by the participation of multiple observers.* This criterion further addresses the tendency of a single reader to find in the text whatever might support the theoretical point at hand. If several readers independently assess a text and come up with similar interpretations, how wonderful! An assumption behind this particular criterion is that agreement among different readers holds more weight than an individual's judgment. What happens when multiple readers disagree? Then a group process in which the readers discuss their interpretations and reach a consensus may help resolve the problem. The adequacy of group process, of course, depends on the readers' ability to communicate in good faith, without the dominance of a single individual (for instance, the principal theorist). Despite this caution, independent readings and group discussion may well improve on a single reader's idiosyncrasies. (At least, so we usually believe when we rely on committees to decide which writings deserve publication, which researchers deserve grants, which books deserve prizes, and so forth.)[30]

g) *If an interpretation is published, a summary of the transcript should precede its interpretation. Within the interpretation, excerpts from the transcript should help substantiate the interpretive arguments. The full transcript should be made available, for instance, as an appendix, on microfilm, or on computer diskette, for the reader's review if he or she is interested.* This eclectic approach to the presentation of transcripts again strikes several compromises. The summary orients the reader without burdening him or her at the start with excessive and/or irrelevant verbiage. Excerpts within the interpretation provide concrete materials based on which the reader can evaluate the interpretation. For the skeptic who wants to check out the full encounter, this technique also tucks away the entire transcript in an unobtrusive location.

h) *If published, the texts and their interpretations should convey accurately the observed variability of content and structure across sampled texts. Of particular interest is the "negative case," in which the elements of theoretical concern either do not appear or are minor features.* This last criterion compels the interpreter to examine critically his or her own theory when presenting texts and interpretations. Predictably, if researchers use systematic sampling to select encounters for analysis, they will find some encounters that substantiate their theoretical positions and others that do not. Rather than permitting a lockstep, mechanical interpretation only for "typical" or "juicy" transcripts, this criterion requires a more balanced picture. Abiding by this criterion, the researchers must present transcripts that prove their points and others that do not. Further, they must try to explain why this variability might occur. To present materials that are both consistent and inconsistent with the theoretical positions at hand injects a certain self-effacing discipline into the research effort. Without such discipline, however, one tries to sell whatever empirical shoes best fit one's own theoretical feet; customers may want to try on some other styles too.[31]

THE METHOD WE ACTUALLY USED

Having offered some general criteria of an appropriate method to study medical discourse, I now show how our method actually shaped up. In describing the method that we ultimately used, I follow the same order that I used to list the criteria in the last section. It must also be obvious that our group did not develop the foregoing criteria in abstraction. Instead, we worked out the criteria about two years before we completed the quantitative study described above and about one year after we began to wrestle with the problems that the in-depth, largely qualitative interpretation of our materials posed to us. The criteria thus emerged through engagement with our own observations. While we revised our procedures to some extent along the way, what follows is what we actually did.

a) *Sampling procedures.* First we selected a large ($N = 336$) random sample of doctor-patient encounters. We wanted to achieve a sample that was representative of the diverse settings in which doctors and patients interact. For this reason, we constructed three "stratified" subsamples that encompassed a variety of practice situations, including both private practice and hospital outpatient departments in two states. Within each subsample, we recruited doctors and patients randomly, through a table of random numbers applied to existing lists of doctors practicing internal medicine and through random selection of patients seeking care from these physicians. Members of the research team recorded on audiotape the full interaction between these doctors and patients; in one subsample, we also recorded all subsequent interactions during a nine-month follow-up period. The doctors and patients answered questionnaires to provide data about their demographic characteristics and attitudes and about elements of their social context (work, family, living situation, and so forth).[32]

It should be clear that we obtained this large random sample of doctor-patient interaction for purposes that were different from the type of textual and contextual analysis that I am attempting here. Specifically, we were trying to meet the sampling requirements for traditional, statistically oriented, quantitative research. Nevertheless, the existence of the large, randomly selected "data base" of recordings proved helpful for the present purposes as well. The random recording of medical discourse in diverse practice settings provided materials that were fairly representative of medical talk. Further, the selection of these materials did not seem to be distorted by the theoretical concerns that emerged.

From this large sample of tapes, we then selected randomly (again, by a table of random numbers) a smaller sample ($N = 50$) for more intensive study. While this sample size was inadequate to meet the statistical requirements of quantitative, multivariate research, it provided textual materials that were sufficient (in fact, nearly more than we could handle) for the in-depth analysis that we wanted to do in this phase of the work. After constructing this smaller sample, we checked and made sure that the characteristics of doctors and patients so chosen reflected a suitable distribution of gender, age, and social class (including occupation and education). By confirming that the sample contained a range of demographic characteristics, we gained some additional assurance that the smaller sample remained representative of doctor-patient interaction in a variety of practice settings.[33]

b) *Primary recordings.* As noted already, the original recordings of medical discourse remain available in a data base, to which other researchers can gain access. Previously, this library of audiotaped recordings has proven helpful for various investigators, who have borrowed tapes to carry out their own research projects on doctor-patient communication.[34] The smaller sample of recordings selected for this phase of our work also stays fully accessible. Costs prohibited videotaping the full sample of encounters, but we did videotape a parallel subset of encounters to provide additional perspectives on nonverbal components of communication. To listen or to look for themselves, skeptics who doubt our transcriptional abilities or interpretive conclusions need only say the word.

c) *Transcription.* After a training period of about three weeks, two transcriptionists used standard rules to transcribe the full recorded discourse from all the tapes in the smaller sample. Developed by others in sociolinguistic research and conversation analysis, these rules explicitly take into account interruptions, pauses, questions, simultaneous speech, changes in tone of voice, and similar features of interpersonal speech. As noted earlier, such nonverbal and quasi-verbal characteristics of speech may prove important in interpreting how contextual issues either do or do not get dealt with in medical discourse. On the other hand, because the fullest elaboration of these features makes transcripts very difficult to read, we have simplified the sociolinguistic conventions somewhat. For instance, these conventions usually require, within transcripts, the specification of such details as the duration of pauses in seconds of time, notations about whether the speaker is inhaling or exhaling, variations in spelling according to intonation, and so forth. Including such details within printed transcripts creates considerable work for the reader, which in our experience rarely contributes to the interpretive task at hand. By modifying the conventions developed previously in sociolinguistic research and conversation analysis, we do not mean to imply that our own rules become better standards for transcription. Actually, we agree with other investigators in this field that even carefully prepared transcripts remain rather poor representations of spoken discourse. In giving our own transcription rules, we merely have stated explicitly our attempt to capture the richness of talk without needlessly burdening the reader. Figure 4.1 contains the simplified sociolinguistic conventions of transcript preparation that we adopted.[35]

d) *Reliability of transcription.* Two research assistants separately assessed the reliability of transcriptions by reading them as they listened to

1. Line Number	001 002 . . . 999 Typescript lines are numbered sequentially from the first line of the transcript.
2. Speaker	D P D is doctor, P is patient. Speaker is noted at the first line of an utterance and at overlap points.
3. Turn/Utterance Location	Each new turn, that is, the beginnings of utterances by speakers in a sequence, generally starts at the beginning of a line in the transcript. Gaps and overlaps are indicated by appropriate markers.
4. Overlap	[If a speaker begins to talk while the other is still talking, the point of beginning overlap is marked by a bracket [between the lines; when a bracket appears below the end of the line or above the beginning of the line, the last word transcribed overlaps the first word of the next line.
5. Silence	. . . . (34) Silences within speaker utterances and between speakers are marked by a series of dots; each dot represents one second. Long pauses are denoted by number of seconds in parentheses. These silences are assigned to the previous speaker if they occur between speakers—that is, they are given the meaning of a post-utterance pause.
6. Unclarity	(cold)/(. . .) Where a word(s) is heard but remains unclear, it is included in parentheses; if words are heard that cannot be distinguished, they are indicated by the notation "(words)"; if there are speaking sounds that are unintelligible, this is noted as dots within parentheses.
7. Speech Features	?/. Punctuation marks are used when intonation clearly marks the utterance as a question or as the end of a sentence. : If a word is stretched, this is marked by a colon as in "Wel:l."

	If a speaker breaks off in the middle of a word or phrase, this is marked by a hyphen -, as in "haven't felt like-."
	((softly)) Double parentheses enclose descriptions, not transcribed utterances.
	.hh, hh, eh-heh, .engh-henh These are breathing and laughing indicators. A period followed by "hh's" marks an inhalation. The "hh's" alone stand for exhalation. The "eh-heh" and ".engh-henh" are laughter syllables (inhaled when preceded by a period).
	Italics or CAPS Italics or capital letters are used if there is a marked increase in loudness and/or emphasis.
8. Names	—— (blanks) To protect confidentiality, blanks substitute for proper names.
9. Deletion in Excerpt	* * * (asterisks) Within excerpts from transcripts, three asterisks signify a passage from the original transcript that has been deleted from the excerpt.

Figure 4.1
Transcription rules adopted for this study, modified from Mishler, Discourse of Medicine, *and West,* Routine Complications, *cited in nn. 5 and 22 below, respectively*

the original tapes of recorded doctor-patient interaction. Each individual marked the transcript where he or she believed that the transcription did not convey accurately what was said and how it was said in the tape itself. The research assistants then met with me, and the three of us decided on a final edited transcript to use for interpretation and later publication. Usually the problems that arose in transcription were minor ones, having to do with how the transcriptionists heard specific passages of speech. For instance, transcriptionists tended to type the technical names for diagnoses and medications incorrectly. From time to time, the research assistants disagreed with the transcriptionists about such details as the positioning of interruptions, simultaneous speech, and pauses. Rarely did they find systematic problems of transcription that occurred more than once. When they did find such problems, however, we notified the transcriptionists to revise their procedures slightly for the remaining tapes yet to be transcribed.

e) *Procedures for interpretation.* For interpreting the transcripts, the two research assistants and I prepared procedures in advance. These procedures derived from our theoretical considerations of ideology and social control in professional-client encounters. Further, the procedures took into account both the content and structure of transcript materials.

Initially, each research assistant was to scan all the transcripts and to note those transcripts that dealt, in even minor ways, with the contextual issues of work; family life and gender roles; aging; sexuality, leisure, substance use, and other forms of pleasure seeking; and emotional problems. In this way, we hoped to accumulate transcripts illustrating the contextual issues of greatest interest. Within all transcripts, each research assistant also was to flag instances when either doctors or patients made statements that conveyed ideologic content or expressed messages of social control. Operationally, we defined ideology rather loosely, following Althusser, as ideas that represented an imagined relationship to lived social experience.[36] Predictably, ideology in medicine would reinforce dominant ideologic patterns in the society. In medical discourse, for instance, ideologic content might comprise a doctor's statement that work would be good for an unemployed worker's mental health, a patient's comment that she expected herself to do housework well despite incapacitating physical symptoms, a doctor's words claiming that men needed to stay sober to take care of their families, and so forth. We operationally defined messages of social control as statements that encouraged people's adherence to norms of appropriate behavior. Examples might include a doctor's refusal to extend certification of disability to a worker who did not want to return to work, a doctor's prescribing a tranquilizer and encouraging acceptance of the situation for a woman who is distressed by marital discord, or a doctor's discouraging sexual activity by pointing out the dangers of sexually transmitted disease and pregnancy.

In addition to flagging these elements of content, the research assistants were to highlight nonverbal and quasi-verbal elements that might clarify a deeper structure lying beneath the surface elements of discourse. Interruptions, other cut-offs, de-emphases, shifts in tone of voice, silence, unresponsiveness to questions, and similar phenomena became special targets for this phase of the work. Here we were seeking the specific points in discourse when contextual issues might arise and how they might be either addressed directly or marginalized. By considering elements that were present, marginal, or absent, the research assistants were to prepare a preliminary structural outline or diagram that depicted how the medical discourse under study processed contextual issues.

f) *Reliability of interpretation by multiple observers.* After the two research assistants independently applied the above procedures to the transcripts, they and I met together for several months to review the annotated transcripts and preliminary outlines or diagrams. The three of us agreed to a surprising extent about the annotations that flagged instances of ideology and social control, as well as about which transcripts best illustrated the contextual issues of work, family life and gender roles, aging, and so forth. On the other hand, we disagreed more about the underlying structures that we felt the transcripts revealed. In our meetings, we brainstormed about our disagreements and explicitly tried to avoid the discussion's being dominated by one person's views (especially my own). We considered various quantitative ways to describe the degree to which we concurred or not; eventually, we decided that attaching a number would not adequately convey either the strengths or the weaknesses in the group process of interpretation at which we had arrived. Suffice it to say, our hashing things out in this way led to a fair degree of mutual satisfaction that we had grouped the transcripts according to which ones illustrated best the contextual issues of concern; that we had analyzed instances of ideology and social control within transcripts as best we could; and that we had made progress toward uncovering at least some underlying structures.

At this point, some practical changes occurred in my own social context that affected this interpretive work rather profoundly. To be both brief and specific, I changed jobs and moved with my family to a different university campus. At my new job, I experienced all sorts of unexpected problems, most of which derived from what I viewed as callous public policies about health services. These problems seriously threatened patients who were seeking care, as well as the clinic and hospital where I worked. Because of these difficulties, I found myself putting my study of medical discourse on the shelf, as I spent time trying to change these public policies so that the contextual situation might improve.[37] These efforts achieved certain improvements, but only at the expense of continuity in the project that I am now reporting. On a more positive note, at my new job I also benefitted from exposure to colleagues who had become influential in post-structuralist literary theory. Their suggestions helped me improve my theoretical analysis, or so I thought, and also made me rethink the interpretive procedures that we previously had adopted.

Why say all this? Sidetrackings and diversions in research seldom surface in accounts of research methods, even though such events—with all their costs and eventual benefits—almost always take place. To present our own methods as a smoothly flowing temporal sequence would misrepresent what actually happened. It also would give little sense of the ways that contextual issues both endanger and strengthen the research process.

To return to the narrative of how the transcripts got interpreted: In a new location, and after three years had passed, I obtained a small grant from my university to help me complete this project. The grant allowed me to hire another, gifted research assistant.[38] The two of us again reviewed all fifty annotated transcripts and spent three further months in preparing a final outline of our interpretations. We focused on instances of ideology and social control within the transcripts, especially as these pertained to contextual issues like work, the family, aging, and so forth. We also examined anew the deeper structures that we thought might be present in the discourse and arrived at interpretive conclusions with which we felt comfortable. Further, we checked out these interpretations with others, including a colleague (my wife) who was using several of our transcripts to analyze medical discourse involving women and a medical resident who was examining medical discourse with elderly patients.[39] Such was the idiosyncratic group process that helped us improve on the idiosyncrasies of our individual interpretations.

g) *Presentation of transcripts and interpretations.* After experimenting with many alternative formats, we took a mixed approach to presenting the transcripts and interpretations. In later chapters, a summary of each transcript appears first. The last research assistant mentioned above and I drafted the summaries after discussion. Within each interpretation, I offer excerpts from the transcript that, at least I hope, help substantiate the interpretive arguments. Finally, the full transcripts are available for skeptical or unusually dedicated readers.[40]

h) *Variability and the "negative case."* We dealt with variability of content and structure in the transcripts as follows. The last mentioned research assistant and I grouped the fifty transcripts according to the predominant contextual arena that the transcripts revealed. That is, we put transcripts focusing mainly on work in one pile, transcripts dealing principally with family life and gender roles in a second pile, those pertaining to aging in a third stack, those alluding to sexuality, substance use, and related gratifications in a fourth, and those focusing on emotional problems in a fifth. Of course, we found some overlap in the contextual territory that each transcript covered. For that reason, we chose for each transcript that pile designating the predominant contextual emphasis of the encounter in question. We also cross-indexed transcripts that we felt manifested more than one contextual dimension. Within each pile, we then selected three to four transcripts that illustrated a wide range of content and structure. To do this, we referred to the annotated transcripts and interpretations that we previously had prepared. While our theoretical orientations clearly lurked behind the choices that we made, it is noteworthy that the two of us differed considerably in theoretical bent, and we both genuinely believed that the range of transcripts selected did reflect the range of content and structure appearing in the materials at hand. Chosen in this way, the transcripts for each contextual arena became the grist for the interpretive mill of the chapters that follow.

From our sorting of transcripts, we also accumulated a sixth stack, containing those in which we could not locate evidence of contextual concerns. This therefore became the stack of negative cases. These transcripts did not yield any appreciable elements of content or structure that reflected the theoretical questions of interest. As required by our criteria of an appropriate method, we needed to look at these negative cases in some depth. For that reason, we decided to devote a later chapter to examining such encounters and trying to explain why they might be "nonproblematic."

I have retraced the sometimes rough trails that I and others have cut in the study of medical discourse. This trek has offered opportunities for self-criticism and reflection on what appear to be rather inherent limitations in previously used methods. From this vantage point, attempts to analyze medical discourse numerically (the quantitative methods) and verbally (the qualitative ones) have led to limited achievements and substantial failings. Toward the end of the excursion, I have arrived at some compromises about a methodical approach to the study of medical discourse, an approach that also takes into account the theoretical concerns of previous chapters.

How well the method works of course depends on applying it to actual texts, which is what comes next.

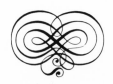

TWO

HOW
MEDICINE
MEDIATES
SOCIAL
PROBLEMS

CHAPTER 5

MEN, WORK,
AND THE
FAMILY

This chapter and the next ask, How does medical discourse deal with personal troubles that derive from work and family life? Because the social issues involved differ substantially for men and women, I organize the chapters according to the patients' gender—men in this chapter and women in the next. Using the methods just described, I summarize and interpret several encounters, drawn from a large, random sample of doctor-patient interaction.[1] These encounters vary in the degree to which work and family life become problematic. Yet they provide an opportunity to see how doctors and patients respond to contextual issues in the workplace and family.

Certain theoretical concerns, as noted earlier, guide the interpretation of these materials. How messages of ideology and social control appear and get processed comprises one theoretical focus. A related concern, influenced by structuralism, looks for deeper structures that may lie beneath the surface details of discourse. From post-structuralism comes attention to elements that are marginal, interrupted, cut off, or absent. By emphasizing these points, I do not mean to imply that the texts do not merit other lines of interpretation from different theoretical persuasions. For readers who want to go another route, or who otherwise doubt the interpretations offered here, the full transcripts are available as a microfilmed appendix (see Preface for details).

For the purpose of orientation, a few words about the format of presenting the encounters may help. A brief summary of the encounter appears first. Some details about the participants' personal backgrounds

then follow; data about the doctors and patients derive from questionnaires that they answered after their interactions were recorded. Then I
interpret the encounter, using excerpts from the transcript for substantia-
tion. In certain instances, I make minor references to lines in the transcript without reproducing the excerpts; the full transcripts contain these
passages. The conventions employed in preparing the transcripts, both
for the excerpts and the complete versions in the microfilmed appendix,
appear as figure 1 in chapter 4.

Another question remains implicit in the pages that follow: Is there a
better way to go? The patients and doctors appearing here do their best to
deal with the problems that confront them. Yet their dialogue reveals
many disquieting features. For instance, I will argue, the structure of
medical discourse tends to marginalize the contextual sources of personal
distress. Further, elements of ideology and social control often encourage
consent to the same conditions that create personal troubles in the first
place. Facing these and other tensions in the encounters, one wonders
what options exist. Speculation about reform then inevitably arises. How
could patients and doctors speak differently, and what changes in social
context would facilitate such improvements? Rather than suggesting
alternatives along the way, I hold the question of reform in abeyance until
the last chapter, in which I grapple more directly with possibilities for
change.

ENCOUNTER 5A: DISABILITY CERTIFICATION

SUMMARY

A man comes to his doctor several months after a heart attack. He is
depressed. His period of disability payments will expire soon, and
his union is about to go on strike. His doctor tells him that he is
physically able to return to work as a radial drill operator and that
working will be good for his mental health. The doctor also prescribes an antidepressant and a tranquilizer.[2]

Here is some information about the participants in Encounter 5A. The
patient is a 55-year-old white male high-school graduate. He is Protestant, Irish, married, and the father of an 18-year-old child. There is no
information available about the patient's wife, who accompanies him
during part of the encounter. The doctor is a 38-year-old white male
specializing in internal medicine and gastroenterology. He is Protestant
and states that his ethnic background is English. The doctor has known
the patient for five and one-half years and believes that the primary
diagnoses are "coronary artery disease" and "severe recurrent depression." The encounter takes place in a private practice near Boston.

Returning to work. The patient's role in economic production be-comes a focus of this encounter. Asking about the patient's work situa-tion early in the interaction, the doctor needs to be reminded that the patient has not returned to work after his heart attack:

DOCTOR: How are things coming at work?
WIFE: He hasn't been to work yet.   75
PATIENT: Well they, you know, they prolonged it, they've
     extended the contract for ten days.
D: Yeah.
P: Which is a good sign.
D: Yeah.   80
P: From what I heard that's a good sign.
D: So when would you be able to, when would they be
  ready to go if they approve a contract?
P: Oh, it'd probably be, well the contract runs out
  the 26th.   85
D: Of this month, that's this Saturday.
P: That's this Saturday.
D: And it's prolonged . . .
P: It'll be a week and a half.
D: Yeah, so if they arrange something, they'll know if   90
  by mid-June.
P: They should.
D: Is that bugging you? The idea of going back to work?
P: Well . . . actually I think I want to go back.
D: Yeah, I think you should go back.   95
P: Actually, I think I want to go back, but then go back
  and go on strike? That seems to bother me.
D: Yeah. But if you go back mid-June it won't,
  won't bother you.
P: No   100

After a long pause, several interrelated issues arise. First, although de-tails are incomplete, it is clear that the patient is receiving disability payments, apparently because of his heart disease. The doctor previ-ously has certified that this disability would end by a specific date:

D: Just strip down to your waist, Mr. ——.
     ((door opens and closes))
D: ((to wife)) What did I say on that form last time,
  I don't remember. Did I say first of June? For
  returning to work.   120
W: On one of the forms you did, you said the first
  of June . . .

D: I thought that's what we decided on, the first
　of June . . .
W: We thought perhaps he could go back, yeah,　　　　　　125
　around the first.

A second problem is an impending strike that the patient anticipates may begin shortly after the disability period ends (lines 96–97 above). The patient worries about a potential scenario in which his disability payments stop, he goes back to work, but then he must go out on strike, thus losing income. Perhaps because the patient does not elaborate, the doctor does not acknowledge this issue explicitly. Instead, he focuses on a third concern, the presumed association between the client's emotional distress and unemployment. According to the doctor, the patient's depression will become worse if he does not return to work:

D: I think he's gotta go back.
W: He is, I told him
　　　　　　[
D:　　　　　　I tell you if this guy stays
　home, he's going to curl up in a ball, you know, he's gonna　　130
　be unreachable.

Later the physician reiterates his view that getting back to work will prove beneficial:

D: I'll check the cardiogram. I would think that
　maybe we would plan on getting you back, say,
　mid-June, you know, to work, which I think is　　　　　　175
　the *best* thing in the world for you, to get
　back to work. Your heart's strong enough, your
　blood pressure's good, there's no reason why we
　can't get you back in the middle of things.

Whether the doctor is oblivious to the financial problems that may arise if the patient returns before the strike or consciously chooses to ignore the issue remains unclear. The overall implication is that working is good for this patient specifically and perhaps for workers in general.

　　This passage illustrates medicine's social control over labor and the transmission of ideologic messages about work at the level of the doctor-patient relationship. Here the doctor controls a working-class patient's role in economic production by withholding the continued certification of illness. Despite some attempts to communicate concern about the timing of his return to work, the patient does not participate actively in this decision. With benevolence, the doctor expropriates the decision-making process regarding both health and work. The patient explicitly states that returning to work in the face of an impending strike "seems to bother me." The doctor invalidates this concern and implies that the strike will be settled by "mid-June," although he could not know this with any certainty. If the patient returns by mid-June, the doctor argues, "it . . . won't bother you." The patient feebly replies, "No," after which a long pause occurs in the dialogue.

Beyond the decertification of illness and loss of decision-making power, the patient receives a strong ideologic message that work is beneficial for his health, which is subtly defined as the capacity to work.[3] In many people's lives, work enhances emotional stability and feelings of personal worth, even if work is alienating and conflictual. The point here, however, is that a professional assumes directive control over the patient's occupational behavior. With medical authority, the doctor mediates the worker's role in production. Despite the pressures of work and contract negotiations, the doctor argues, the patient will feel better, mentally and physically, if he is working than if he is idle. From the theoretical perspective developed in earlier chapters, such ideologic elements reinforce the society's dominant ideologic conceptions about work and economic production. In Gramsci's terms, for instance, these ideologic elements help shape individuals' roles in work and thus contribute to the broader "hegemonic" impact of ideology in society.[4] Such micro-level communications, which tend to reproduce macro-level relations of production, are quite common in doctor-patient interaction, although the participants rarely perceive that these messages contain broader social import.

Emotional disturbance and psychiatric technology. While the patient remains quite concerned about the contextual issue of work and its discontents, the doctor marginalizes the social context by focusing on the patient's emotional disturbance, which then becomes amenable to technical intervention through drugs. As a post-structuralist reader might note, the text moves work from a central focus to a marginal one.[5] Here the switch takes place through an abrupt shift of attention initiated by the doctor. Specifically, the marginalization of social context becomes apparent as the doctor cuts off discussion of the forthcoming strike and invokes a need for psychotropic medication:

P: Actually I think I want to go back, but then go back
   and go on strike? That seems to bother me.
D: Yeah. But if you go back mid-June it won't,
   won't bother you.
P: No   100
D: I think if you're going to take anything,
   you ought to take the Mellaril. We ought to
   maybe add some Elavil. 'Cause I think most of
   your symptoms are depression and frustration
   right now.   105

Thioridazine (Mellaril) is a medication for psychosis; amitriptyline (Elavil) is an antidepressant. The doctor shows these actors to the stage immediately after the patient voices concern about a script that dictates returning to work in the face of an impending strike.

In his verbal behavior, the patient gives no evidence of psychosis; his statements seem appropriate, grounded in reality, and without bizarre or incomprehensible features. On the other hand, the patient is clearly upset and perhaps suicidal, although he expresses his feelings laconically. One revelation is the patient's terse statement of suicidal thoughts:

D: Uh, uh, what are you taking for medication now?
P: Well, I don't know. I take Mellaril. Some days I take four, I
    take six, I'm right at a point now I don't know if I should   5(
    take Mellaril, Librax
                    [
W: Librium
P: um, Librium . . . or poison.
D: You're just all wound up now. . . . You want to take poison?
P: Jeepers, I don't know what, I don't know what to take. I'm right   5
    at a point now, I don't know what would do any good.

This danger signal about poison leads to a brief question by the doctor, apparently intended to assess the patient's suicide potential. Quickly, however, the issue of suicide disappears from the conversation, as the doctor refocuses attention on medications.

The doctor does not attempt to explore the patient's distress in depth. Instead, two professional interventions occur, neither of which encourages the patient to seek the roots of his depression in psychodynamics or in the social environment. First, the doctor offers technologic assistance in the form of drugs. To manage the patient's emotional problems, the doctor uses polypharmacy—a variety of medications without clear-cut pharmacologic rationale. Prescriptions include: (a) Mellaril, a major tranquilizer whose indication is schizophrenia or other serious psychosis; (b) Librium, a minor tranquilizer intended for relief of anxiety and/or neurosis; (c) Librax, a combination of Librium and an antispasmodic for emotion-related gastrointestinal disturbances; and (d) Elavil, an antidepressant. The literature of psychopharmacology sheds doubt on the usefulness of any of these agents for this patient, whose distress seems to derive in large part from the social situation, especially work, and from concern about heart disease. Moreover, when suicide is a possibility, the danger of overdose from these drugs, especially in combination, is severe.[6]

Despite these quibbles, the point here is not to criticize the doctor's medical judgment but to see how this judgment communicates an ideologic message. Specifically, polypharmacy converts a socioemotional problem to a technical one. Drug treatment objectifies—or reifies, to use Lukács' term[7]—a complex series of psychologic and social questions. Symbolically, scientific medicine shifts the focus to the physical realm, depoliticizes the social structural issues involved, and mutes the potential for action by the patient to change the conditions that trouble him.

A second intervention concerning emotional distress involves the medicalization of work. A rosy picture of work's psychic benefits diverts attention from its physical, socioemotional, and economic hazards. The patient voices concern (though not too articulately) about these hazards, but the doctor portrays idleness as a root of psychic disaster and re-employment as a mode of adjustment if not cure. Voiced with the authority of medical science, this ideologic message reproduces the worker's place in the relations of production. The professional's words convey the promise of happiness, or at least relative happiness, in work as currently organized.

Patterning family life. While the medical encounter reinforces the structure of work, it patterns family life as well. In this interaction, the doctor decides not only how and when the patient should work but also under what conditions the patient may relax, travel, and enjoy himself. The doctor argues that too much leisure time is bad for physical and mental health. On the other hand, after the doctor says that the patient should return to work, the patient carefully seeks permission to travel:

P: Well, what do you think about going to Maine,   180
   down and back in one day?
D: How long a drive would it be?
P: Be twelve hours and fifteen minutes, twelve and a half.
D: So long as you stop the car every hour and get
   out and take a little walk around, keep the   185
   circulation going, fine, no problem.

Just as the doctor states the date for return to work, the patient questions if a trip to Maine would be acceptable. The patient does not ask for a long vacation, just a one-day excursion. In response, the doctor requests information about how long a drive this would involve. The doctor then approves a twelve- to thirteen-hour trip, as long as the patient stops every hour to walk. Perhaps the physician's concern here is the possibility of blood clots in the patient's legs if he remains seated for too long. It is worth noting, however, that the patient is more assertive about his desire for this drive to Maine than about any other stated goal in the encounter except reduction of smoking. His wife reiterates the patient's request later and again receives conditional approval (lines 206–12). This couple do not indicate what other activities give them pleasure. The leisure they do seek, however, is subject to medical regulation.

Although, as Foucault might point out, professional surveillance of the family occurs here, the encounter nonetheless maintains an uncritical stance regarding family relations.[8] The participation of the patient's wife in the encounter is striking but not unusual. The interaction allows certain inferences about family dynamics and the doctor's reinforcement of them. While the patient is the economic breadwinner, he emerges as a relatively helpless person, unable to care or even speak for himself without his wife's assistance. The wife elaborates at length on the patient's emotional disturbance, sleep problems, disability certification, and desire for a pleasure trip. She and the doctor hold side conversations between themselves, both in and outside the patient's presence. Although the doctor encourages the patient to become more active by returning to work, he subtly colludes with the wife in retaining the patient's day-to-day helplessness within the family. In but one example, while the patient is undressing in another room, the doctor invokes military imagery, depicting his own struggle, perhaps in alliance with the wife, to control the patient's problems:

W: Well, he feels it's all the cigarettes.
   But if it isn't one thing
                      [
D: it's something else.
   You knock down one soldier and another one pops up,   13∎
   you know?

The doctor and the patient's wife thus become presumed allies in the war against internal enemies within the patient. Their collusion extends from agreement about the emotional impact of idleness, to diminishing the patient's concern about smoking, to instructions about drug dosages (lines 194–206). Further, the patient himself voices no objection to this pattern of communication. Although the doctor recognizes depression as one of the patient's two major medical diagnoses, he does not explore the family's dynamics. To the extent that psychologic problems in the family exist, the medical encounter reinforces the status quo.

Ideology and structure. Throughout the interaction, technical knowledge occupies a minor place, in comparison to the ideology and symbolism of scientific medicine. The doctor asks a few questions from the standpoint of cardiology (regarding chest pain, lines 27–32), inquires about the use of a cardiac medication (nitroglycerine, lines 62–66), discusses gauze and nail care (lines 140–55), performs a brief physical exam, and orders an electrocardiogram. Otherwise, it is difficult to find evidence in this encounter of scientific medicine per se. On the other hand, the doctor offers a series of pronouncements about work, leisure, and emotional difficulties. These utterances contain little or no scientific rationale, yet their impact derives from the symbolism of scientific knowledge and technique. Carrying the authority of medical science, the doctor dominates the interaction.[9] In this sense, the professional assumes control over major areas of life inside and outside the medical realm.

What are the underlying structural elements of this encounter? Let me return now to the points made toward the end of chapter 3. To reiterate: The contextual issue of greatest concern here involves the patient's work (A). Depression is a personal trouble that the patient experiences, partly in anticipation of a return to uncertain employment (B). In the medical encounter (C), the patient expresses concern about returning to work while his union intends to go out on strike (D). The doctor, however, interrupts him or otherwise de-emphasizes the patient's worries about what will face him when he returns to work (E). Instead of pursuing the contextual problem, the doctor reassures the patient and the patient's wife that work will benefit his mental health. Moreover, the doctor uses the technical resources at his disposal to prescribe a tranquilizer and an antidepressant medication (F). After the patient leaves the encounter, he presumably continues to prepare himself for a return to work. Figure 3.1 presents a diagram of this structure.

The discourse in this encounter does not empower or provide autonomy for the client in any apparent way. The doctor offers little technical information but many ideologic messages. Much of the communication mystifies the social roots of distress with the symbolism of scientific medicine, as the professional assumes decision-making control over wide areas of the patient's existence. In all of this, the patient acquiesces. The doctor truly cares for the patient, the patient appreciates the doctor's concern, and for all the participants' conscious intents and purposes, this is probably an excellent doctor-patient relationship. That the encounter may reinforce the social sources of discontent in the workplace and family escapes notice entirely. Such are the puzzling anomalies of a caring relationship between doctor and patient in this society.

ENCOUNTER 5B: OCCUPATIONAL ILLNESS

SUMMARY

A man with diabetes sees a doctor for the first time because of pain in the back and neck. The pain becomes worse with physical movements at work, but the patient finds it difficult to rest at home because of the demands of his job. In response, the doctor prescribes pain relievers, a neck collar, heat, and other measures to relieve muscle spasm. He advises the patient to rest as much as possible.

In Encounter 5B, the patient is a 41-year-old man who works as an assistant food operations manager in a hotel. He is Catholic, black, divorced, a high school graduate, and the father of three children. The doctor, a 43-year-old white male who practices general internal medicine and endocrinology, states in his questionnaire that he is a Mormon by religious persuasion and "Danish Scottish English German" in ethnic background. In this encounter, the patient and doctor are meeting for the first time in a suburban practice near Boston. According to the doctor, the patient's primary diagnosis is "acute muscle spasm."

Pain and work. The verbal content of this encounter, which again focuses largely on the impact of physical symptoms on work and vice versa, appears more routine and prosaic than that in Encounter 5A. Presenting with musculoskeletal pain, the patient's complaints rank among the most common problems for which patients see doctors. The patient's motivations about continuing on the job also seem different from those of the last patient. Rather than seeking exemption from work or certification of disability, the patient in Encounter 5B wants help so that he can continue to work despite painful symptoms that worsen on the job.

Leading into a series of questions about the patient's neck and back pain, the doctor very early connects the themes of work and health:

D: All right. And you're working somewhere?
P: At the ———— . . . (words)
D: What is your job there?
P: I'm the assistant food and beverage manager.   3⦁
D: All right. Are you a healthy man basically?
P: I am.
D: Any chronic diseases?
P: I have, uhm, they call it, um, mature diabetes.
D: Do you take medicine for that?   3
P: No. I control my weight.
D: Good.

The doctor juxtaposes questions about where the patient is working and whether he is "a healthy man basically." This simple connection, however, conveys the subtle message that healthy men work. Performance at work thus becomes a routine question that doctors learn to ask, with the assumption that work capacity is linked to general health status. The basis of this assumption remains unexamined. As noted earlier, however, the ideologic notion that tends to define health as the ability to work pervades the history of twentieth-century medicine and health policy.[10] From this perspective, the healthy man is he who works. (The next chapter considers medical ideology and *women's* work.)

Work rather than family remains the encounter's chief contextual focus. The patient mentions family ties only twice. First, in response to the doctor's routine question about marital status, the patient responds that he is divorced (lines 21–22). Much later, in describing his neck pain, the patient alludes to a woman friend:

P: My girl was rubbing my neck at, uh, the   171
    first part of the week, and there was actually a *knot* up
    there.

In neither instance does the doctor or the patient pursue any discussion about the patient's family. For this male patient and his doctor, work becomes the contextual issue of concern, and family matters receive little or no attention.

    In contrast to Encounter 5A, the patient in this encounter wants to continue working and views his physical symptoms as an impediment, since exertion on the job makes his pain worse:

D: And were you working this morning?
P: Right.
D: Hm hm. And was it worse when you got up or worse after   80
    you were at work?
P: Well, I think it got worse when I got to work.

While the patient and doctor acknowledge that muscular strain at work exacerbates the problem, the patient sees some difficulties in staying home or even cutting back on job-related physical activity. These difficulties center on some pressing engagements and the inability to obtain coverage for his work responsibilities:

D: I want you to   255
    get a heating pad if you don't have one, and you lie on it.
    You go home, and you may not be able to work today. Um, is
    the whole Sheraton Hospital [*sic*] chain gonna stop if
    you weren't working today?
P: Well, see the thing is, the food and beverage manager is gone, he   260
    won't, he won't be coming back until Tuesday night, and we
    have the Seagram's auction of (word) and
                                 [
D: Yeah, and you're the
    liquor man for Seagram's.
P: Right. And plus the fact that this is (words) tonight,   265
    and
    [
D: Well
      [
P: this afternoon, and
       [
D: you've got to compromise. Ideally, you ought to go home

and lie on a heating pad. You probably can't do that, because   27◦
  (words). I will give you some other pains, other pills for
  pain. And this will be codeine. Can you take it?
P: Yes.

In short, the patient is experiencing pain that derives from physical exertion at work, but he finds no way to stop working in the near future. The doctor suggests a temporary break from the job and jokes about the patient's sense of responsibility ("Um, is the whole Sheraton Hospital [*sic*] chain gonna stop if you weren't working today?"). However, the patient notes that the food and beverage manager, who presumably might substitute for him under other circumstances, is away, and a liquor auction needs attendance. The doctor imputes ambivalence to the patient ("you've got to compromise"), noting that the patient should rest but feels that he cannot, apparently because of expectations at work. For that reason, the doctor offers codeine, a narcotic, to provide pain relief while the patient continues working.

Occupational barriers to rest. A central dilemma in this encounter, quite a routine one in the medical encounters studied, centers on the conflict between work demands and therapeutic rest. Here, the doctor and patient seem to share a view that work is beneficial, or at least necessary. The patient does not seek exemption from work or certification of disability. On the contrary, the doctor urges the patient to take some time off on a temporary basis, presumably to hasten the recovery process. The patient is reluctant to do so, however, and the doctor responds by modifying his treatment recommendations. Because the patient cannot, or will not, rest at home, the doctor prescribes a narcotic, heat, and a collar:

D: No irritation from that, huh. Ah, this is strong. It may
  make you a little bit dizzy, some people are. But the back.   27.
  If you can't, will you have any time during the day that you
  can lie down, even on the job, lie on a heating pad?
P: Well, once I get this bar set up this afternoon, I think
  basically they should (words) me on leave.
D: Well, I would like to have you away as much as possible. At   28◦
  home, lying down on a *flat* bed. Don't lie down on a hammock.
  Make it a flat bed, and if it's not very flat, lie on the
  floor. And put the heating pad on the floor and lie on it.
  Put a couple towels. And first don't burn yourself, but
                                                  [
P: Right   28.
    [
D: leave it as the cloth. And do that for an hour
  or two. And then some warm clothing over your back, so it

doesn't, uh, get chilled after. And the final thing is, that
you will benefit by a collar. Wearing a high collar around
your neck. Even though the pain is a little bit lower than   290
that right now, you've got neck residual distress here at the
side muscles, and if we can hold that immobile, you can work
with the collar on.

P: Right.

By choosing these objective treatments, the discourse reifies a complex
set of social relations that the patient faces at his job. In this way, doctor
and patient select a less desirable therapeutic option: continuing on the
job under conditions that may worsen the patient's physical condition.

The point here is not whether the doctor's and patient's decisions are
helpful or harmful, but rather that a major thrust of their encounter
pertains to the patient's ability to function at work. The patient develops
a physical symptom that either derives from occupational exertion, worsens due to this activity, or both. Such a condition actually defines an
occupational illness, for which by law an employee becomes eligible for
compensation and medical benefits.[11] Neither doctor nor patient, however, mentions the scenario of occupational injury or disability—again in
marked contrast to Encounter 5A. Instead, the participants in the encounter follow what seem to be the patient's preference for meeting his
work responsibilities under adverse circumstances. The patient vaguely
alludes to the possibility of being placed "on leave" (line 279), but no
definite plans get made. Although the doctor shows some discomfort
with the patient's continuing to work, he stretches his imagination to
accommodate treatment to the patient's job requirements. Thus, the
doctor reasons, the patient can wear a collar and rest with a heating pad,
despite the obvious difficulties of lying down on the job.

In mediating the work process, the discourse of this encounter tacitly
accepts the conditions of work as currently organized. While the doctor
urges the patient to take time off to rest, he does not push too hard on this
point, even though he recognizes that continuing to work exacerbates
the physical problem. For instance, the doctor does not offer to write a
note to the employer or to intervene in other ways. On the contrary, the
doctor with some reluctance modifies his statements about appropriate
treatment to help the patient stay on the job. When the doctor jokingly
asks if the patient's company is "gonna stop if you weren't working," this
joke conveys an innuendo that the patient's internal sense of responsibility has become misguided under the present circumstances. Thus,
the doctor implies, the patient should have the good sense to take time
off to heal and places the responsibility for leaving work on the patient's
shoulders. Rather than taking more initiative on this score, the doctor
uses rather nondirective comments to encourage rest. Because of external
job requirements and internalized sense of responsibility, however, seek-

ing exemption from work because of illness sometimes proves not at all simple.

Dark humor. At several additional points in the encounter, the doctor assumes the jokester role. In this and in other encounters studied, doctors frequently crack jokes or use humorous imagery. Humor may release tension in medicine, although the position of jokes in doctor-patient dialogue has received little attention.[12] This doctor's joking imagery conveys the themes of the military, strength in military (or at least maritime) duty, masculine strength versus weakness, and physical violence.

In short, the humor becomes rather dark. A maritime theme arises at the beginning of the encounter, as the doctor misinterprets the patient's address and the patient clarifies his military background:

D: What's your permanent address?
P: Well, I, I'm living in ——, apartment ——, Home from
   the Sea.
D: Does that mean you *are* home from the sea, you've been a seaman?
P: No, no, no. That's the apartment, the name of the   10
   apartments. (words) name, I swear (words) a cartoon.
D: That's an elegant name. I just wondered if you
   were a retired seaman. Hh heh ha.
P: I (words) Air Force.

This former military man thus is not home from the sea, just living in the Home from the Sea apartment complex. A military man, one would think, ought not complain about minor aches and pains. So the doctor jokes:

P: This morning when I woke up I just, I just couldn't
   even lift up off the bed, I had to (word) up.
D: The toughest men are the biggest sissies.   7
P: Heh ha ha.

The conversation then proceeds to a series of questions and answers about the patient's military service. Although the doctor's purpose in these inquiries about military experience remains unclear, the sequence concludes with another dark joke:

D: What'd you do in the service?
P: I was a procurement specialist.
D: In what?
P: Uh, purchasing contracts (word)   12
                            [
D: Navy, Army, Air Force?
                                           [
P: Air Force.

D: So, much the same kind of work.
P: Right.
D: But you can have a bigger mustache now.   130
P: Oh, yeah, .Hh heh heh ha.
Woman's voice: .Hh heh heh ha.
D: You don't have to wear a wig on your off-duty hours.
                                        [
P: No. No.
D: You haven't been retired too long, have you?   135
P: No, May '72.
D: '72. All right, well if I can't cure you, do I have
    permission to shoot you?
P: No, no, please.
D: A horse gets this way, I don't waste much time on him.   140
    Is it more on the right side?
P: Right side. Nothing up there. Thi- There.

The patient laughs at the doctor's joke that his mustache can grow longer
in civilian life. The laughter somehow stops, though, when the doctor
asks the patient for "permission to shoot" him, as he might shoot a horse
in pain.

    Although the doctor then switches to a more technical mode, as he
offers his thinking about future diagnostic studies and treatments, other
dark jokes appear. The first alludes to death:

D: And for
    my peace of mind, I wish you would call me Friday.
P: Right.   305
D: Okay, just tell me how you're doing.
P: Okay. Where do I get this collar
                             [
D: or your widow can call me,
    okay.

As the encounter ends, the doctor again resumes a joking, quasi-military
posture as he writes down a note that presents a list of doctor's orders so
that the patient will not forget. These orders initially include: (1) codeine,
(2) a neck collar, and (3) heat. The fourth, fifth, and sixth orders are as
follows:

D: Um, fourth thing is a flat sleeping surface. And if your   350
    bed really is too soft, you may want to put your mattress on
    the floor and sleep on your mattress on the floor tomorrow
                                                   [
P: All right
   [

D: and later we can get a bed board and put it under. And five,
   you can swear all you like. It might make you feel better.   355
   And sixth, you're gonna call me.

By including the written "order" that the patient can "swear all you like,"
the doctor again invokes the image of the sailor or soldier, swearing as
expected at the physical inconveniences of work.

Ideologies of work. To summarize: In this encounter, patient and
doctor confront an acute physical problem that work has caused or
worsened. Much of the technical content of the encounter focuses on the
diagnosis and treatment of muscle spasm. The patient's other chronic
illness, diabetes mellitus, receives attention only in passing. Instead,
doctor and patient concentrate here on the relation between work and
pain. While the doctor believes that rest away from work might help, the
patient notes that the demands of his job would make that option difficult. Then the doctor initiates a series of measures intended to relieve
pain while the patient continues to work. The patient does not request
disability certification, nor does the doctor offer it. Although the doctor
alludes jokingly to the patient's sense of responsibility for staying on
the job while in pain, he does not explore the concrete difficulties of
taking time off and does not offer to intercede with the patient's employer. Meanwhile, the doctor's dark humor conveys imagery of masculine strength under adversity. The patient departs with a makeshift
collection of concrete and reified remedies that may help him stay on the
job by reducing his pain.

How does the encounter reproduce ideologies of work? Through humor, the doctor does voice a critique of job expectations that demand
continuing physical activity in a situation that worsens the problem at
hand. However, this critique subtly questions the patient's attitude about
work, rather than actual job conditions. After the patient mentions his
problem of getting proper coverage for an auction, the doctor diminishes
this concern by joking that the corporation will not cease operations if the
patient stays home to rest. Concerning work, the doctor's interpretive
achievement is to convert a problem of external job demands to an
intrapsychic problem. From this view, it is not so much the job that is
creating the difficulty, but rather the patient's overly compulsive attitude
that leads him to tough it out despite job-induced pain.

An ideology that internalizes work-related problems thus enters the
discourse of the medical encounter. This ideology commonly holds that if
people do not adjust smoothly to the demands of their jobs, it is their own
fault. Such a teaching, which places the responsibility for unhappiness on
the individual worker rather than the work situation, pervades the occupational system in the United States and probably in similar industrialized

societies. Others have referred to the emotional suffering that this internalization causes as a "hidden injury" of social class.[13] In the discourse spoken here, the doctor senses and the patient confirms that taking time off work to rest because of an occupational illness may not be easy. Instead of questioning critically a work situation that engenders rigid job expectations, however, the doctor shifts the burden to the patient. It is the patient's ambivalence about resting from work that has become problematic, the doctor implies, rather than the demands of the job itself.

Further, the doctor marginalizes the patient's contextual concerns by belittling them subtly in humor. After all, it is laughable for the patient to feel that his corporation will stop functioning if he does not attend a liquor auction. In this way, the patient must take responsibility not only for working in a pain-inducing job situation but also for overcoming intrapsychic conflict about taking time off to rest. If the patient cannot cope smoothly with such pressures, it is nobody's fault but his own. The doctor's humorous way of moving the contextual issue of work demands to the margins of the discourse reinforces an ideologic message: adjusting successfully to the requirements of the job—even if this means taking some time off—remains the responsibility of the individual worker.

Ideology and structure. The underlying structural elements of this encounter appear to be the following (figure 5.1). As a key contextual issue, the patient's job situation demands physical exertion that causes pain, exacerbates it, or both (A). This troubling symptom leads him to seek help from a doctor (B). In the medical encounter (C), the patient describes the pain and its relation to the work context (D). In response, the doctor suggests time off from work for rest. When the patient mentions job expectations that make it difficult to rest, the doctor marginalizes this tension by joking about the patient's sense of responsibility and intrapsychic ambivalence (E). In this way, the discourse reproduces the ideology of individual responsibility for job-related difficulties. The doctor offers a series of technical suggestions, intended to reduce pain and to help the patient continue working. Critical attention to the demands of the job remains absent from the encounter (F). The patient presumably returns to work, consenting to conditions that may worsen his occupational illness.

Acute, work-induced illnesses like muscle spasm commonly receive attention in medical encounters. On the surface, they seem very routine. While some patients seek exemption from work through disability certification, many do not, as they adjust to their job expectations with medical help. In responding, doctors may encourage rest, but absence from work often proves inconvenient or otherwise undesirable from the patient's perspective. Under these circumstances, doctors' technical sug-

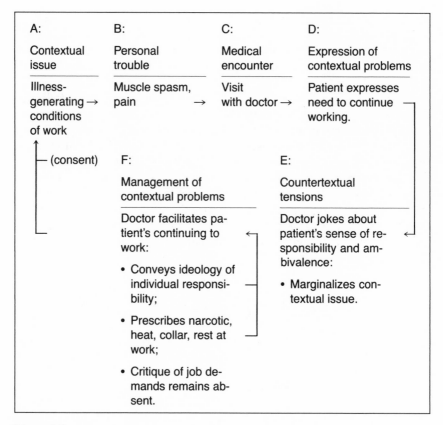

Figure 5.1
Structural elements of a medical encounter with a man who presents with a job-related musculoskeletal disorder

gestions become compromises that help patients adjust to work conditions that may worsen the physical problem.

Further, musculoskeletal disorders comprise only one of many occupational illnesses that doctors and patients process in this way. Much more serious work-related problems (such as occupational lung disease, exposure to cancer-causing chemicals or radiation, jobs with high risk of accidents or violence, and so forth) also become the focus of dialogue in medical encounters. When workers find no alternative sources for their livelihood, they often must continue to expose themselves to illness-generating conditions.[14] In that case, doctors see little option but to ease symptoms so that workers can return to the same conditions that cause or worsen their physical problems. Aiding this accommodation to illness-generating conditions at work then becomes another of the strange contradictions that characterize modern medicine.

ENCOUNTER 5C: SUCCESS IN WORK, STRESS IN THE FAMILY

SUMMARY

A man with hypertension comes to see his doctor for a regular blood pressure check. Doctor and patient engage in lengthy discussions about the recent death of the patient's mother-in-law and about the current challenges and stresses of the patient's job. Noting that the patient's blood pressure has risen, the doctor attributes this change to the patient's emotional situation. They make plans for a follow-up visit to check the blood pressure again.

The patient in Encounter 5C is a 58-year-old man who works as a physical therapist. He is married, has no children, considers himself a Catholic, and states that he is Italian. His professional education consisted of schooling in physical therapy. The doctor here is the same one who appeared in Encounter 5A; he is a 38-year-old specialist in internal medicine and gastroenterology, whose religion is Protestant and whose ethnicity is English. According to the doctor, he has known the patient for about three and one-half years. The encounter takes place in a suburb of Boston. From the doctor's viewpoint, the patient's main diagnoses are "moderate essential hypertension" and "moderate to severe chronic anxiety."

A death in the family. A personal trouble, the death of the patient's mother-in-law, comes up right at the encounter's beginning:

D: How are you feeling, first of all?
P: Fine
    [
D: are ya?
    [
P: fine, I'm OK. Yeah, nothing unusual, no,
    the same . . .   5
D: The same old nudgy things, eh?
P: Yeah, well we, uh, uh, we buried, I buried my mother-in-law
    three weeks ago.

Responding to the doctor's general question about how he is feeling, the patient first replies, "Fine," then equivocates somewhat, and then pauses. The doctor breaks the pause with a metaphor for the emotional. "Nudgy things" apparently conveys a cue to the patient that the doctor expects to hear some further emotional content. Taking this cue, the patient immediately begins a colloquy on his mother-in-law's death:

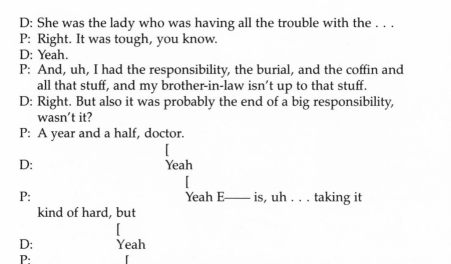

D: She was the lady who was having all the trouble with the . . .
P: Right. It was tough, you know.   10
D: Yeah.
P: And, uh, I had the responsibility, the burial, and the coffin and
all that stuff, and my brother-in-law isn't up to that stuff.
D: Right. But also it was probably the end of a big responsibility,
wasn't it?   15
P: A year and a half, doctor.
                 [
D: Yeah
                 [
P: Yeah E—— is, uh . . . taking it
kind of hard, but
         [
D: Yeah   20
P: [
I think she'll pick up. She has to.

Here the patient complains about the stress that he has endured, especially by taking on the funeral arrangements. The patient's shift of pro-
nouns reflects the burden that he has felt ("Yeah, well we, uh, uh, we
buried, I buried my mother-in-law three weeks ago"). A brother-in-law,
who may have been a more appropriate candidate for these responsibilities, perhaps because of a blood relation to the deceased, apparently
was not able to handle these tasks ("isn't up to that stuff"). The doctor
strikes a more upbeat note, observing that a burden has been lifted and
that grieving by the patient's wife (E——) will reverse itself eventually.

Although the doctor then tries to cut off the discussion of socioemotional context by questioning directly about physical symptoms, the
patient persists in the funereal voice, again implying that he has shoul-
dered more than his share of the burden:

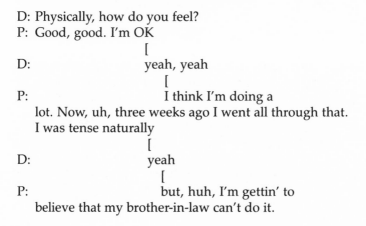

D: Physically, how do you feel?
P: Good, good. I'm OK
           [
D: yeah, yeah   30
           [
P: I think I'm doing a
lot. Now, uh, three weeks ago I went all through that.
I was tense naturally
        [
D: yeah
        [
P: but, huh, I'm gettin' to   35
believe that my brother-in-law can't do it.

D: Yeah

   [

P: You know I used to, I've always had the feeling,
   well, I could do it.

D: Yeah.   40

P: Of course I'm the kind of guy who says it has to be
   done

      [

D: Yes

      [

P: even if you're not up to it.   45

                           [

D: Yes

                           [

P: It has to be done.

D: Yeah.

P: Some people just bow out. Maybe they can't do it. I don't
   know, I shouldn't criticize, you know. I don't criticize.   50

D: Yeah.

P: It's just, uh, I could use a little help.

                         [

D: Yes

                         [

P: You know what I
   mean, doctor?   55

D: Some people, uh. (. . .)
   Yeah.

P: But it seems as though "Let N—— do it."

The doctor shifts emphasis away from the socioemotional realm by asking, "Physically, how do you feel?" In the lines that follow, the patient's emotional conflicts play themselves out in a series of inconsistent and contradictory statements. The patient demands a great deal of himself, as he carries out responsibilities that he does not relish. He at once feels that he should take on such familial responsibilities, perceives another family member as not carrying his load, wants to complain, feels he should not complain, yet complains nonetheless. Such language conveys psychic conflict, doubtless an underpinning of what the doctor diagnoses in this patient as "chronic anxiety."[15]

Accomplishments at work. After another brief cut-off alluding to the patient's medications, the doctor then moves from familial context to the world of work. In introducing the discussion of work, the doctor again focuses quickly on the patient's emotional responses:

D: Tell me something. What are you taking for medicine now,
   N——?   60
P: Six (. .) tablets a day.
D: No, I didn't mean that.
   (. .) anything else?
P: No, no.
D: You still working like a crazy man?   65
P: Oh yeah, yeah, I'm havin', uh . . . I'm havin' a lot of nice
   things happen to me.

Again, the technical information exchanged here about medications
takes little time, compared to the discussion of work that follows. After
the brief questions and answers about drugs, the doctor asks a strikingly
ambiguous question, "You still working like a crazy man?" On the one
hand, this question implies that the doctor has not viewed the patient's
work habits as altogether sane. On the other hand, the question also
connotes admiration for diligence on the job. In fact, the patient seems to
hear the more positive meaning of the simile in the doctor's question.

For the patient, "nice things" at work have to do with some accomplishments and gratifications he sees in the physical therapy that he is
giving to a young woman who has suffered a severe head injury in a
motor vehicle accident. Throughout the passage that follows, the patient's role subtly shifts to that of a professional colleague, and the
doctor's role changes to that of a consultant. The patient describes his
work experiences almost as though he were making a case presentation.
In response, the doctor asks questions not about the patient, but about
the patient's patient:

D: What's, uh, happening?
P: Well, I'm rehabilitating a girl who had a severe head
   injury in an auto accident, S——'s automotive store's   70
   daughter?
D: Oh, Jees.
P: Uh, five months in the hospital in B——
                                          [
D: God
                                          [
P: Two   75
   months of therapy; no progress. She come to me, I
   got her hand open.
D: Good. Is she paralyzed?
P: Uh, couldn't open it with a pair of pliers. She's
   doing this now.   80
D: How old a kid is she?
P: Eighteen.
D: Eh.

D: Was she racin' or something?
P: On a dune buggy.   85

Patient and doctor then explore the psychologic dimensions of this challenging problem in physical therapy. Just as they previously had discussed the physical therapist's socioemotional problems in his own family, they now focus on socioemotional problems in the family of the paralyzed patient whom the patient is attending at work:

P: Passenger, yeah. The, uh, the mother feels responsible.
   She, she . . It's the same story "Why did I let her out?"
                                                            [
D: Yeah   95
   [
P: "If I had watched her . . . "
                    [
D: Sure, grief, yeah. Guilt.
P: Right, guilt, doctor.

Here the patient returns to the theme of responsibility, such a powerful force in his own family relationships. Attributing the feeling of responsibility to the mother of the young paralyzed woman, the patient presents a scenario in which the mother criticizes herself for not supervising her injured daughter more closely. The doctor then adds two technical labels oriented to psychiatry—"Sure, grief, yeah. Guilt." Agreeing with the doctor's diagnosis at a distance, the patient seems to derive pleasure from his ability to share with his doctor these psychodynamic speculations about another patient's socioemotional context. That this case bears certain parallels to his own familial context (grief, guilt, and so forth) escapes explicit attention.

Further details follow about the technical challenges that this brain-damaged young woman offers. In this passage, partly in response to the doctor's questions and comments, the patient describes how he has diagnosed a problem in the young woman's gait that her own physicians apparently had missed (lines 100–127). Such an in-depth account of an occupational experience creates an unusual scene of collegial give and take, especially since the dialogue does not pertain directly to the patient's own medical problem of hypertension. Eventually this collegial discussion about work ends with a cut-off by the doctor, asking the patient to prepare himself for a physical exam:

P: Yeah, quad strengthening, that's right.
D: Let's . . . you sound like you're OK. Let's look and see
                                                          [
P: Yeah
                                                           [
D: if you really are.   130

P: Yeah, yeah.
D: You know where the room is, why don't you just go on in
   and strip down to your waist then.

During and after the subsequent blood pressure check, patient and doctor discuss the current level of pressure and also review the patient's medications.

Blood pressure, the family, and work. In the midst of the blood pressure check, the patient again begins to talk about family matters. He does so by asking about the doctor's family, by emphasizing his view of the family's importance, and by describing an upcoming excursion when he, a childless man, will see a musical performance by two nieces:

P: How's the family?
D: Good. Very good.
P: Hey, that's what counts, boy. I'm going to John Hancock   145
   Hall to see my two little nieces perform.
                                    [
D: Yeah
                                    [
P: I called
   off patients and just to see them.
D: What do they do?   150
P: A little dance recital.

To this patient, the family is "what counts." The patient indicates that family problems, like those he has described concerning his mother-in-law's death, do not detract from this basically positive picture. Returning to the family theme, the doctor asks about headaches that the patient's wife had been experiencing:

D: Breathe in now. Out . . . . breathe slowly . . . OK. Did your
   wife ever go into the headache clinic?
P: No, doctor. I, uh, thought maybe you'd you'd like to have   160
   her go to see that D—— ——, is it? The neurologist.
D: He's a neurologist. Yeah, I'm sure she could see him.
P: He'd talk to her about headaches?
D: Yeah, well sure, you know he's a neurologist.
                              * * *
D: Let's have you sit up now . . . Stand up please. ((Blood   172
   pressure)) 160 over 100 . . . which is, that's passable,
   you know.

One wonders if this conversation about the wife's headaches creates the most favorable conditions for an accurate blood pressure reading. Indeed, the doctor does find a blood pressure level higher than previously observed, in the midst of this talk about the ups and downs of family life.

Later, the dialogue returns to family and work as potential causes of the patient's worsening blood pressure. Discovering that the pressure is higher today than in the past, the doctor invokes imagery that might prove less than reassuring:

D: Well, 160 over 100 isn't (. .)
P: For me it is.   210
D: It isn't necessarily going to kill you, uh, 160 over 100.
   I would like to see you a little lower.
                      [
P: Yeah
                      [
D: just a *little*
   lower. If we could get that 100 down to 90, I would be, uh,
   happy as a clam.
          [
P: I understand.
              [
D: Breathe deep . . . . again.   218

The patient's pressure, though higher than before, remains in the range of "mild" hypertension.[16] A not too calming image ("It isn't necessarily going to kill you") here is combined with the doctor's metaphorical treatment goal (he would be "happy as a clam" if a somewhat lower pressure were achieved). Shortly thereafter, the patient explains his view that the rise in pressure may be an artifact of his encounter with the doctor—not because of the doctor, that is, but because of the patient's sense of internal motivation:

P: I think doctor that, uh, in about a half hour, I'll   225
   probably be 150 over 90. . . .
   No, no, I don't believe it's you. It's just Nature trying to
   say to me "I hope I get a good reading."

The doctor then adds a comment that refers vaguely to the patient's backward movement. In response, the patient interprets this comment as referring to familial stress as a precipitating cause:

D: And then get yourself going backwards.
P: I think it's that. For God sakes. What I did with my
   mother-in-law and . .
D: I'll tell you what let's do. Before I do anything, since   235
   you've had this episode. Why don't you come in in a month,
   and let E—— take your blood pressure.

From the patient's viewpoint, then, "going backwards" derives from the stress of dealing with his mother-in-law's death. In response to the doctor's nonspecific comment, the patient infers that the doctor is alluding to an emotional cause for worsened blood pressure, a cause which the patient finds in the family.

After he discusses medications briefly, the doctor reinforces his rationale for treating hypertension through a combination of drugs and emotional change.

D: Yeah, we'll see. Uh, the other thing is that, uh, the eyes,   260
   as you look in the eyes, your blood vessels look normal.
   [
P: Yeah
   [
D: Your heart's normal. So you know if there's no
   evidence that this has taken its toll in your blood
   pressure, you know, you can treat it with a little less   265
                                  [
P: I understand
   [
D: worry and fear.
P: Sure.
D: But you can't treat it so cavalierly that you just say,
   "Oh, you know, I'll take the pills or I won't" . . .
P: No, I've been taking them faithfully like you told me.

The doctor focuses here on "worry and fear" as a factor that contributes to the patient's hypertension. He tells the patient to "treat" his blood pressure with "a little less" of these emotions, as well as several pills each day. The image evoked again places the patient in the role of the health professional, taking part in his treatment by partialing out to himself less of this emotion or that one. How can the patient accomplish this task of emotional modulation? The doctor gives no clue. True, the doctor does allow the patient to emote at length about the events in his family that have been troubling him. Perhaps the doctor assumes that this verbal expression will provide a cathartic release which may prove helpful to the patient. Outside the encounter, given the patient's keen sense of responsibility, feeling "a little less" worry and fear may prove easier said than done. While he permits some emotional release within the encounter, the doctor advises emotional change without providing a methodology to accomplish this goal. On the individual level, the doctor does not mention therapeutic approaches to deal with the patient's psychodynamics. Nor do the patient and doctor discuss alternative role relationships in the family that might ease the patient's psychic burden. Concerning the family, the discourse identifies a source of stress but remains unclear about how the stress might be reduced.

A similar ambiguity remains in the final discussion of work that appears in this encounter. Here the doctor reiterates his plan to check the patient's blood pressure again in one month:

D: And I'll plan on seeing you in September. And in a month
   when you come in, just let E—— check your blood pressure.
   Don't pick a good day. And don't pick a day that you're
   rested . . .   315
P: Sometimes I go by when I'm makin' my rounds, doctor. That's
   what I usually do.
D: Yeah, that's what I want.
P: It's a funny thing this morning I didn't do too much—I
   thought maybe you'd have a . . . To me it doesn't, it doesn't   320
   make any difference. I don't believe it's the work.
D: No, I think it's minimal
                            [
P: I think it's me.

The doctor seems to be driving here at the point that one should check
blood pressure under typically stressful circumstances. He instructs the
patient not to "pick a good day," agrees that an appropriate day would be
when the patient was making work rounds, and thus implies that the
patient's work may entail stress which may worsen blood pressure. The
patient understands the implication and denies it by saying: "I don't
believe it's the work. I think it's me." That is, one presumes, the patient
believes that some other, more intrinsic quality of his personality exacerbates his hypertension. The blame thus shifts from a potential external
source in the social context to an internal source within the patient
himself.

Since the patient dwells at other points on work and its responsibilities, both physical and psychological, one may expect that physical
therapy involves tasks that for him are stimulating but also emotionally
taxing. The doctor refers indirectly to this possibility, while the patient
describes the challenging details of his work as "good things" that are
happening to him. Although the patient doubts that work worsens his
blood pressure and implies that his professional activities are not particularly stressful, his preoccupation with work becomes evident, despite
his emphasis on pros rather than cons. Venting the emotional content of
work within the medical encounter might help the patient temporarily.
As in the case of familial stress, however, neither doctor nor patient raises
the possibility of alternative arrangements. Whether work brings happiness, grief, or some combination of the two, the conditions of work as
such do not receive critical attention.

Ideology and structure. In the final instance, the patient internalizes
responsibility for adverse changes in blood pressure as his own problem,
rather than as a reflection of work or family demands. As in Encounters
5A and 5B, the ideologic underpinnings of attitudes toward work become
clear. Work leads to "good things," despite its sometimes grim details.
Likewise, the importance of close-knit family relations gains emphasis; as

the patient notes, "that's what counts." Whatever the problems that work and the family present, responsibility for accommodating to these difficulties remains an individual matter. This ideologic assumption within the discourse of a professional-client encounter reinforces a broader, hegemonic ideology in the larger society concerning work and the family. Despite—from Foucault's perspective—the professional surveillance of work and the family, doctor and patient do not explore how these contextual stresses might change, nor even how the patient might react differently to them in concrete ways. These omissions, or deemphases, occur although both participants explicitly recognize a psychologic component in high blood pressure.

Certain structural elements of the discourse therefore become apparent (figure 5.2). In the social context of the encounter, stressful conditions in the family and work have arisen (A). Stress in the family has become particularly troubling to the patient, who has more than his share of responsibilities. He also reports work activities involving cognitive, emotional, and physical contributions that are both gratifying and demanding. The patient feels some emotional conflict and anxiety about these contextual issues (B). During a routine medical encounter to check his blood pressure (C), the patient expresses these contextual problems, going on at length about familial stress and professional challenges. The doctor takes what might be called a humanistic tack, encouraging the patient to emote about these difficulties and facilitating the discussion of the social context through questions and comments about family and work (D). Although he permits the expression of contextual concerns to a degree, the doctor eventually uses several cut-offs to return the dialogue to a technical direction, concerning the patient's physical symptoms, medications, and the physical exam (E). Both doctor and patient recognize that emotions related to the social context, in the family and to a lesser extent at work, may worsen hypertension. The doctor tries to manage contextual problems by allowing the patient to emote about them in the encounter and by recommending a reduction of certain emotions like "worry and fear." Without considering concrete changes in family or work that might lessen stress, doctor and patient apparently accept an ideologic assumption that internalizes responsibility for such difficulties at the individual level (F). Throughout, the patient consents, often enthusiastically, to the contextual conditions at home and at work to which he returns.

By encouraging, or at least allowing, the patient to emote about difficulties at work and in the family, this doctor doubtless performs a psychotherapeutic function. For many doctors in primary-care specialties like internal medicine and family practice, the psychotherapeutic role has emerged as a substantial part of the medical task. About one-third of patient visits in these fields entail problems that derive in large part from

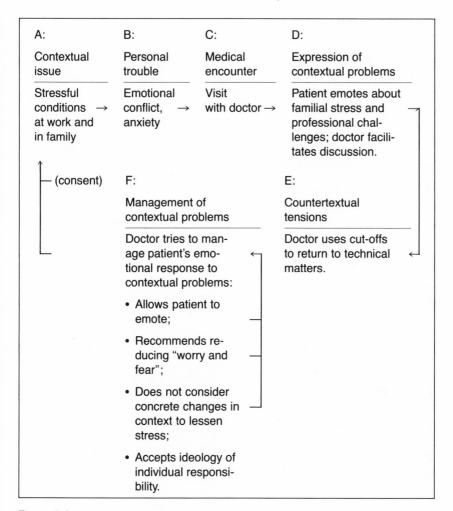

Figure 5.2
Structural elements of a medical encounter with a man whose problems include hypertension and anxiety

socioemotional disturbance.[17] With many or most of these patients, formal psychotherapy with a psychologist or psychiatrist does not prove feasible, because of financial barriers, patients' preferences, fear of psychiatry and psychiatric labels, language differences, or other constraints. Under these circumstances, emotional fallout from the social context frequently appears within the discourse of routine medical encounters, sometimes guided by a growing literature on how to do psychotherapy in general medical practice.[18] Through this psychotherapeutic function, medicine comes to mediate the contextual stresses in such spheres as work and the family. As in the present case, the option of change in the social context may not arise at all. Rather, the individual may return to stressful conditions, perhaps more fortified but at least readier to cope.

MEDICAL MEDIATION OF WORK
AND THE FAMILY FOR MEN

These three encounters deal with work and family life in different ways but presumably with similar outcomes. The patients keep working under circumstances that, to varying degrees, remain problematic. Family life also goes on for these men, without change or critical examination. After a heart attack and before an impending strike, the patient in Encounter 5A expresses reluctance about returning to work with such financial uncertainty. As a response, the doctor concentrates on the patient's depression, prescribes psychotropic medications, ends disability certification, and argues that work will prove good for the patient's mental health. In the family, although the patient continues to occupy the role of breadwinner, he maintains toward his wife a relatively helpless and dependent demeanor. In Encounter 5B, burdened by the pain of muscle spasm that grows worse with physical activity at work, the patient nonetheless feels an obligation to stay on the job. The doctor somewhat reluctantly goes along with the patient's working under illness-generating conditions, as he prescribes several remedies to ease the patient's pain. The patient in Encounter 5C reports gratification from work that is physically and psychologically taxing, along with emotional difficulties in the family. From the doctor's viewpoint, the patient's anxiety may exacerbate his high blood pressure. By allowing the patient to emote at great length about these concerns, the doctor apparently helps the patient continue to function adequately under stress.

Ideologic content arises in all three instances. In Encounter 5A, the doctor argues that work will have beneficial effects on mental health, despite the patient's concern about an impending strike and its financial impact, and makes the point that work is preferable to idleness. The doctor in Encounter 5B humorously interprets the patient's difficulty in arranging coverage at work as an intrapsychic problem. In doing so, he reinforces an ideology that places the blame for occupational maladjustment on the individual worker, rather than on the work situation itself. In Encounter 5C, when the patient voices his strong sense of commitment to his work and his family, the doctor responds positively in a collegial way, despite the possibility that stress is contributing to worsened blood pressure. Again, the doctor makes the patient responsible for improvement in anxiety, the emotional component of illness here, without examining how stress might change in the family or at work. From the theoretical perspective of earlier chapters, ideologic messages emerge in these encounters that in one way or another reinforce dominant ideologies of the wider society.

For these male patients, medical discourse focuses extensively on work, but not in a critical way. The diverse occupational details that arise in encounters like these converge toward a common pattern. When patients describe personal troubles pertaining to work, the structure of medical discourse tends to convert a contextual issue to a physical and/or psychological problem. Doctors sometimes respond humanistically by encouraging patients to emote. Alternatively, the discourse may reify the contextual issue, as doctors offer technical responses, designed to ease pain and suffering. Negotiations about disability, leaves, and other types of time off also frequently take place. When dealing with work, medical discourse generally encourages workers to adjust to the vicissitudes of the workplace using attitude changes, medications, relaxation, or other limited maneuvers. If adjustment appears unfeasible, disability can be certified.

Although the family figures less prominently in these encounters with male patients than does the workplace, a similar lack of critical appraisal becomes apparent. For two of the three patients, family relations raise certain problems. While the physical therapist in Encounter 5C complains about stress as he extols the family's virtues, the heart attack victim in Encounter 5A assumes a position of dependency and passivity toward his wife. Both these men experience emotional difficulties that attract therapeutic comments from the doctor, and some of these difficulties may spring from how the patients get along in their families. Yet current family relations do not receive critical attention in any of the encounters. The discourse seems to accept these men's roles in the family as given, or at least alternatives to existing patterns do not suggest themselves.

Because there is little room in medical discourse for a critical examination of the social context, problems in work and the family tend to become marginalized. From the standpoint of post-structuralist theory, superficially marginal elements of context in medical discourse take on crucial importance. In these dialogues, devices of language that include interruptions, cut-offs, and de-emphases move contextual matters to the margins of discourse. In the process, the option of changes in work and the family to improve the consequences for health and mental health receives scant attention.

Could this scenario be different? Whether medical discourse *ought* to deal more critically with work and the family then becomes the question. Some responses to this question appear in the last chapter. The answer is not simple, since increasing doctors' involvement in the occupational system and family life also runs a risk of further medicalizing social problems. That is, any call for a more critical discourse in medicine needs to consider the limits of the medical role, both in this society and in others.[19]

Meanwhile, medical discourse continues to do its part in mediating the often troubling conditions of work and the family. In Foucault's terms, professional surveillance of social context occurs during medical encounters, with generally conservative outcomes. After seeing their doctors, some patients return to their jobs, perhaps better able to function. Others gain exemption from work for varying lengths of time, possibly with financial compensation. Most return to the same family relations. Patients in these instances can feel satisfied that they have benefitted from the expertise of doctors, who—within the limits of the discourse available—have tried to help as best they could.

CHAPTER 6

WOMEN, WORK, AND THE FAMILY

When women talk with their doctors, family life often enters the conversation. Work does also, although usually to a lesser degree. Women's roles in the family and at work entail certain typical problems. When such problems arise in the social context of the medical encounter, women may speak about these difficulties with health professionals, sometimes directly, sometimes in passing. How the discourse of medicine mediates women's roles in work and the family is the question here.

As patients, women see doctors more than men do, and the communication that occurs in such encounters may be less than ideal, to say the least. About two-thirds of outpatient visits in primary care involve women patients. Among the many complaints that the medical profession has received from women and the women's movement, difficulties in communication have figured among the most common. These complaints have focused on sexism, professional dominance, and emotional insensitivity. Research studies have confirmed specific communication barriers that arise when female patients and male doctors try to talk with each other. While such difficulties may diminish as the proportion of women physicians increases, there is doubtless still a long way to go in describing and then improving these communication patterns.[1]

Outside medicine, the importance of gender in discourse also has become something of a burning issue. Influenced by the women's movement worldwide, feminist scholars have criticized male-oriented patterns of thought that have dominated not only social life in general, but also a host of intellectual disciplines. Feminist studies have emphasized

107

the ideologies that affect women. Research efforts have clarified how these ideologies manifest themselves in literature, history, the natural sciences, and the social sciences. Taking into account structuralist and post-structuralist theories, feminist scholarship also has focused on omissions, silences, contradictions, and marginal elements in literary and nonliterary discourse. In such details of discourse, the ideologies that affect women become apparent. Among its goals, feminist interpretation looks for the ways that language reinforces male dominance. Such efforts also aim toward changes in discourse, linked to broader changes in the social relations between men and women.[2]

The three encounters that follow illustrate in distinct ways how medical discourse mediates work and family life for women.[3] Because contextual elements predominate in the first encounter, this interaction requires more comment than the second and third. The interpretation of these encounters again emphasizes elements of ideology and social control, as well as a possible underlying structure beneath the surface details of discourse. How medical discourse does or does not deal with contextual issues of work and family life becomes a central concern, especially when these issues pertain to the personal troubles that patients report.

ENCOUNTER 6A: MARITAL CONFLICT

SUMMARY

A woman comes to her doctor for a routine checkup. She has separated from her husband and suffers from depression. The doctor reviews the patient's history of gynecologic problems and her current contraceptive practices. In a lengthy discussion, doctor and patient explore the socioemotional situation, including her work, suicide potential, alcohol use and smoking, social support network, and alternatives for psychotherapy. Afterward, the doctor also does a brief physical exam, recommends a follow-up visit four months later, and orders laboratory tests.

Some relevant background information comes from the questionnaires that the patient and doctor filled out after their recorded interaction: The patient is a 37-year-old woman who works as an educational consultant for a large corporation. Originally from Italy, she has received a college education, reports her religion as Roman Catholic, and lives in a suburb of Boston with her three children, who are twelve, ten, and seven years old. The doctor is a 39-year-old white male, of German ethnic background and Episcopalian Protestant religious persuasion, who practices general internal medicine. According to the doctor, he has known the patient for five years and believes that her diagnosis is "situational depression."

Work, money, and relationships with men. The patient's work situation comes up right at the beginning of the encounter and at one later point. In contrast to the discussions of work involving male patients in the last chapter, however, the conversation here treats work in a rather peripheral way, compared to more fundamental concerns about the family. As the encounter opens, in response to the doctor's question, the patient reports that she is still working in the educational division of a large corporation, although she mentions a thwarted desire to teach Italian:

D: OK, so this year you're 37.
P: Right.
D: An::d are you still with, uh, ((corporation name)), huh,
P: Yes, hm hm.
D: Uh, that's the educational division   5
                                    [
P: Right, uh huh
                                                    [
D: is it not, yeah.
P: Yeah, I'm going
              [
D: Are you using your Italian in that, uh?
P: A::h, no.   10
D: Not.
P: No. I was tempted to go back teaching Italian, because of
   what you just said, you know, teaching Italian it means
   speaking the language,
                                            [
D: Yes   15
P: very important for me, I don't get much of a chance, uh, I
   haven't found (words)
D: OK, so you're at least still
P: Ah, yeah, still in ((corporation name))
              [
D: staying, ((corporation name)), OK. The events of   20
   the past year, I guess the most significant probably relates
   to your hysterectomy.

Internal conflict concerning work remains unexplored throughout the rest of the encounter. The patient has not fulfilled her professional aspirations to teach Italian, which she apparently has enjoyed in the past. Here the doctor cuts off the discussion of professional goals with an abrupt turn to gynecologic matters. Even though occupational frustration may bear on the emotional troubles that the patient reports later, her career aspirations here move to the margins of the dialogue, as the doctor shifts attention to a hysterectomy (to be discussed later).

From the doctor's perspective, work also becomes a good place to meet men. Later in the encounter, when doctor and patient explore the dimensions of her current depression and discuss her social support network, the doctor inquires if the patient has started to date and suggests men at work:

P: And I, I don't find being with other men is the right thing.   29
  At least in terms of
D: Hm hm, no. Can you find that you can date, or that there're
  either coworkers, or other associates that you
                        [
P: Well, it's difficult, it's just   30
  a very touchy situation because a lot of people I know are
  married, and it gets into a sticky mess and I work and I'm at home
  with the children so much, I don't get a chance to see anybody,
  and it's just one of those vicious circles.

For the patient, work is not fertile ground for establishing new relationships with men. From the doctor's view, despite the patient's dissatisfaction with the content of her work life, work becomes a vehicle to reestablish a heterosexual relationship.

Work does not provide financial stability either. The patient reports that both her own and her husband's jobs have become insecure. Immediately after bringing up the issue of marital stress, the doctor asks about the husband's work situation:

D: Um, with
  reference to the second problem, or the related problem here,   9
  the marital stress. What's the status of that, now?
P: That, uh, well, I, ah
D: You still separated?
P: Yes, right. And there should be a divorce in the fall.
        [
D: An:y   You're filing,   10
  or he?
P: I'm filing.
D: Mm hm. And he's still with, uh, —— Press?
P: Well, no. He's, ah, he's gone from —— Press.
D: Mm hmm. What's he doing now?   10
P: Um, presently he's doing consulting, and he's looking for
  another job.

By focusing on the work role of the husband, who relies on irregular consulting arrangements as he seeks a new job, the doctor clarifies an unstable financial situation. Despite this instability, the patient depends on the husband financially, since he contributes to her and her children's living expenses. As the encounter evolves, the patient's financial difficulties become clearer. Because of business losses during the past year, the company for which she works apparently will cut back her own employment. Therefore, she must look for a new job. Her uncertainty about employment thus combines with her husband's occupational instability to create a severe financial problem, which even interferes with her ability to obtain psychiatric services:

D: uh, and certainly through family service, or —— Clinic,   370
    there's some very capable psychiatric social workers and such,
    who, you know, appreciate the financial commitment that's
    necessary if you want to get into private psychiatry, there are
    some extremely capable people there, too, that have, at least
    helped a lot of people see their way through   375
        [
P: I'm, I'm sure would benefit from it enormously, but,
    financially we are in a very bad situation right now, and I have
    to find a new job and all sorts of very bad things went on last
    year (words) certain business in the hole, it's, ah, so I have
    to just limit (word)   380
        [
D: Well, through ——, —— Clinic, they
    will scale it according to income and ability and so forth, and
    nobody's going to (word), so uh
        [
P: All right.

Despite a possible sliding scale according to income, financial barriers to psychiatric services nevertheless remain. While the doctor expresses optimism, he cannot be sure that a social service agency will circumvent these economic difficulties.

The doctor ends the discussion about finances and psychiatric consultation with a cut-off that leads into a technical discussion:

D: So, again, it's not the, it's not the whole
    panacea, but it, uh, it may help, and uh:h
P: I'll keep it in mind.
D: At least knowing that opportunity is there, and uh, and
    through family service and such and, uh, there we're   405
    fortunate at least
    [

P: I'll keep it in mind
[
D: at least knowing that there are some alternatives to,
   uh, going to the poor house.
   OK, the, uh, questions of animal fat in the diet here   4
   are of, ah, you're obviously aware of the dieting factors and
   we've talked about the cholesterol and such in the past, less
   urgent in a woman than a man, but your cholesterol's always
   been good, and, uh, worth knowing about.

Here the doctor expresses a hope that some social service agency will intervene with the patient and provide counseling at a reduced fee. He relies on the patient to take the initiative in seeking this help, and the patient responds that she will consider this option. After the poor house image, the doctor abruptly shifts to the biochemical level and deals with nutritional methods of lowering cholesterol. Eating less animal fat seems fairly simple, in comparison to the complexities of the financial context. As the conversation moves away from and finally marginalizes the contextual issues of jobs, money, and psychotherapy, it is unclear if the finances that the patient and her estranged husband can generate will actually keep poverty from overtaking her and her children. As the doctor mentions, such "alternatives" to the poor house indeed are not "the whole panacea."

Female problems. The physical concerns which receive most attention in the encounter center on the female reproductive organs. This dialogue starts immediately after the doctor establishes that the patient is still working. What begins as a technical discussion of an abnormal pap smear moves swiftly to sexual and psychiatric concerns. Because her pap smear previously has revealed a premalignant pathology, her primary-care physician and gynecologist have considered recommending a hysterectomy. However, the pap smear has returned to normal after a non-surgical procedure, cauterization of the uterine cervix. For that reason, the gynecologist is simply repeating the pap smear every six months. After reviewing these events, a recent vaginal infection, and her menstrual periods, the doctor introduces the issue of contraception, whose psychological and sexual ramifications become rather complex.

Contraception, it seems, has become intertwined with depression and the meaning of marital dissolution. Separated from her husband, the patient does not feel much need for contraception. When the need does arise, a diaphragm or the birth control pill is available. Furthermore, despite previous headaches and fluid retention, the patient mentions that she sometimes uses the birth control pill as a tranquilizer and/or antidepressant agent, to quiet her moods:

D: And contraception, what are you using?

P: U::hm, on and off I've used the pill, and, uh, I've used a
diaphragm also, but I don't use it that much, because, well, for   55
one thing, I'm separated right now, uh, there isn't that much
need, but when there

                    [

D: so

   [

P: is need, it's either the diaphragm or, I have taken the pill.
As a matter of fact, last winter, January or February, I was   60
very depressed, and not because of intercourse, because I find
the pill calms me down, it's a very strange thing. I took
the pill for a month. The pill does things. It makes
my feelings even, over the month. I used to get very upset
just before   65

      [

D: Uh huh

          [

P: my period. Very, very upset, very nervous
and very tense. I find that that helped a little bit.

The patient thus reveals that she has been using birth control pills as a
psychotropic medication. When depressed, especially during menstrual
periods, she has taken the pill to reduce emotional tension.

The well-meaning discourse here not only achieves, from Foucault's
perspective, a professional surveillance of female sexuality; the conversation also reveals a tendency that some have called the "hysterization" of
social problems.[4] From this perspective, medical language transforms
important social problems facing women—family roles, occupational
aspirations, sexuality, childrearing, and so forth—into objectified disorders of the sexual and reproductive organs. Further, a desire for more
favorable social conditions, which remain lacking, translates into genital
dysfunction. In this encounter, doctor and patient use gynecologic language to begin discussing the contextual problem of marital dissolution,
with all its emotional and economic fallout. Genital organs and social
context thus become linked. The doctor's only current diagnosis, given in
a separate questionnaire, is "situational depression." That is, the doctor
does not view any of the gynecologic problems—abnormal pap smear,
vaginal discharge, or birth control—as major diagnoses. Nonetheless, he
introduces the theme of marital dissolution with the technical details of
gynecology. In this case, rather than illuminating the entire social stage,
medical discourse spotlights the genitals.

The problem list. Another way that the discourse maintains focus and
control amid a welter of psychosocial issues involves the use of a "prob-

lem list."[5] This doctor's references to a list of numbered problems take on the characteristics of interruptions or cut-offs, which steer the discourse by returning to an orderly medical voice, away from the loose, chaotic, and difficult-to-control details of the patient's story. Right after he asks about the patient's work, for instance, he focuses on the gynecologic problem as "the most significant probably"—in short, problem number one (lines 20–22 above). The "second problem" is marital stress (lines 94– 96 above). After eliciting some troubling information about child custody and the husband's intention to contest the divorce, the doctor quickly shifts back to the problem list, this time concerning diseases in the patient's family:

P: Uh, I have temporary custody of the children unless there was a
                                                                        [
D: Yeah, so
  [
P: court battle, unless—you know, I don't know.
D: You don't—do you expect that he will
                                              [
P: No, I don't   14
                                           [
D: contest it?
P: Oh, yes. Definitely. He'll protest everything, but, uh,
   he has no reasons
  [
D: But, at least he
    [
P: right now.   14
D: OK. Now, um. All right. Let's just go over your list here
   for a minute. The other areas that we have looked at in the
   past, there was the concern about, although they were all benign
   tumors, that the, your father had the benign brain tumor, your
   mother had the benign breast tumor, sister fibroids; anything   15
   more in terms of changes in family history in the past year?
P: Not at this point. Not at this time, you know.

The doctor then reviews other problems presumably on his list: weight and diet (lines 157–90), eyesight (lines 191–94), smoking (lines 194–202), drinking (lines 206–24), urination at night (lines 225–31).[6] During the discussion of dieting, the doctor notes that the patient has lost fifteen pounds and reassures himself that the patient's diet is adequate (lines 180–81). Then he moves briefly through the problem of urination at night to the problem of depression (lines 225–40), after which, as noted already, the doctor again uses the problem list to effect an abrupt transition to the problem of animal fat and cholesterol.

    Throughout the encounter, then, the problem list provides convenient

markers en route that guide the discourse toward and away from contextual sources of personal trouble. Processed via the list, the difficulties
themselves take on a quality of reified, narrowly defined, objective phenomena. The formality of numbered problems assists the technical voice,
seeking to create professional order from the contextual chaos of the
patient's personal story. While this approach converts the discourse into a
coherent format, especially for record-keeping purposes, the narrative
reads as choppier and more disjointed than it otherwise might. By switch-
ing among problems to cover the list at hand, the doctor gains control
over the flow of a conversation full of explosively charged material.
Through the problem-oriented approach, which seems so reasonable to
so many, the doctor segmentalizes the patient into many small components, rather than letting her story run its full, perhaps more frightening
course.

Elements of depression. What are the elements of the patient's depression? First, her frustrated professional aspirations may contribute, although this possibility receives short shrift in the dialogue. A more
prominent element involves the patient's role in her family. Although her
estranged husband continues to provide financial support, he mainly
emerges as a cause of distress.

Marital estrangement and its impact on depression appear early in the
encounter, when the doctor asks about the "second problem" of "marital
stress." When the doctor then questions about her husband's current
work and the patient's contact with him, she responds with a negative
picture:

D: Mm hm. Do you have any significant stressful contact or
   nonstressful contact with him, now?
P: Ah, it's dormant stressful contact, in the sense that he   110
   desperately wants to get back, and I just, uh, it would be
   just suicide for me to get back with him, because it would
   just be repeating the whole thing all over again,

Although the husband wants to reconcile, the patient sees no way; to do
so, she says, would prove quite destructive for her. Her reference to
suicide does not attract comment here but remains as a red flag to which
the doctor later returns. The patient has previously dealt with the husband's alcohol problem, which apparently has improved (lines 114–15).
Doctor and patient then turn to the patient's three children (lines 116–
45). According to the patient, their reaction to the separation is "not bad
at all," because they "get along with their father," who "comes over all
the time." The husband's involvement with the children, including frequent suppers together, "makes it very difficult for me, but it's been very
good for the children," who are not yet aware of plans for divorce. As
noted earlier, the patient reveals uncertainty about retaining custody of

the children if a legal dispute develops. In short, the patient's family situation gives her plenty of cause for depression.

At this point, the doctor switches to the next problem on his list, a family history of benign tumors, but the theme of depression again subtly arises in a discussion of weight. Since the patient has lost fifteen pounds, the doctor asks, "What do you account for that?" The patient replies, "Not eating." The patient reveals pleasure from losing weight (line 170): "I feel so good when I'm a decent weight, I really do." Perhaps recognizing that weight loss is a so-called vegetative sign of depression, an indicator of depression's seriousness, the doctor asks whether the patient is "really starving yourself" and is "not talking about absolute starvation" (lines 180–90). In response, the patient replies:

P: No, no, no. I eat salads, and I, I drink
   my glass of wine, and, uh, I eat strawberries and,
   but very very very little of what I eat, you know
   [
D: OK, OK, but it's fairly strict restrictions and being very
   cautious, OK
            [
P: almonds, I treat myself to mushrooms and whatnot.

Salads, wine, strawberries, almonds, mushrooms, and whatnot—the patient's diet at least is not starvation-level. When she states how good she feels at a "decent weight," the patient expresses more enthusiasm than at any other point in the encounter.

The patient conveys the image of a thin body as desirable, while a fat one is not. The preoccupation with being overweight, of course, concerns many if not most women in modern society, reflecting strong cultural preference. Such emphasis on thinness creates widespread grief, even for those women whose weight is normal. This is one reason, as some have argued, why "fat is a feminist issue."[7] Further, for many women, depression and desire for weight loss become closely linked, as they do for the patient in this encounter.[8]

While she succeeds in losing weight, the patient fails in her attempts to cut back on smoking and drinking, and the doctor explores whether these lapses also may reflect her depression. Previously, the patient had stopped smoking entirely, but now she has resumed the habit, at about half a pack per day. The reason, she says, is because "it's always when I stop dining I start smoking" (lines 198–99). Doctor and patient indulge in one of their two episodes of laughing, when the doctor jokes, "I guess what you can, you know, get down to 130 and stop smoking. Hh heh ha" (line 202). The patient then confides that she drinks more alcohol when she is avoiding food. In response, the doctor gingerly questions about whether this behavior is leading to alcoholism:

D: No, it's just that somebody offers it's not that you're   220
    [
P: No, uh uh
    [
D: coming home and pouring yourself a double before you go to
    bed or anything
    [
P: No, I never drink alone, I, ah, I never drink alone, no.

Although the patient diminishes the importance of these changes in
eating, smoking, and drinking, a picture emerges that on the whole
shows a troubled descent into self-destructive habits.

After a brief diversion to the problem of urination at night, the doctor
turns to further discussion of "the questions of depression and, uh,
problems at home." The patient responds that she believes her depression is "something physical, I think it's something a little bit physical,
too, because it's pre-period depression, it's really bad" (lines 232–44). In
reply, the doctor raises the issue of suicide risk. Initially, he uses as a
euphemism the term "something dramatic" to refer to suicide and juxtaposes this possibility with the option of getting "some help":

D: Uh huh. Have you really, you know, gone to the depths of   245
    depression, that you thought, you know, I've got to either do
    something dramatic or get some help
                                     [
P: Yeah, I have
    [
D: in the past year?
P: Yes I have.

At this point, by saying yes, the patient seems to refer to the question
about seeking help, rather than the image of doing "something dramatic." The patient goes on to say that she and her husband had seen a
doctor for joint therapy, because "I thought I could save the marriage."
Although this approach did not lead to successful dialogue about the
marriage, the patient states, "It could have helped me, as a person but,
uh, it's too expensive, I can't afford it" (lines 251–62).

Later the doctor moves away from euphemism to ask directly if she
has considered suicide. In reply, the patient answers affirmatively but
notes that the presence of her children prevents her from acting on this
thought:

D: Yeah, OK. And have you ever been so depressed that you thought   280
    that, you know, well, the only out is suicide or something
    like that?
P: Yes, but not having, I, I, I have. (words) probably I have, but

not that strongly, I mean, but there are times when I thought
that after all the children are growing up, and they really
won't need me that much more, and unless there is some cheerfulness in my life, unless there is warmth and love, you see,
it's, I miss my family a lot now, I don't have anybody around.

                 [

D: Yeah, they're all, yeah your
    (word) are dead, and your sisters, where?

P: Well, you see, I have an enormous family back home, but, uh,
    ((husband's name)) won't let me go.

D: Mm hm, mm hm.

By her stuttering answer to the doctor's direct question ("I, I, I have"), the
patient reveals the depth and conflict of her suicidal fantasies. While she
has considered suicide, the children stand in the way. As she recalls both
their cheerfulness and their need for her, she shifts the mental timing of
her possible suicide forward to the future, when the children are grown.
She also refers to isolation from her family in Italy and claims that her
husband will not allow her to return, presumably because he wants
continuing contact with the children.

In effect, the patient sees herself living for her children until they are
grown. Ironically, the children give her life meaning yet severely limit her
options. From this vantage point, the children require constant sacrifice,
not the least of which is allowing her husband to stay in her life. Because
of the children, she does not travel to her homeland, change jobs, move,
or make any other major change that might alleviate the symptoms of her
"situational depression." In short, as critical analysts of the family from
Engels onward have suggested, this patient's reproductive role in childrearing overshadows all other concerns.[9]

During the next part of the encounter, the doctor inquires about the
patient's social support network. Concerned with her well-being, the
doctor seeks ways to help her cope with emotional distress. As noted
earlier, he suggests dating men at work. Then he asks if she has turned to
anyone else, such as a clergyman or a friend. While acknowledging that
"I should perhaps, find someone," she says that she has not yet done so
(lines 311–17). She looks forward to another difficult winter and again
refers to her inability to return to Italy because of the children. The doctor
explores a number of options for professional help, including those available at low cost. These lengthy and sensitively phrased suggestions
include counseling, medication, psychiatric social work, private psychiatry, and group therapy (lines 350–409). Although the doctor admits the
limitations of these alternatives, he argues that they at least would reduce
the possibility, euphemistically, of "doing some things very dramatically":

D: But at least it may help you to deal with it, and I would think, you know, before you get so overwrought that you really start thinking of doing some things very dramatically, or start to plan ways to do yourself in, it would probably be worth, uh, worth a phone call anyway to say, you know, how much farther down could you go before you go up? So uh   360

P: You mean, like uh, I should have a name, somebody's name here.

Recognizing the importance of rapid access to help for a person contemplating suicide, the doctor mentions himself,[10] a family service, and a mental health clinic as resources in case of emergency. When he sees a red flag of distress, in short, the doctor does what he can to provide therapeutic options.

The doctor's words imply that a dramatic outcome like suicide is undesirable, compared to the control resulting from professional surveillance. While the option of therapy provides less drama, it also entails financial sacrifice and may not offer fundamental solutions. The tensions of this approach become clear through the ambiguities that remain. For instance, one does not know whether the patient will seek help, if she will attempt suicide, how the marital separation will proceed, and so forth. Furthermore, although the doctors' comments become quite directive regarding strategies to help the patient cope, a number of more basic alternatives do not arise. The doctor is careful not to criticize the patient's husband, or to suggest legal assistance, or to question the patient's commitment to her maternal role, or to encourage a return to her family abroad, or even to suggest changes in current financial arrangements. To enunciate options such as these would move beyond what would seem appropriate content for even the most humanistically oriented medical discourse. Could a doctor presume to advocate basic changes in social context? Even if these interventions might alleviate personal suffering to a greater degree than undramatic options like therapy, their mention would probably seem intrusive, overly controlling, and inappropriate within the customary talk that doctors and patients expect to exchange.

Return to the technical. Through the incoherencies of the encounter's conclusion, the constraints of medical discourse also become apparent. After their extensive dialogue on depression, suicide, and financial barriers to mental health services, the doctor cuts off the contextual issues by returning to the technical question of dietary fat and then performs a brief physical exam, which he begins by listening to the heart ("So, let's see if you're still ticking," lines 415–16). As the encounter ends, he orders a chest x-ray, says that an electrocardiogram is not necessary, compliments the patient on her weight loss, and expresses a preference to schedule a follow-up appointment in four months:

D: I'm delighted to see the weight loss and, uh, I think
   what we might do is just schedule a follow-up in say about four
   months or so, maybe in October, just to sort of touch base and
   see how things are going. If uhm, if there's a concern, uh, if   48
   you're feeling perfectly well and things are rosy, simply
   call and cancel it, but I think just to at least have that,
   uh, uh, it may be that at that
                              [
P: OK.
   [
D: time that either, intervening with some medication or something   49
   is appropriate.
P: OK.
D: If so, we'll do it. OK, so I'll write the slip for the lab
   and the, uh, x-ray and, uhm, you can go down.
P: Thank you very much.   49
D: OK, right.

In requesting a follow-up visit several months later, the doctor also
implies optimistically that "things" might become "rosy" enough by that
time for the patient to cancel the appointment. If not, a psychotropic
medication, or a vague "something," may help (line 490). Finally, the
doctor shows the patient out with a slip of paper required for lab tests and
a chest x-ray. Such papers are what doctors and patients expect to exchange, as concrete and reified symbols of the body's scientifically ordered reality, in contrast to the disorder of the contextual environment.

The doctor's rapid shift from social context to cholesterol, followed by
the physical exam, marginalizes the troubles that comprise the patient's
major diagnosis, situational depression. Through this shift, the doctor
tips his hat to medicine's technical expectations. For the patient, problems of the heart are not those of cardiac dysfunction, yet the doctor feels
he must use a stethoscope to hear if a physical heart is "still ticking." As
he proceeds through an uneventful exam, the doctor conveys an impression of physical normality amid psychosocial chaos. By returning to the
physical realm and finding nothing wrong, the doctor's technical routine
somehow may provide a reassuring center for the disordered contextual
elements, which now move to the margin.[11]

Ideology and structure. While the dialogue deals so strikingly with the
private troubles of this woman's life, it does not offer any sort of critique
concerning the social relationships that seem to cause her depression.
Further, the discourse reinforces ideologies of women's appropriate role
in work and the family. Even when marital strife creates disturbing
emotional, occupational, and financial problems, there is little room for

basic change. A woman's primary responsibility remains toward her children and their stability. Likewise, tolerating a husband's visits, accepting professional frustration, and enduring isolation from family roots all emerge as sacrifices to be accepted in fulfillment of a woman's reproductive responsibilities. Discussions of social support and therapy aim toward avoiding the dramatic possibility of suicide through professional surveillance. These options help the patient cope with the present social context. As the patient leaves the doctor's office, little has actually changed in her life. The ideologic assumptions requiring personal sacrifice for the sake of family remain intact.

To summarize, the encounter shows a number of underlying structural elements (figure 6.1). In the social context, expectations that govern women's roles in the family and at work create troubling emotional and financial circumstances for a woman who is going through divorce (A). As a result, she suffers from depression and suicidal thoughts (B). When she enters the medical encounter (C), she responds to a series of supportive and humanistic questions from the doctor, concerning her marital strife, professional frustration, and emotional distress (D). The doctor introduces order into this discourse by following a clearly defined problem list, which leads him to interrupt the dialogue at several points by returning to technical problems. Toward the end of the encounter, he cuts off and marginalizes a discussion of contextual issues by asking about gynecologic matters and diet, and by performing a brief physical exam (E). The doctor tries to manage the patient's problem by suggesting low-cost counseling or psychotherapy, by encouraging social activities such as dating other men, and by offering himself and other social service agencies to provide professional surveillance through emergency contacts. By focusing on gynecologic abnormalities and contraceptive behavior, the conversation tends to transform contextual problems into disordered function of the genital and reproductive organs. While the patient's childrearing responsibilities create considerable burdens, the ideological assumption that such responsibilities are a necessary part of woman's role in the family receives no critical attention (F). After the encounter, the patient presumably consents in returning to her previous role, as a dedicated mother and aspiring teacher who is trying as best she can to deal with the depressing conditions of her existence.

In this and similar encounters, medicine mediates difficult social problems by helping a patient to cope. All in all, the doctor here shows a humanistic orientation. True, his problem list and need to do something technical sometimes lead him in rather inscrutable directions. But he spends considerable time and energy, listening to and trying to help the patient as she deals with marital conflict and depression. Such psychotherapeutic practices are becoming more common in primary-care prac-

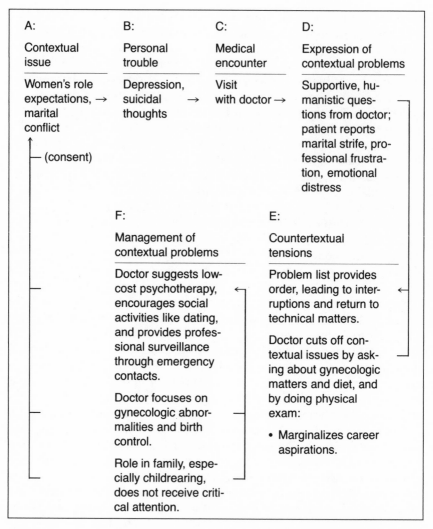

A:

Contextual issue

B:

Personal trouble

C:

Medical encounter

D:

Expression of contextual problems

Women's role expectations, → marital conflict

↑
— (consent)

Depression, suicidal → thoughts

Visit with doctor →

Supportive, humanistic questions from doctor; patient reports marital strife, professional frustration, emotional distress

F:

Management of contextual problems

E:

Countertextual tensions

Doctor suggests low-cost psychotherapy, ← encourages social activities like dating, and provides professional surveillance through emergency contacts.

Doctor focuses on gynecologic abnormalities and birth control.

Role in family, especially childrearing, does not receive critical attention.

Problem list provides ← order, leading to interruptions and return to technical matters.

Doctor cuts off contextual issues by asking about gynecologic matters and diet, and by doing physical exam:

• Marginalizes career aspirations.

Figure 6.1
Structural elements of a medical encounter with a woman experiencing marital conflict

tice, and this particular doctor measures up well to current standards governing the assessment and treatment of situational depression.[12] This skillful approach allows catharsis and develops options for other types of support, if a patient takes initiative and can afford them financially. That the patient after such an encounter returns to an essentially unchanged social context, however, receives little if any notice.

ENCOUNTER 6B: SUBURBAN SYNDROME

S U M M A R Y

A woman visits her doctor because she is "not feeling well." She complains of multiple symptoms, including exhaustion, pains in various parts of her body, loss of appetite, frequent urination, and itchy skin. In describing her problem, the patient notes that she is extremely busy with social activities. The doctor diagnoses her problem as "suburban syndrome." He recommends rest and—after a brief physical exam—prescribes a tranquilizer.

Information about the doctor and patient is available from the questionnaires that they filled out after their encounter. A 30-year-old college graduate, the patient is married, has two children (ages 5½ and 3½), is Jewish, and gives "housewife" as her occupation. Together with her family, the patient has recently moved from a different area of the country. A 47-year-old white male who practices internal medicine in a suburban private practice near Boston, the doctor denies religious preference and gives his ethnic background as Russian. Patient and doctor have known each other about seven months. The diagnosis, according to the doctor, is "acute and chronic (anxiety and) depression."

Many complaints. As doctor and patient begin their dialogue, the patient complains about a variety of physical symptoms:

D: Talk to me. Why are you here?
P: I'm here because I'm just not feeling well. I, uhm, I feel
    exhausted lately, I've been running around doing lots of
    things entertaining and lots of committees and so forth, and   15
    lots of social butterfly stuff, and I'm just exhausted.
    Everything hurts me. I don't know whether I have a cold in
    my body, my back, muscles. My shoulders hurt, my arms, my
    fingers, my wrists. When I wake up my legs hurt and my feet
    hurt, and I haven't been walking during the night. And, uhm,   20
    going along with it I just feel sort of nervous on and (word)
    on and off. Loss of appetite at times, frequent urination . . .
    tired. I (words, very softly), and uhm, oh. Occasionally I
    get this very itchy feeling on my skin when I take my clothes
    off. Whether that's due to some kind of nerves or not, I   25
    don't know. And even last week I felt I was hyperventilating
    a little bit, which, uh, stopped after a few minutes, but I
                        [
D: You know enough

You know enough about that I take it . . . You've done that
before (word).   30
P: I'm not really terribly depressed or anything, I'm just sort
   of tired and uptight about things, irritable a little bit.
D: You have a pretty good insight, huh? Haven't you?
P: Well,
D: Hmm?   35
P: Insight into what?
D: Your story that you give me almost gives the answer with
   it, doesn't it?
P: What I'm going through a housewife syndrome?

It does not take much to unleash a torrent of words from the patient
about her symptoms and activities. She is seeing the doctor because she
is not feeling well, and not feeling well means many things. First and
foremost is fatigue, which she says comes from too extensive social
activities. Furthermore, aches and pains arise in various parts of her
body. She also is experiencing problems with dietary intake, urinary
excretion, itchy skin, and respiration. At one point she mentions a possibility that at least some of these difficulties may be due to "nerves." In
short, much is going on. Although one expects that the patient might
continue this soliloquy for some time, the doctor interrupts her in the
middle of a sentence (line 27).

Through the interruption, the doctor breaks the litany of complaints
and uses a variant of Socratic methodology in leading the patient to
diagnose herself. Initially he refers to the patient's self-knowledge and
ability to understand her diagnosis. When the doctor mentions that the
patient has "done that before," he apparently is referring to similar
problems in the past. Taking this cue, the patient denies that she is
depressed, as she probably has been previously. Instead, she refers to her
fatigue and irritability. In responding that she has "pretty good insight,"
the doctor encourages her to come up with some other interpretation of
her symptoms, that is, to provide an "answer" for her own "story." What
the doctor hopes to reveal through insight initially eludes the patient
("insight into what?"), but she soon voices a hypothesis about "housewife syndrome."

Discussing suburban syndrome. In the dialogue that follows, the doctor elaborates and modifies this self-diagnosis. First, he refines and para-
phrases the patient's "story" by depicting it as a vicious cycle of activity
and fatigue. While the doctor alludes to too much activity, the patient
worries about the opposite, since a lack of social contacts previously has
brought on her depression. She also returns to her physical symptom of
"achiness":

D: Well, I don't know if that would express it. With the   40
    story that you give me certainly, uh, you're telling me that
    you're doing too much and you ache and you feel so, push
    yourself, and keep going. And you keep going and then you
    feel more tired and then you keep going-
P: Well, at first I didn't think, I think it's better for me   45
    to keep going than to just be very docile in the house,
    because then I get depressed, doing that. But, uhm, it just
    started with this achiness and I *thought* at first that I had
    a cold and that's why I wanted to come to you initially,

Through a subsequent series of questions, the doctor clarifies that the symptoms started about one week previously, came on gradually, and arise in association with social activities away from home. The patient then refers again to the busy life-style that she has developed since moving to the area, after which the doctor gives a more definitive modification of the diagnosis that he had led the patient to make previously:

P: We're, you know, we're fairly new to the area, too, and I've
    become involved in certain things. Trying to limit it, not
    to, you know, join everything and be in everything. But it
    just happens that I guess in the springtime lots of things are   70
    going on and they climax around this time of year, and sort
    of taper off during the summer.
D: ——, and you're learning something very interesting. It's
    not the housewife syndrome, it's called the suburban syndrome.

The Socratic method thus has revealed that the diagnosis is not "housewife syndrome," as the patient had supposed, but "suburban syndrome," whose characteristics and treatment the doctor will soon explain in more detail.

    Although these syndromes do not appear as traditional diagnoses in medical textbooks,[13] and although he may be defining the terms on the spot, the doctor indicates a clear distinction between the two conditions. The housewife syndrome involves doing too little outside the family, it seems, while the suburban syndrome involves doing too much. Treatment for the suburban syndrome requires saying no. Responding to the patient's lament about difficulties in limiting her social involvements, the doctor reinforces the importance of setting limits and again alludes to the patient's "insight":

D: And what you have to learn is something that you learned many   75
    years ago, that is how to say *no*. Because once there's a
    willing worker, you then, starting from Welcome Wagon on,
P: Hm hmm.

D: all sorts of religious, religious, political, and social
   groups are just going to be knocking on your door. And, uhm,   8(
   I think you're, you're just going to go through cycles like
   this. It's perhaps a little horrendous what people go through,
   and I think that, uhm, your insight, this is what I'm talking
   about, it's right. You know *damn* well what you're doing.

Suburban syndrome, thus, consists of social overload. From the doctor's viewpoint, the multiple involvements expected from this woman,
and presumably from similar women who live in suburbia, create stress
and exhaustion. To make progress under such circumstances, a patient
needs considerable self-awareness and the ability to create firm boundaries between oneself and the expectations of others. The doctor expresses confidence that the patient's "insight," to which he has led her
through Socratic technique, will assist her in doing what is necessary,
although some might question the delicacy of his tone.

Rest and tranquilization. Unfortunately, treating the suburban syndrome is not simple. One ought to be able just to say no, but that often
becomes hard to do while staying in one's customary environment.
Although she recognizes the importance of slowing down, the patient
also wants some help in doing so. The help she seems to want involves a
tranquilizer. She subtly introduces the theme of psychotropic medication
through an indirect, conditional statement about what happens when
she uses such medication:

P: And even if I take something, like a Valila, Valium, (words)
   (mumbled words). You know, if I feel nervous for a day
   or two, uh, and take one of those, there just (mumbled words)   95
   I've just been living on Bufferin, I think, for the past week
   just because of the achiness that I have.

"Even if" she takes Valium, she still feels physical pain and needs to take
Bufferin, a medication for pain, as well. At this point, the doctor does not
pick up on the reference to Valium, a tranquilizer.

Instead, he emphasizes that a long vacation may prove necessary to
help the patient's cycle of overactivity and fatigue. Suggesting that a brief
rest seldom proves sufficient for fatigue of this magnitude, he argues for
an extended holiday in the sun. Based on her experience with shorter
getaways, the patient is not so sure that this approach will calm her
down:

D: And yet the treatment
   certainly *would* be the one you mentioned, namely, *stop.*
   Don't do anything. Not just quietly relax, but you know,   110
   one week in Florida sunshine would cure so many of our
   diseases.

P: Well, you know, my husband and I went away for a weekend
    about a month ago, and I was so wound up that the weekend
    didn't put me at ease at all. I felt like I should have   115
    been doing something, ((quietly mumbling)) and I couldn't
    even (words).
D: That's, this is what's wrong with the weekend. This is why
    it takes, you know, have you ever been on a month vacation?
P: Hmm nn.   120
D: Do you know how long it takes to really calm down? It
    takes quite a long time.

The doctor's travelogue sounds appealing; he may want to do something
like that himself. From the patient's perspective, though, empty time
feels as though it should be filled up by activity. The anxiety that she
experiences during excursions away from home can become quite unpleasant, and she suspects that during a longer vacation she also would
get "wound up."

After considering the doctor's suggestion of a vacation, the patient
returns to the tranquilizer theme, when she describes her previous
depression and points out the contrast between the present and the
past:

P: Uhm, there's such a contrast in my
    life in Dallas, where we just moved from around, about eight
    months ago, to here. Uhm, in Dallas I just hated it and did
    nothing. Wouldn't join anything, wouldn't do anything, and   135
    as a result I was very depressed and, uhm, I went through a
    depression for a while, it was just terrible, I was even on,
    uhm, Triatol [*sic*], you know, for a while, and I was on
    it quite a long time, and since I've been up here I certainly
    haven't taken any and yet it's been sort of a reversal. I've   140
    really gotten back into the swing of things,

In Dallas, the problems included social isolation and depression. Having
taken a psychotropic medication previously, she returns to the theme of
tranquilization, when the doctor expresses an inability to treat the unpleasant "feeling" that the patient describes:

P: Okay, but what do I do about this feeling, you know?
    I've got   185
    [
D: Ignore it.
           [
P: No, I can't, I mean I'm
              [
D: I have no way of treating you. My answer to you is very

simple. Rest and Bufferin if you want it, or ignore it, or
a hot sauna, or a hot bath, or stay in bed all day, but I   190
don't find anything organic, I mean (word).
P: Well is there some kind of sedative or tranquilizer you
can give me?

Here the patient starts to push more explicitly for a tranquilizer, after the
doctor voices, perhaps from exasperation, a series of somewhat contradictory, rapid-fire therapeutic alternatives. Lacking a technical diagnosis
or a technical cure, the doctor offers nonpharmacologic alternatives to
achieve relaxation, but to no avail.

As the patient keeps pushing, the following negotiation takes place,
which converts a complex social reality into an objective, reified, technical response—a medication that will take the edge off the patient's con-
textually based distress:

P: I mean I sometimes feel really really nervous
and want something that'll settle me down. And I feel that
if I take a drink, which you know, you would think would   195
pep me up, it works the opposite way.
D: You don't need that. Why should you need it? Why should
you need it? You are a *very* healthy person, with
very normal reactions. They'd be very, it would be
                         [
P: You're not making me happy.   200
D: No, I'm not. Because I know you're pushing me to a
tranquilizer, and I don't want you to have one.
P: Well, I don't want to be dependent on one either but I
                         [
D: All right.
Then you and I are talking the same language.   205
                         [
P: But I don't, but
if I'm *stuck* one day, and really need one, I want to be
able to have one.
D: All right. If you're gonna use it very sparingly, and under-
stand that it isn't going to cure any of your problems.

The doctor leaves little room for doubt about his preferences in the
matter; he does not want to prescribe a tranquilizer. However, the patient's plea wins out. She will take the medication, she argues, only
under real necessity. In response, the doctor reluctantly concedes, although he notes that to tranquilize is not to resolve the patient's contextual difficulties.

By the encounter's conclusion, the doctor not only concedes to the patient's request for a tranquilizer but also allows her to refill the prescription without contacting him:

D: ((laughs)) But look,
    it's renewable. If you need it, just renew it. If you
    don't feel good, (words)
P: Okay.   255
D: Bye bye.
P: Bye bye. Thank you.

Some might question the rationale for a refillable prescription of a tranquilizer, especially when the purpose is not entirely clear.[14] On the other hand, from the doctor's perspective, such a concrete approach to socioemotional distress might reduce the future frequency of such face-to-face negotiations.

Physical versus psychosocial. Throughout the encounter, a tension arises between the patient's expressed concern about her symptoms and the dialogue about psychosocial causes, which the doctor usually initiates. At the beginning, as noted earlier, the patient mentions a variety of physical complaints, possibly tied to exhaustion from social activities. It does not take very long for the doctor to offer the diagnosis of suburban syndrome, even though he has neither fully explored the patient's bodily symptoms nor performed a physical exam.

While the patient recognizes a psychologic component in her nervousness, she does not seem to accept the doctor's implication that her overactivity explains all her symptoms. For instance, just after she first introduces the tranquilizer theme by mentioning Valium, the patient quickly returns to her bodily discomfort and, in response to the doctor's question, gives some possible diagnoses that she herself has considered:

D: What do you think it is?
P: I thought it was a cold.   100
D: What are you worried about? . . . . You think it's more than a cold?
P: Hm hmm. I suppose some things run through my mind.
D: Okay, what?
P: Oh, I don't know, pleurisy or, hmm, maybe anemia, or maybe
    something worse, I don't know.   105

The doctor then explains all these problems as manifestations of exhaustion, and he recommends a Florida vacation. That does not seem to satisfy the patient, for she returns to her somatic symptoms just as the physical exam starts. Mentioning that her husband came to see the doctor less than a month earlier with "this achiness in his shoulders," she notes that now "I've got the same thing," and that "that's too much of a coincidence" (lines 149–53). The doctor reassures the patient that her husband is "a very healthy man" and proceeds with a very brief examination of the lymph nodes, chest, neck, thyroid, and mouth, which he reports as normal (lines 154–75). He then suggests that the patient make an appointment for a "complete physical" and comments:

D: But I think your symptoms right   175
    now are *very normal* and very nice as a matter of fact I think
    you'd be a *manic* if you did what you did without feeling what
    you're feeling. I mean *this* is the *price* you pay.

Here the doctor implies that the patient's symptoms become a sort of payment for bad decisions about social activities, rather than a physical disorder.

   Even with such reassurance, however, the patient returns once more to her physical symptoms and concern about organic disease, just before the encounter ends. Here she mentions that she was expecting a blood test and that her mother suffered from anemia. Immediately the doctor cuts off this line of inquiry with a flourish:

P: That's what I thought maybe you would give me a blood test
    today, see if I was anemic.   235
        [
D: For what? Nah, (words)
                [
P: I sometimes feel
    light-headed.
D: I know.
P: And my mother, and my mother tends to be anemic.   240
D: Don't choose a diagnosis out of the blue. Buy a medical
    book and get a real *nice* diagnosis. Well, and you, I'll
    order them. Which drug store do you use?

While the tone reflected in this statement deserves further comment later, its implication is clear: the patient's search for an underlying physical disorder is, from the doctor's perspective, fruitless.

   The diverse symptoms that the patient describes do fit the pattern of a "somatization" disorder. According to psychiatric theory concerning this type of trouble, people who are unable or unwilling to face their emotional problems consciously may "convert" them into unpleasant bodily sensations. This conversion then becomes a psychic defense against the problem itself. Patients with somatization disorders can present diagnostic and therapeutic challenges for primary-care physicians, who frequently find that their skills in handling such difficulties prove inadequate.[15] In the present situation, the doctor concludes very rapidly that the patient's physical symptoms reflect troubles in her social context, more than pathophysiology. Yet his attempts to persuade her on this point never quite succeed. Despite the diagnosis of suburban syndrome, the dialogue repeatedly moves from contextual matters to concrete, re- ified symptoms and speculations about objective, physical causes.

Context and tone. Certain details of the contextual issues that may contribute to the patient's distress remain notably absent from the dia- logue. In contrast to the last encounter, there is no mention of work, possible marital conflict, child care, the financial situation, or support from friends and family. A college graduate with young children at home, the patient does not refer at any time to her own work aspirations or to her children, nor does the doctor ask. For the present and indefinite future, one assumes, her work consists of the housewife's duties. Refer- ence to the patient's husband enters the conversation at only two points: when the patient describes a tense weekend getaway and when she notes the similarity between her husband's "achiness" and her own. Both patient and doctor attribute the major source of stress to social obliga- tions imposed by the suburban life-style. They do not explore other contextual sources of distress that might prove emotionally charged.

Whether further investigation, on a less superficial level, might reveal additional troubles remains unclear. Based on her chronic and recurring emotional distress, one could predict that the patient may be coping unsuccessfully with issues that do not arise explicitly in this encounter. Rather than inquiring in depth, the doctor limits and marginalizes the range of contextual difficulties to be discussed. According to the doctor, the social demands of suburban living comprise the problem, rather than unexplored difficulties closer to home.

The verbal and nonverbal tone conveyed in the dialogue also contrib- utes to this marginalization of contextual issues. While not fully depicted by the transcript, the doctor's tone of voice in the recording frequently becomes blunt, gruff, or even sarcastic. This tone appears when the doctor says such things as, "You know *damn* well what you're doing" (line 84), and "Don't choose a diagnosis out of the blue. Buy a medical book and get a real *nice* diagnosis" (lines 241–42). As he apparently becomes more exasperated about the patient's somatic complaints, the doctor engages in some colorful repartee when the patient points out a contradiction in his advice:

D: I, I don't
    say slow down, I think that
                         [
P: But you said slow down.   180
D: Well, only if you bitch. And if you don't bitch, don't slow
    down. If you're lovin' it and enjoyin' it, don't let it
    worry you one bit.

The patient may not find this advice reassuring, since she immediately asks, as noted above, what to do about this uncomfortable "feeling" (line 184). How she interprets the meaning of "only if you bitch" cannot be known. Does the phrase convey the meaning of the verb, to bitch, as it says, "only if you feel like complaining"? Does it also express the meaning of the noun, bitch, to connote something about the doctor's appraisal of the patient? Either way, the tone does not exactly convey respect for the patient's plight.

On the other hand, the patient's tone moves from the above tense description of bodily complaints, to nervous laughter, to inaudible mumbling. At several points, she laughs in the midst of emotionally charged material. Laughter accompanies her statement that "I need something now" (line 85) and that the contrast after her move from Dallas "overwhelmed me" (lines 142–43). She also laughs as she refers to the similarity of her husband's "achiness" and notes "that's too much of a coincidence" (lines 151–53). Especially when she alludes to psychic distress, the patient's voice sometimes trails off to mumbling, the content of which cannot be heard. This tendency occurs when she mentions the tranquilizer, Valium (lines 93–95), and again when she describes the tension she felt during the weekend getaway with her husband (lines 115–17). Judged by the verbal material with which they are associated, laughter and mumbling emerge as defensive, nonverbal devices that seem to offer protection from emotionally troubling features of the social context.

Ideology and structure. This encounter, then, manifests several structural elements (figure 6.2). The key contextual issue involves familial role expectations affecting women (A). These expectations have led to stressful conditions for a college-educated person with young children who recently has moved to a new geographical area. The social demands that she faces have resulted in several personal troubles, including exhaustion and emotional irritability; a variety of physical symptoms that she experiences also may derive from psychic distress (B). Because of these troubles, she visits her doctor (C). When he asks the reason for the visit, she expresses the contextual problem by describing her exhaustion, social overload, bodily discomforts, and nervousness. After a brief discussion and without a physical exam, the doctor gives a contextual diagnosis: suburban syndrome. The doctor points out the importance of insight into the problem, presents his own interpretation of how social responsibilities in the suburbs can become stressful, and encourages rest (D). Despite the contextual diagnosis, potentially important contextual issues arise in the conversation either marginally (as in the brief allusions to the patient's husband) or not at all (as in the case of work aspirations, child care arrangements, and social support network). The doctor's tone further marginalizes the range of contextual difficulties discussed. In the

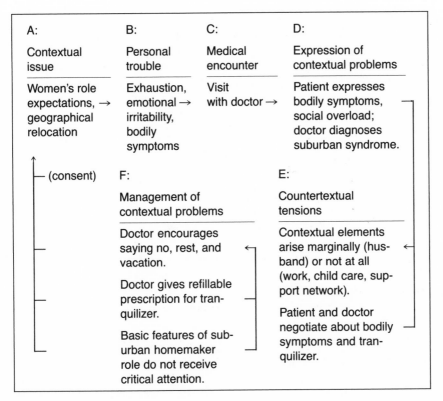

Figure 6.2
Structural elements of a medical encounter with a woman diagnosed as having "suburban syndrome"

dialogue, tensions arise as doctor and patient negotiate about physical symptoms and a tranquilizer. At least in part, these tensions reflect the participants' inability or unwillingness to explore contextual problems on other than a superficial level (E). Nevertheless, the doctor tries to manage the patient's contextual difficulties by encouraging rest and a long vacation. With some reluctance, he also prescribes a tranquilizer and makes the prescription refillable. While the doctor encourages the patient to "say no" to some social activities, the more basic features of her social role do not receive critical attention, even though they may contribute to her distress. As a result, the patient presumably continues to accept the ideologic assumption that her current social role as suburban homemaker is the proper one for her, perhaps ameliorated by rest and tranquilization (F). She thus returns and consents to the same social context as before, now with the benefit of medical advice and pharmacologic assistance.

While the last two encounters vary in the approaches of the physicians involved, the second encounter leads to similar results as the first: little if anything changes. Again, the ideologic assumptions that govern women's familial and work roles remain unexamined. Questions that could initiate a critique of suburban syndrome (regarding work advancement, male-female relations in the family, provisions for child care, and so forth) do not get asked. Instead, contextual tensions are converted to irritating bodily symptoms requiring tranquilization—the technical and reified help that medicine proves able to provide.

ENCOUNTER 6C: PHYSICAL DIFFICULTIES WITH HOUSEWORK

SUMMARY

A woman visits her doctor because of irregularities in her heart rhythm. She complains that palpitations and shortness of breath are interfering with her ability to do housework. The doctor checks an electrocardiogram while she exercises, changes her cardiac medications, and congratulates her in her efforts to maintain a tidy household.[16]

Some characteristics of the participants, known from the questionnaires that they filled out, are as follows. The patient is 50 years old, white, married, Roman Catholic, and "English-Irish-French" in ethnic background. She attended some college, has four children, and reports her occupation as "wife." The doctor is a 39-year-old man who practices general internal medicine. The encounter takes place in a Boston suburb. According to the doctor, the patient, whom he has known for five years, has "rheumatic heart disease with mitral insufficiency" and "menopausal syndrome."

Technical content. The highly technical orientation of this encounter distinguishes it from the relatively nontechnical orientation of the last two. (Partly for this reason, the interpretation of Encounter 6C will be briefer.) In fact, Encounter 6C contains more content based in scientific medicine than any other of the fifty transcripts randomly selected from the larger sample of doctor-patient interactions. The patient suffers from rheumatic heart disease that affects principally the mitral valve. In the past she has endured episodes of congestive heart failure and irregularities of heart rhythm. She takes at least two cardiac medications: hydrochlorothiazide (Hydrodiuril) to reduce fluid accumulation and propranolol (Inderal) to control rhythm disturbances. Although the patient has been able to manage fairly well with limited physical exertion, her heart disease is serious enough that the doctor is contemplating heart surgery with valve replacement. In addition, the patient has menopausal and hearing problems.

A large part of the interaction deals with technical issues of diagnosis and treatment (lines 1–170, 235–467). The doctor asks questions about exercise tolerance, compliance with medication schedule, symptoms of heart failure (pain, shortness of breath, ankle swelling), menstrual symptoms, and ear symptoms. He does a partial physical exam and an electrocardiogram. He then spends considerable time explaining his notion about the relation between the patient's symptoms and her irregular heart rhythm. Since he apparently believes that her rhythm abnormality may have returned because she decided on her own to reduce her medication, he requests that she use the prescribed dose and check with him before making further changes.

The patient takes an active role in the technical discussion. When confused about the doctor's explanation or instruction, she asks frequent questions. The doctor confirms her competence, when she describes her previous reaction to digoxin, a cardiac medication:

D: The digoxin slowed you too much   340

             [

P: Yeah. Except that
   not that extreme. But it would just get very very
   feathery and very very tired.

D: Yeah, well I know you're sensitive and a good
   observer, I   345

      [

P: And when I cut it back to one, everything seemed to be so much better

Despite this compliment, he suggests that she not modify her medications independently. That the patient does understand is clear from her response to a question in the interview after the medical encounter. The questionnaire asks: "Did Dr. —— say that anything was wrong with you? What did he say?" She replies: "Bigeminy [coupled extra heart beats] has returned with exercise. We will attempt to control it with increased medication." Regarding the technical basis of the encounter, the doctor seems eager to share full information with the patient and to encourage her autonomous participation. Although the doctor's professional knowledge remains a basis of asymmetry in the relationship, he communicates this knowledge in a straightforward way. He thus reduces the inherent inequality of the relationship and avoids domination in the encounter. Interestingly, these positive features of the interaction seem to stem in part from its focus on predominantly technical issues relating to the patient's physical illness.

Household work and physical limitations. Against this background, the messages of ideology and social control that the physician does convey are noteworthy. Although the interaction in this encounter appears very egalitarian, the overriding goal is still the client's adequate functioning in work: in this case, the occupation of "wife." The patient's physical symptoms are problematic mainly insofar as they interfere with this occupation. Exertion in housework triggers the patient's symptoms of irregular heart rhythm. This experience makes her unhappy and even guilty:

P: But if you really feel my pulse, it's not, uh,
   it just seems like a normal pattern.
D: Is it fairly regular? Or does it seem to be skipping?
P: Well, if I'm doing anything at all, it gets irregular.
D: Mmm hmm.
P: I can cook the dinner and wash the clothes, but you
   know, any sweeping, cleaning that I do, that kind of
   sounds like an excuse, but it really isn't.
D: ((laughs)) Yeah. No, I . . .
P: It's just when I used to do it, like in fifteen or twenty minute
   intervals, and then sit and relax for five or ten minutes,
   then I could carry on. Now I can't do that. It's sort
   of maddening,

The patient hopes for a way to improve her physical capacity to perform the labor that her household chores require.

At this point, the doctor has several options. He could try to explore and to ease the patient's guilty feelings about her physical limitations. Also, he could suggest alternative social arrangements, including greater division of labor in housework. Instead, he opts for a pharmacologic solution, increasing the dose and frequency of a medication to suppress irregularities in heart rhythm. He views this technical intervention as a desirable alternative in dealing with physical or emotional demands:

D: Yeah, well it seems that the irregularity is when
   you place, you know, when there is either increased
   tension or increased stimulation to your heart or
   more demands on it because you're starting to work
   more. And that
                  [
P: What worries me is that the demand
   is such a little thing
                       [
D: Yes.
P: That I, I cut out so many things, that you have to do.

D: Oh, absolutely. And you see what we wanted you to do
   is allow you to do those things without, without having
   the tendency to the irregularities or the poundings,
   and if we can suppress, you know, the intent of the
   Inderal, uh, or propranolol, is to, it blocks, if you   370
   will, some of the extra, you know, some of the extra
   beats. So that when your heart is being pushed by
   any sort of external or internal influence, this can
   slow that down.

An extraordinary expression of this attitude is the doctor's encouraging
comment as he instructs the patient to exercise more strenuously during
the electrocardiogram:

D: . . . I guess that showed it as being absolutely regular,   270
   and what we'll do is, I'm just going to have you
   exercise a little bit and let's just run the, uh,
   run the machine. OK. Could you do some sit-ups
   for me? Just put it on, you're on lead two.
NURSE: Yes.   275
D: Just, do them a little bit faster. You can stop it
   now and then. And, uh, OK. Just do about, uh,
   try to get yourself a little bit short of breath . . .
   Try it again . . . . Just scrub one more room.

Through this possibly humorous instruction, the doctor indicates that he
is trying to replicate the physical demands of housework, so that the
electrocardiogram can record any resulting rhythm abnormality. By applying the technology of electrocardiography to the problem of physical
distress in housework, the discourse reifies a complicated contextual
issue and converts it to a more objective disorder, amenable to professional manipulation. Presumably, the purpose here is to make technical
adjustments, informed by scientific observations, so that the patient can
keep on scrubbing.

The implicit ideologic message is that the woman's role in housework
is worthwhile, desirable, and necessary. Again, alternatives remain ambiguous. It is hard to fault the doctor for seeing as his main task the
optimization of the patient's physical capacity. Struggling against sexism
perhaps would be too much to expect in such an encounter. Questioning
or challenging the patient's work at home might upset her deeply; on
some level, the doctor may be aware of this dilemma. Yet the doctor
reinforces this woman's household activities, and even her troubled
feelings about them. Such work by women—as Engels and innumerable
later analysts of the family have pointed out—is crucial in reproducing
the relations of economic production.[17] Here a well-intentioned doctor

contributes to this socioeconomic arrangement. There is no critical appraisal of any aspect of the woman's role, even those physical demands that exacerbate symptoms of heart disease.

The husband's work. That the woman's continuing ability to reproduce her husband's economic role is a major goal also becomes clear from the doctor's inquiry about life stress. This topic would seem a reasonable one for a concerned physician to initiate. Notably, the doctor's question about stress addresses the work of the patient's husband:

D: Yeah, OK . . . . The areas of pressure and stress. Your
   husband is, now . . .
P: He's employed and he's in state
                              [
D: He's employed now
                              [
P: and as far as   17
   [
D: And . . . liking it better?
P: Well, he makes anything interesting. He really does
   it all out, you know, better than anybody else could
   do it.
D: Yeah, yeah, sure.   18
P: Um, but his comment on it is "Any high school kid
   could do it." Well I don't think they really could.
D: No, no.
P: They might basically understand some of it, but
   they couldn't meet with the engineers and   18
                              [
D: Well, he
   takes a lot of pride I think in the fact that, you
   know, that he can, obviously is pretty competent.
P: And he always cuts himself down ((laughs)), so . . .

The conversation implies that the husband has found a job after a period of unemployment, is happier than he previously was, works hard, yet feels dissatisfaction because his work lacks challenge. Although the doctor praises the husband's competence, the patient reports that her husband denigrates himself.

While the physician here shows understandable concern about stress, the revealing feature of this concern is that it focuses first and foremost on the economic role of the patient's husband. The caring doctor hopes that such stress will not take its toll on the patient, and also that the patient's physical condition will not impede her ability to maintain the breadwinner's home. Doctor and patient seem mutually to desire these outcomes; alternatives escape critical scrutiny. The encounter subtly affirms that stress related to the husband's occupational role is a necessary part of social life and that medicine's goals include satisfactory adjustment to this stress.

Family tensions and pleasures. Similarly, the physician tries to learn about and to manage other tension-laden experiences in the family. Early in the interaction, the patient mentions a possible relation between irregular heart rhythm and emotional conflict with her daughter:

P: So I decided to, you know, try to rest. Maybe I had done
   something or something had gone wrong. My daughter had
   been home one weekend and I, maybe there had been a   20
   conflict, emotional conflict
                                [
D: Yeah, yeah
                                [
P: because, I don't
   know why it would do it so suddenly,

The doctor drops the subject but returns to it later, when he asks about the children. Again the patient alludes to problems she anticipates when her daughter returns to work as a lifeguard. That the daughter's presence is a source of anxiety is clear from a laughing claim that the patient is trying not to worry now:

P: Well, uh, my daughter's going to be home, after
   school. She's been away for three weeks, and she's   200
   coming back this weekend to do lifeguarding and
   teaching at the pool in town.
D: Mmm hmm.
P: And I'll take that when it comes. ((laughs))

Also in response to the doctor's question about whether the children will be home, the patient briefly refers to her oldest son's military training (lines 206–08). The reasons for the doctor's professional surveillance of family life are not entirely evident. Apparently, he again wants to do what he can to reduce, or at least to investigate, sources of emotional stress that may affect the patient's physical health. Perhaps because no acute problems seem present, he does not offer concrete suggestions.

The medical management of leisure and pleasure also occurs in this encounter. Planning for a summer vacation is the background for the doctor's questions about the patient's children (lines 196–98). The doctor then asks if the patient will "get away this summer." She replies about a possible trip by car to visit her mother-in-law in St. Louis. Despite the patient's concern about finances, the doctor encourages her to fly. He inquires whether she will be spending some time at the beach and implies that this would be a good idea. However, the patient replies that her husband is "not a beach loller" (lines 209–34). The doctor perhaps may have some concern here about the physical effects of long periods of sitting for a patient with heart disease. On the other hand, he seems to imply that relaxing at the beach may be more pleasurable than a "long haul" by car to visit one's mother-in-law. Although the doctor remains nondirective, the partial medicalization of leisure and pleasure, within an otherwise technically oriented encounter, is striking.

Ideology and structure. In this encounter, as already noted in chapter 3, a number of structural elements emerge (figure 3.2). Women's social role in the family again comprises a problematic contextual issue (A). The patient tries to perform her household work—an important activity in reproducing her husband's economic role. Physical symptoms and emotional distress arise because her cardiac symptoms interfere with housework (B). In the medical encounter (C), the patient expresses this concern (D). The doctor responds supportively and tries to address the problem through technical means. Specifically, he performs an electrocardiogram during exercise and, by asking her to "scrub one more room," replicates the physical demands of housework. Through this maneuver, more basic questions pertaining to the woman's role expectations and possible alternatives move to the margin of the conversation, as both participants attend to scientific observations (E). In managing the contextual problem, the doctor intervenes technically by changing the patient's cardiac medications. By this adjustment, he encourages her efforts to maintain a tidy household. The ideologic assumption that a woman should maintain her reproductive work in the home therefore goes unquestioned, even though such activities entail a certain risk (F). After a largely technical dialogue, the patient continues consenting to the challenge of housework despite serious heart disease.

Again, the communication seems admirable. Both patient and doctor maintain a strong orientation to the technical details of the patient's physical illness. The doctor shares information openly. The patient participates actively. They convey an impression of mutual respect and cooperation. Nonetheless, themes of ideology and social control arise, albeit to a lesser degree than in the first two encounters. A primary goal of the encounter is the client's ability to function in economic reproduction within the family. By not examining the problematic features of women's role, the discourse implicitly supports it. Difficulties in family life, when questioned, are amenable to technical intervention, stress reduction, and adjustment rather than to contextual change. Medical mediation also arises in the realm of leisure and personal pleasure. Aside from the positive communication that occurs, the encounter still reinforces things as they are.

MEDICAL MEDIATION OF WORK
AND THE FAMILY FOR WOMEN

In these encounters, patients and doctors confront some of the contextual issues that trouble women. For the patient in Encounter 6A, marital conflict has created frustration on several fronts: social isolation, geographical immobility, blocked career aspirations, financial problems, and conflicts concerning child care. Although the doctor encourages the patient to talk about these difficulties and about her emotional distress, the available therapeutic options do not point to clear avenues of improvement in any of these arenas. The woman in Encounter 6B suffers from an overload of social responsibilities as a suburban housewife. A tranquilizer provides a technical means of coping with a variety of bodily and emotional discomforts. Meanwhile, very little if any attention gets paid to children, career, marriage, or other contextual issues that are pertinent. In Encounter 6C, doctor and patient focus on the technical details of the patient's disabling heart disease. During their discussion, they seek to preserve the patient's functional capacity to perform housework, despite disturbances of cardiac rhythm induced by exertion. Again, alternative social arrangements do not receive consideration.

Passivity is a striking element in these encounters. Explicit anger is absent. The first two patients, according to the doctors' diagnoses, are depressed, and the third is concerned about her physical limitations in housework. Although the first patient seems intent on pursuing divorce, the most active course taken in the three encounters, even she sees little possibility for change in the contextual issues that have become most troubling for her. As judged by the words they express, all three patients internalize their feelings and focus on the body. The women's activities in life and conceptions of self center on supporting and reproducing the economic activities of men. These reproductive commitments involve such pursuits as homemaking, childrearing, and socializing. To varying degrees, the women suffer long-term effects of expectations attached to women's role in the family; their personal struggles have taken some toll. Yet they do not question very deeply, nor does medical discourse provide a framework for doing so.

As gender-role patterning creates problems for women, the doctor-patient encounter provides one place for the expression of such troubles. Tensions that derive from women's roles in the family and at work lead to emotional disturbances, as well as difficulties in achieving role expectations when physical illness occurs. Sympathetic doctors voice caring concern and offer remedies such as drugs and counseling. Yet, in general, medical discourse tends to marginalize the contextual issues of greatest concern. For example, social roles in the family rarely are open to critical analysis, even when contextual conditions become the principal source of a client's distress. While focused intervention occasionally becomes necessary (as in physical abuse)[18] medical discourse usually assumes that the social context of family life will continue more or less unchanged. Personal adjustment and consent to the social context remain the norm.

The doctor-patient encounter rarely elicits a critical analysis of troubling social patterns affecting women, let alone strategies for change. Medical management of psychic distress generally involves an intervention—medication, advice, or even the permitting of negative comments and emotional catharsis—that facilitates clients' adjustment to troublesome circumstances. A health professional may ask questions about family life or work and may make limited suggestions. But major structural alternatives—sexual equality in housework, child care options, employment opportunities, divorce, children's emancipation, and so forth—seldom become suitable recommendations. The ideologic impact of the medical encounter thus tends to be conservative. Although reduction of stress may seem desirable, major modifications in social relations elude serious consideration. Lacking a critical thrust, medical discourse helps reinforce women's roles in the family and at work—roles that reproduce so much else that goes on in society.

Is there a different way to go? The last chapter will raise some possibilities. Meanwhile, it is enough to say that the answers are not simple. For instance, doctors and others sympathetic to patients' plights might argue that a critical examination of family relations in medical discourse would create more harm than good. Without the ability to intervene and to orchestrate other kinds of social support, initiating a critique of the family might well add to patients' emotional distress, while not providing any palpable assistance. A patient then would be left high and dry, perhaps more critically aware but no more able to change contextual arrangements. Further, is doctors' involvement in such matters appropriate anyway? The critique of medicalization holds that the medical management of social problems in some ways can become worse than the problems themselves.[19] Doctors' intrusion into family and work relations then might subtly put such problems under professional control, rather than under the control of women seeking autonomously to restructure their social roles. A medical discourse that heightens critical awareness, offers concrete options for change, yet does not take control over the process— constructing such a discourse remains easier said than done.

Pending the clarification of such questions, women continue to mention contextual problems as they talk with their doctors. When personal troubles arise that have roots in the family and work process, doctors respond as best they can. In doing so, however, the constraints of medical discourse limit what both patients and doctors can hope to accomplish as they speak.

CHAPTER 7

AGING

How do patients and doctors deal with the process and problems of aging? To ask this question addresses a large part of what medicine is becoming in advanced industrial societies. Here, the age distribution of the population is changing drastically, so that more "seniors" stay alive and comprise an ever-increasing proportion of medical practice. While medicine no doubt contributes to such increases in longevity, medical technique does not necessarily assure a pleasant quality of life. In such countries as the United States, social policies to help the elderly leave many of their needs unmet. As a result, older people confront a strange contradiction: although modern medicine can provide the technical means to keep them alive, life at an advanced age frequently becomes burdensome and unhappy. Further, medicine creates this mixed achievement at great financial cost.[1]

When elderly people talk with their doctors, the social problems that they face almost inevitably enter the conversation. Such contextual problems derive from bereavement, financial insecurity, isolation and loneliness, declining physical capacity, dependency, inadequate housing, lack of transportation, and a host of other issues. These issues may arise directly, as patients bring them up or doctors explicitly ask about them. Alternatively, such problems may appear indirectly, in passing, or marginally, as doctors and patients focus on technical concerns. Certain programs in geriatric medicine use multidisciplinary teams, including social workers, to help with such problems; whether these interventions can improve the conditions facing senior citizens remains to be seen.[2]

Meanwhile, many elderly people continue to consult medical practitioners for whom the social context may not seem pertinent or interesting. Yet the social context affects these patients and doctors as they talk. How their discourse does or does not deal with contextual problems becomes the question that I consider here.

The following three encounters involve doctors and elderly patients who face somewhat different contextual issues. As before, the interpretation emphasizes elements of ideology, social control, and an underlying structure that may not be immediately apparent.[3]

ENCOUNTER 7A: INDEPENDENCE AND PHYSICAL DECLINE

SUMMARY

An elderly woman visits her doctor for follow-up of her heart disease. During the encounter she expresses concerns about decreased vision, her ability to continue driving, lack of stamina and strength, weight loss and diet, and financial problems. She discusses her recent move to a new home and her relationship with family and friends. Her physician assures her that her health is improving; he recommends that she continue her current medical regimen and that she see an eye doctor.

From the questionnaires that the patient and doctor completed after their interaction, some pertinent information is available: The patient is an 80-year-old white high school graduate. She is Protestant, Scottish-American, and widowed, with five living children whose ages range from 45 to 59 years; she describes her occupation as "homemaker." Her doctor is a 44-year-old white male, of German and English descent, who gives no religious preference. He states his specialty as internal medicine. The doctor has known the patient for about one year and believes that her primary diagnoses are atherosclerotic heart disease and prior congestive heart failure. The encounter takes place in a private practice in a suburb of Boston.

Vision, mobility, autonomy. Right at the beginning of the encounter, the patient complains about her vision and its implications. Although her cardiac symptoms apparently have improved, she still feels "rocky," by which she refers to visual difficulties:

D: You say you're feeling better.
P: I am better.
D: Yeah.
P: But I:: feel kind of rocky.

D: You are (word).
P: My eyes are bothering me. I can see perfectly, read signs,
   but R—— [friend] said she wondered if I was eating right, and
   if I, a little vitamin A or something would, ah, when I go back,
   turn back from a bright lights, it looks dark to me, although   15
   I can see. What I mean, ah, after it clears I can see all
   right. But my eyes don't feel right.

In the passage that follows, the doctor expresses doubt about vitamin A
and states a preference that the patient consult an ophthalmologist (lines
19–48). Just before leaving, the patient again presses the doctor for a
prognosis regarding her sight:

P: What about my eyes? Do you think those will straighten out?
D: I think they will, yeah.
P: Doctor —— says he thinks I might need glasses. (words)
D: Yeah. Well, you're gonna see him again.   390

The patient's reiteration of concern about vision, which frames the encounter at its beginning and end, reflects a troubling preoccupation. Yet
the dialogue remains ambiguous about the implications of visual loss.
The doctor does not check the patient's vision, nor does he examine her
eyes. Instead, he withholds an opinion as he reinforces her plan to
consult an eye specialist.

Why does vision preoccupy the patient? At several points in the
encounter, she attaches importance to eyesight as a critical aid for mobility and autonomy. At age 80, the patient still drives a car and wants to
continue to do so. She emphasizes the link between vision and transportation immediately after the doctor agrees with her intention to visit a
specialist. As she introduces the subject of driving, the doctor banters
with her about speed and safety:

P: I drove my car yesterday, down Arlington Heights
   [
D: Oh, dear. Eighty miles an hour again.   50
P: No, I didn't. I went thirty.
D: Thirty.
P: Yeah, down Mass Avenue.
D: Well, that's the first time in years you've ever slowed
   down to thirty.   55
          [
P: Nope
   Hm hmm.
       [
D: Yeah. Ha haa.

* * *

P: And parked my car. And I hadn't taken it out till yesterday,
   and I made my (word) my mind I have just got to push myself a
   little bit. So I went out, and I don't feel like walking too
   far. I did walk from the project up to —— Street the other
   day, I made myself do that. Well I got my car, and I says
   "Well now I'm going down and get my sticker."
D: Mm hmm.

Despite a joking demeanor, the patient gets the point and reassures the doctor that she has reduced her speed in line with community standards. She also mentions her determination to take initiative in mobilizing herself. Because she does not "feel like walking," presumably because of weakness, she has committed herself to using her car and completing legal registration requirements. By associating vision and driving, the patient subtly expresses anxiety that physical decline, involving the use of her eyes, will interfere with her mobility. Throughout this part of the encounter, when he is not joshing the patient about her driving techniques, the doctor enunciates a series of noncommittal conversational fillers ("Yeah," "Mm hmm," and so forth)—neither encouraging the patient's automotive escapades nor explicitly discouraging them.

Driving is not just for pleasure, however; it is also a matter of surviving with autonomy in the face of approaching death. The patient depends on her car for a variety of functional necessities and social contacts. She indicates a few of these concerns in a later passage, just before she returns to the discussion of vision that concludes the interaction:

P: It's all right for me to drive a little bit if I feel like it?
D: I guess we're not gonna stop you.
P: Well, no, that isn't the question. It's whether you feel my-

    [
D: I, I think it's all right, yes.
P: Like going (words)
   shopping center on Baker Street.
D: Yeah, I know.
P: If I feel like it.
D: I think the main hazard these days is other drivers. You
   gotta watch out for them.
P: Oh, I don't know. I'm not too perfect myself.
D: Well, I think you probably-
P: Still, I tell you, I go (word) right hand turns. (words)
   lights. And there are ways that I can get to these places
   without too much hassle.
D: Yeah.
P: (word) driving, I went to a funeral (words)
D: Yeah. Well, I don't if you use your judgment that way, sure.

The negotiation about driving here expresses several themes, which objectify and (to use Lukács' term) reify the complex social conditions facing this elderly person by converting them into a concrete professional decision about physical capacity to use a car.[4] First the patient requests the doctor's approval for her continuing to drive. His response proves much less than enthusiastic, as he uses the royal "we" to note that he will not invoke his legal responsibility, as a doctor, to prohibit driving for patients whose physical incapacities predictably might interfere with safety. As the patient begins to reply that the doctor's stopping her "isn't the question," she begins to clarify the question, but the doctor interrupts (line 367). The doctor gives tentative approval, noting his view that other drivers have become the "main hazard." Then the patient alludes to the importance of using the car to go shopping and also for social responsibilities like a recent funeral. Her car thus becomes her means to buy the necessities required for independent living, as well as a way to fulfill her social obligations—among which the funerals of friends and relatives figure prominently for people at her age.

For the patient, who lives alone long after her husband has died and her children have departed, autonomy in activities of daily living has become an ever-increasing struggle, in which modest success emerges as a source of personal pride. The mobility that her car provides becomes just part of a story about independent function that the patient spontaneously narrates. For instance, she also expresses pleasure in her ability to do housework, to cook, to feed herself, and to maintain her wardrobe:

P: Now I'll tell you what I did yesterday. Uhm,   120
          I did all my own work, and I've been, been doing a fair amount
          of vegetable cooking, getting better meals for myself.
D: Mm hmm.
P: I managed to get a whole tomato down this week.
D: There you are.   125
P: And a whole banana. Ha! Kidding. Well, . . . ah, I took the
     car out, then I came home, and I said, "Well I've got (word),"
     so I ironed.

Later she alludes to gratification in buying groceries on her own.

P: Still I'm getting better, I can, I can move around pretty well.   215
     I went ramblin', picked a (word), oh I have two, three weeks
     ago, all my groceries myself.

While the patient uses a humorous and ironic tone, she clearly takes such accomplishments quite seriously. Again the doctor punctuates the narrative with brief fillers, which seem to support the patient's efforts to preserve autonomous daily function.

The pride that the patient expresses about independence in such activities also may reflect the fact that homemaking comprises her stated occupation. Presumably, for many years, the patient's work has centered on the maintenance of her home. She thus has involved herself conscientiously in reproductive concerns, as she has raised a family and taken care of feeding, clothing, cleaning, and nurturing others in addition to herself. The dedication and initiative that she brings to independent function in old age carry forward a work role through which she at least partially has defined herself as a woman. Anxiety about the loss of functional capacity then centers on the same responsibilities that she has discharged as wife and mother.

Social support, family life, and the meaning of home. Although the patient values her independence, she also tries to maintain a social support network, which she again describes spontaneously to the doctor without prompting. Such allusions to a social support network usually arise within this medical encounter as marginal features, which the patient mentions in passing and which the doctor does not pursue in depth.[5] Among her social contacts, R——, presumably a friend, appears the most central. The patient tries to see R—— regularly for lunch and other get-togethers. Socializing with R—— brings her pleasure, advice, and support. For instance, when she describes her current nutritional status and medications, she says:

P: And I'm trying hard to eat a banana once in a while, trying to eat some tomatoes, and
D: uh
P: I ate a, R—— took me to lunch, and I had an elegant lobster salad sandwich.

3

As a source of advice, R—— has raised a question about vitamin A as a factor in the patient's visual symptoms (lines 13–15). The patient also mentions that R—— has helped her move to a new home (line 230) and has discussed her plans to buy new dresses (line 298). In a medical encounter, these frequent and unsolicited references to a friend indicate the importance of a social contact for an elderly woman trying to live independently.

Family members figure less prominently as sources of support and also create some rather burdensome obligations. Apparently, most of the family have moved to other geographical areas. The patient keeps in touch by telephone and mail, especially for birthdays, but she finds herself unable to do as much as she might like, partly because of the number of people involved:

P: Well I should- now I've got birthday cards to buy.
I've got seven or eight birthdays this week—month. Instead

of that, I'm just gonna write 'em and wish them a happy
birthday. Just a little note, my grandchildren. 100
D: Mm hmm.
P: But I'm not gonna bother. I just can't do it all, Dr. ——.
D: Well,
P: I called my daughters, her birthday was just, today's the third.
D: Yeah. 105
P: My daughter's birthday in Princeton was the, uh, first, and I
called her up and talked with her. I don't know what time
it'll cost me, but then, my telephone is my only indiscretion.

At no other time in the encounter does the patient refer to her own
family, nor does the doctor ask. It seems that family members remain
largely at a distance. The patient does her best to maintain contact with
them, even though she does not mention anything that she receives in
the way of day-to-day support.

Compounding these problems of social support and incipient isolation, the patient recently has moved from a home that she occupied for 59
years. The reasons for giving up her home remain unclear, but they seem
to involve a combination of financial factors and difficulties in maintaining it. Her reactions to the move include both pluses and minuses,
although one suspects that her sense of loss might be greater than she
cares to admit. She first mentions the move quickly but then moves on to
a pleasant visit with R—— and her shopping accomplishments:

P: And of course I'd been awful busy changing addresses, 'n-
D: Yeah.
P: And today, I've been to lunch with R——. And I've done all 80
my week's shopping. And here I am.

During the physical exam, the patient spontaneously returns to the
move. Here she mentions more details about the loss of possessions and
relationships with previous neighbors, along with satisfaction about certain conveniences of her new living situation. Further, as the patient
speaks, the doctor asks a couple of clarifying questions about the move,
as well as a series of his usual pleasant fillers, before he cuts off this
discussion by helping the patient from the examination table.

P: Yeah . . . . ((moving around noises)). Well, I sold a lot of my 225
stuff.
D: Yeah, how did the moving go, as long as (word)
       [
P: Oh, finally rid of-
I thought I'd never out with it. And I was so but you know
they wouldn't let me do any lifting and R—— and B—— and my 230

neighbor across the street there in Arlington did
it all.

D: No.

P: And y'know take forty ni- fifty nine years accumulation. Boy,
and I've got cartons in my closet it'll take me till doomsday   2:
to, ouch.

D: Gotcha.

P: But I've been kept out of mischief by doing it. But I've got
a lot to do, I sold my rugs 'cause they wouldn't fit where I
am. I just got a piece of plain cloth at home.   2٠

D: Mm hmm.

P: Sometimes I think I'm foolish at 81. I don't know
how long I'll live. Isn't much point in putting money into
stuff, and then, why not enjoy a little bit of life?
[

D: Mm hmm, (words).   2٠

P: And I've got to have draperies made.

D: Now, then, you're (words).

P: But that'll come. I'm not worrying. I got an awfully cute
place. It's very, very comfortable. All electric kitchen.
It's got a better bathroom than I ever had in my life.   2٠

D: Great . . . . . . Met any of your neighbors there yet?

P: Oh, I met two or three.

D: Mm hmm.

P: And my, some of my neighbors from Belmont here, there's Mrs.
F—— and her two sisters are up to see me, spent the afternoon   2٠
with me day before yesterday. And all my neighbors, um, holler
down the hall (words) . . . years ago. They're comin',
so they say. So, I'm hopin' they will. I hated to move,
cause I loved, um, I liked my neighbors very much.

D: Now, we'll let you down. You watch your step.   2٠

In the passage that follows, after the doctor mentions briefly that the
patient's heart "sounds good" (line 264), he and the patient go on to other
topics. They do not return to the patient's loss of a home, despite the
importance that the patient attaches to this move through her extensive
narrative during the physical exam. The doctor's cut-off and his return to
the technical assessment of cardiac function therefore have the effect of
marginalizing a contextual problem that involves loss of home and community.

For the patient, the move seems to hold several meanings. First, in the
realm of inanimate objects, she has gained some and lost some. Her new
living situation, apparently an apartment (line 257 mentions a hallway),
contains several physical features that she views as more convenient, or

at least "cute." The "all electric kitchen" and the "better bathroom" represent improvements over her prior home. On the other hand, she apparently has sold many of her possessions, which carry the memories of fifty-nine years in the same house. Further, she feels the need to decorate her new home but doubts the wisdom of investing financial resources in such items as rugs and draperies at her advanced age (lines 242–44). In her ambivalence, she also believes that she should enjoy her surroundings while she is able and denies that such decisions about physical objects are causing her to worry.

Aside from physical objects gained and lost, the patient confronts a loss of community. Her previous neighbors helped her move and have promised to visit her. In response to the doctor's question about meeting new neighbors, the patient says that she has met "two or three," including some who have visited her and others who make their presence felt "down the hall." Yet she states her feelings clearly: she "hated" to move, because of the affection that she held for her prior neighbors. Describing her attachment, she first mentions that she "loved" them and then modulates her feelings by saying that she "liked them very much." It is as if the patient is censoring herself, trying not to admit how much she misses them. Whatever the pain that this loss has created, the full impact remains unexplored, as the doctor cuts off the line of discussion by terminating the physical exam and returning to a technical comment about her cardiac condition. The problems of the heart that are most on the patient's mind, however, are not physical ones, and the doctor's technical reassurance may not go very far in assuaging her sense of loss.

Throughout these passages concerning friends, family, and the loss of a home, until a rather abrupt termination, the doctor supportively listens. Both from his brief words and his tone of voice on the tape, one gets the impression of a humanistic, caring professional, who genuinely involves himself in the patient's concerns. The doctor lets the patient talk, asks short questions about her social context, and enunciates a series of fillers that encourage her to keep talking. He makes no specific comments or suggestions to help the patient in these arenas, nor does he guide the dialogue toward deeper exploration of her feelings. While he appears to empathize with the patient, he also functions within the traditional constraints of the medical role. When tension mounts with the patient's mourning a much-loved community, the doctor returns to the more comfortable realm of medical technique.

Financial problems. Worries about money come up at several points in the encounter. As already noted, she has sold many of her possessions, and economic considerations are constraining her decisions about decorating her new home. Further, desire to maintain mobility and autonomy by driving a car also creates financial stress. Facing unpaid bills, the patient expresses some ambivalent regret about the additional expenses that her car creates:

P: So, uh, I shan't do anything about buying something for myself
   until I get my bills paid. So, and I suppose I was awfully
   foolish to put my car on the road this year.
D: Will it help, if you want to do it, that's all right.
P: Well, I know that, but there comes a, it's a question of   31
   what to do, what's right to do.

Driving a car thus increases some financial pressures while reducing her dependency on other people.

Even more than the expenses of housing and driving, however, the costs of medical care have become a burden. Noting that her insurance coverage remains incomplete, the patient describes a hospital bill that is causing consternation. This bill has affected her ability to make other needed purchases, for instance, of clothes:

P: So I told R——, I said I'll go and get a dress at a time. I
   got a nice bill from —— Hospital yesterday. Two hundred
   and forty-one dollars. ((sniff))   3(
D: Was that, uh,
P: That was the tail end, that is the, the, uh, whole itemized
   account. I only got a hundred and twenty four dollars out
   of ((corporation name)), and I can't understand it.
D: How about Medicare?   3(
P: I::'ve got, you see I didn't have Medicare D [sic], Doctor.
   A—— didn't think we needed it. And I was so, well, negligent I
   should have had it. But I am registered for it the first of
   July.
D: Hm.   31

Apparently the patient has received services at a hospital that neither private insurance nor Medicare would reimburse. She mentions that a corporation, probably the one for which her deceased husband worked, has paid a small part of the bill through a private insurance policy. In reply to the doctor's question, the patient notes that Medicare will not cover the bill because she and her husband had not signed up under the appropriate section of Medicare regulations. Like many other seniors, she regrets that she had underestimated the need for insurance;[6] she hopes to correct this problem by registering for added Medicare coverage during the next fiscal year.

The dialogue about these very typical financial problems again remains rather asymmetric. The patient initiates consideration of such issues. The stimulus for her doing so seldom becomes completely clear, as one association seems to move to another. For instance, the discussion of medical expenses follows a description of weight loss, the need for a new wardrobe, and the constraints that inhibit her from buying new clothes. The doctor punctuates the patient's narrative with supportive filler and a few clarifying questions. Continuing such lengthy comments about the social context, the patient consumes a great deal of time and frequently takes the initiative in calling attention to these contextual issues. While the doctor seldom interrupts the contextual narrative, his style remains nondirective. He has a job to do, after all, and intervening in the social context does not seem to be part of it. As a result, the patient's contextual difficulties remain unengaged and ultimately marginal elements of the discourse.

Physical decline and approaching death. The patient knows her age and its implications. She wonders about the wisdom of decorating her new home when the duration of her ability to enjoy it may not be very long (lines 242–44). Further, after mentioning her difficulty in keeping up with birthdays in her family, she assumes one of her more pessimistic tones:

P: I don't care, I never go to the movies, and I very seldom watch
   movies on television even. So, . . . uh (word) oh, if I could
   only (word) with my own self
                              [
D: ((cough))
   [
P: and go like I used to. But what can you expect when I'm,   115
   when I'm, when you're almost, when you're gonna, going toward
   81?
D: Well, but you've gained some strength back, if you (words)
                              [
P: Oh, I've
   gained a lot. Now I'll tell you what I did yesterday.   120

The patient then proceeds to recount her accomplishments of the day before. She realizes, however, that her functional achievements have taken on a temporal quality, as physical decline runs its course.

A scenario of deterioration also appears in an extensive discussion about weight loss and its impact on the patient's wardrobe. The patient introduces this topic:

P: Well, . . ah, I took the
   car out, then I came home, and I said, "Well I've got (word),"
   so I ironed. I had three dresses, which I'll never wear because
   they're about that wide and I'm about that wide. If you want
   to see something, come here, look at me.   130
D: Uh huh.

P: Look, look at that.
D: Well, you've lost a little weight, huh?
P: A little? I've lost about twenty pounds.

After the doctor questions about her diet and performs a brief physical exam, the patient later returns to the impact of weight loss on her wardrobe. In this passage, the patient alludes to her continuing attempts to sew clothing for herself, a skill that the doctor seems to reinforce positively through his questions:

P: Well, my goodness, you should see the bra I got me, I can
   laugh at home. But I haven't had time to go spend by myself
   to go, and you know, with this moving deal. I
D: Do you do that sort of sewing yourself?　　　　　　　　　290
P: Well, I, no, not uh, not taking in undergarments like bras or
   anything like that.
D: How about the dress?
P: Oh, the dress, good Lord, I've made my clothes for years.
   And I'm heart broken because I had a couple of nice summer　　295
   dresses that I made myself, and, they're miles too big.
D: Yeah.
P: So I told R——, I said I'll go and get a dress at a time.

In short, the patient is experiencing distress about changes in her body and her image of it. As her body shrinks, she no longer is able to clothe it as she once could. The dresses that she has sewn for herself, which have served as trusted and well-loved companions, now have become strangers to her. Her "heart broken" feelings at the loss of such clothes blends with the effects of her various other losses.

The technical meaning of weight loss remains ambiguous, as the patient never questions the doctor explicitly about this, nor does he offer an explanation. Apparently the patient attributes some degree of mystery to her change in weight, as she claims that she is continuing to force herself to eat well. In his silence, the doctor must be considering a differential diagnosis to explain the weight loss. Some possibilities include insufficient nutrition, successful treatment of fluid accumulation associated with prior congestive heart failure, fluid excretion caused by medication (the patient is taking chlorothiazide, a diuretic), infection, cancer, and depression.

Although the doctor addresses the first three possibilities through discussion and the physical exam, he and the patient do not deal with the last three. In particular, the well-known association between cancer and weight loss remains absent from the conversation, even though this explanation probably has already occurred to a person as intelligent as this patient. Further, while the patient has experienced a series of losses and verbalizes a few depressed emotions, she does not mention the word "depression"; likewise, the doctor neither asks about depression nor lists it as a possible diagnosis, despite a well-recognized association between depression and weight loss in the elderly.[7]

Throughout this dialogue, then, impending death hovers in the background. When the patient obliquely refers to the end of her life, the doctor does not encourage exploration of her feelings or plans about dying. When she occasionally requests prognostication, he responds with reassurances that remain necessarily vague. In all this, the patient stoically observes her own physical deterioration, and the doctor listens supportively as she describes her attempts to transcend the sadnesses of physical aging.

Ideology and structure. Dialogue concerning the socioemotional context of aging predominates in this encounter. Typically, the patient initiates such topics; the doctor listens and enunciates brief verbal fillers that convey interest and support. Technical content occupies a relatively small part of the dialogue, involving brief discussions of weight loss (lines 133–73), ankle swelling (lines 202–14), blood pressure (lines 219–24), cardiac status (line 264), and medications (lines 322–36), as well as the patient-initiated accounts of visual symptoms that frame the encounter at its beginning and end. Such technical details give way in most instances to extensive conversation about the experiences of aging. These contextual issues concern mobility and autonomy of day-to-day function; loss of family, social support, home, and valued possessions; financial difficulties; and physical decline leading to impending death. Patient and doctor engage in warm and mutually respectful dialogue, as they both confront troubling issues that presumably remain beyond the reach of medicine.

Several ideologic assumptions thus become apparent. Coping with the vicissitudes of aging remains a matter of individual responsibility. This ideologic orientation emphasizing individual responsibility is quite consistent with the dominant ideologic pattern in United States society.[8] The rugged individualism that the patient describes, spunky and admirable as it is, has become difficult to maintain. As the patient doubtless values her independence, neither she nor the doctor raises the possibility of alternative arrangements that would enhance her physical and social support. Further, preserving her ability to execute those functions that are typical features of women's social role—homemaking, shopping, cooking, feeding, sewing, and so forth—remains a high priority. Despite a professional responsibility in social control, which involves the monitoring of unsafe behavior like reckless driving, the doctor passes the buck to an eye specialist who can examine the patient's visual capacity. He thus encourages her continuing efforts to maintain independent, though possibly unsafe, function. Further, in the face of impending death and physical deterioration, the dialogue reinforces the patient's stoical attempts to cope as an individual, with very little help from others.

In line with the theoretical approach developed in previous chapters, this encounter shows several structural elements that appear beneath the surface details of doctor-patient communication (figure 7.1). A number of contextual issues affect the patient, as they do many other elderly people. Such issues include social isolation; loss of home, possessions, family, and community; limited resources to preserve independent function; financial insecurity; and physical deterioration associated with the process of dying (A). Because of these contextual difficulties, the patient experiences loneliness, frustration, and anxiety, in addition to the physical troubles of heart disease, visual symptoms, and weight loss (B). In a visit with her doctor (C), she expresses concerns about contextual problems at great length. The doctor listens supportively, allowing the patient to describe her situation in detail and to emote about it (D). The doctor does not intervene to improve any of the contextual difficulties that the patient presents, nor apparently does she expect him to do so. Nevertheless, tensions in the discourse arise that reflect medicine's presumed inability to affect the contextual issues that most trouble the patient. Facing these tensions, the doctor cuts off a discussion about loss of home and community and deflects concerns about the impact of visual symptoms on independent function by referring the patient to another specialist (E). To manage the patient's contextual problems, the doctor reinforces her efforts to maintain independent function, despite some questions about the patient's ability to drive safely. Through supportive listening, he also encourages her efforts to coordinate her own social support network, her grieving process following the loss of a home and community, her plan to reduce financial insecurity by registering for Medicare insurance coverage, and her nutritional efforts to resist physical deterioration. In these ways, the discourse maintains ideologic assumptions that value individualism and stoical attempts to cope with adversity. Critical exploration of alternative arrangements to enhance her social support does not occur (F). After the medical encounter, the patient returns to the same contextual problems that trouble her, consenting to social conditions that confront the elderly in this society.

That such structural features should characterize an encounter like this one becomes all the more disconcerting, since the communication seems so admirable. At an advanced age, the patient has retained a keen intellect and takes initiative to lead her life with independence and dignity. She shows no hesitation in voicing whatever questions and emotions seem pertinent. Likewise, the doctor manifests patience and compassion, as he encourages a wide-ranging discussion of socioemotional concerns that extend far beyond the technical details of the patient's

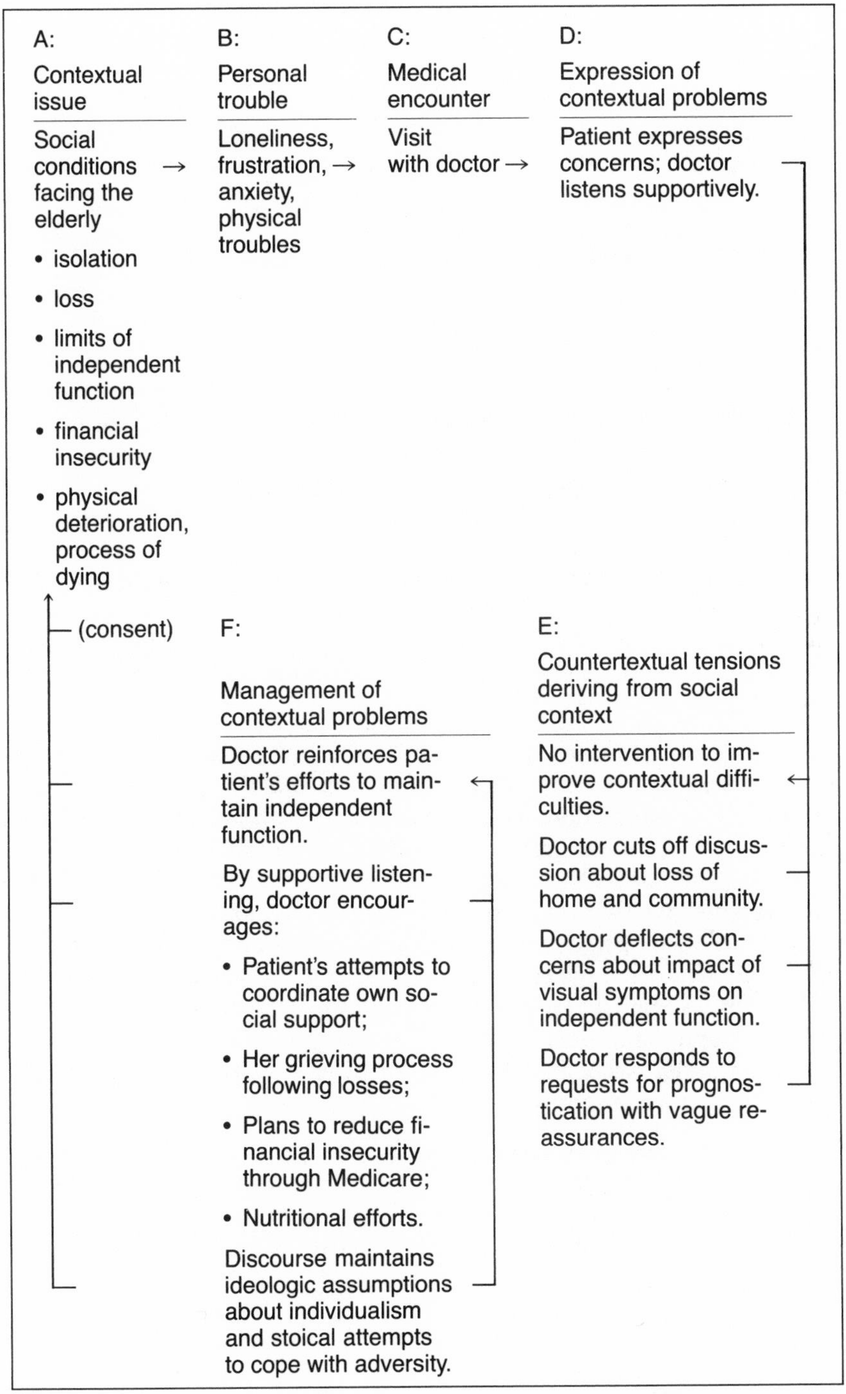

A: Contextual issue	B: Personal trouble	C: Medical encounter	D: Expression of contextual problems
Social conditions facing the elderly → • isolation • loss • limits of independent function • financial insecurity • physical deterioration, process of dying	Loneliness, frustration, → anxiety, physical troubles	Visit with doctor →	Patient expresses concerns; doctor listens supportively.

— (consent)

F: Management of contextual problems	E: Countertextual tensions deriving from social context
Doctor reinforces patient's efforts to maintain independent function. By supportive listening, doctor encourages: • Patient's attempts to coordinate own social support; • Her grieving process following losses; • Plans to reduce financial insecurity through Medicare; • Nutritional efforts. Discourse maintains ideologic assumptions about individualism and stoical attempts to cope with adversity.	No intervention to improve contextual difficulties. Doctor cuts off discussion about loss of home and community. Doctor deflects concerns about impact of visual symptoms on independent function. Doctor responds to requests for prognostication with vague reassurances.

Figure 7.1

Structural elements of a medical encounter with an elderly woman trying to maintain independence in the face of physical decline physical disorders. Yet the discourse does nothing to improve the most troubling features of the patient's situation. To expect otherwise would require redefining much of what medicine aims to do.

ENCOUNTER 7B: DEPRESSION AND PHYSICAL ILLNESS

SUMMARY

Accompanied by his wife, a man comes to his doctor for a routine visit. His main complaints focus on hoarseness, a dry throat, and coughing up strange material. The doctor reviews the patient's medications, which include an antidepressant that the patient reports has helped him. The patient mentions pain in his groin, which he thinks reflects disease of an artery. When the patient gets undressed for a physical exam in another room, the doctor discusses the patient's depression with his wife. During and after the physical exam, the doctor talks about the throat symptoms with the patient and his wife, and he refers the patient to an ear, nose, and throat specialist.

Some pertinent information about the patient, doctor, and setting of the encounter comes from the questionnaires that the participants filled out after their interaction. The patient is a 69-year-old white male who lists his occupation as "retired." He reports a high school education, Protestant religious identification, and English ethnic background. He and his wife have two children, whose ages are 39 and 32. A 38-year-old white male who specializes in internal medicine and gastroenterology, the doctor states that his religious preference is Protestant and his ethnic background is English. He has known the patient for about one year. The patient's main diagnoses, the doctor believes, are "depressive reaction" and "arteriosclerosis obliterans." This encounter takes place near Boston, in a private practice setting.

A *"gob of matter."* In response to the doctor's opening question, the patient immediately calls attention to bothersome symptoms of the throat and upper airway. Exploration of these difficulties occupies a large portion of the encounter that follows. Here is part of the initial dialogue:

D: How are you feeling?
P: All right. So far hoarse.   5

* * *

P: Throat's bothering me.   12
D: How's it botherin' you, Mr. ——?
P: Dry.

* * *

P: About a month ago I cleared my throat and there was a gob
   of matter come up as big as half a dollar.   20
                                        [
D: Yeah.
WIFE: Looked like a piece of flesh.
P: Piece of flesh with, uh, gray matter and blood in it.

According to the patient, he has experienced hoarseness and a dry throat.
But the most worrisome event for both the patient and his wife involves
his coughing up an unusual and unpleasant substance. The metaphorical
language by which these two observers describe the expectorated material paints a foul and ominous picture.

It is not just the symptoms, however, that bother the patient and his
wife; it is also their diagnostic meaning. Hoarseness, coupled with such a
foreign-appearing substance from the throat or airway, has raised the
specter of a potentially life-threatening cause. Among the frightening
possibilities, one disease raises the most apprehension:

D: Yeah, did you? . . You know when —— saw you, did he look at
   your vocal cords and so forth.   25
P: He looked down there and he said . .
                        [
D: He pulled the tongue way out
   and really gagged you?
P: He looked down and said there was no cancer I think.
D: This has been of concern to you . . . I'm sure . . . cancer, is that   30
   right?
W: That's what he was thinking of.
P: Yeah, that's what I thought.
D: Are you taking any medication now?

Immediately after his clients graphically describe the gob of matter, the
doctor makes sure that the patient has received a thorough examination
by an ear, nose, and throat specialist who is capable of accurately performing the rather difficult evaluation of the throat and airway. The
patient then expresses his fear very directly, when he alludes to the
specialist's comment about cancer. Despite the specialist's apparent judgment that cancer is not present, uncertainty remains, as the patient
qualifies his account of the specialist's reassurance by adding the words,
"I think." After the doctor very briefly confirms that cancer indeed comprises a major concern for the patient, he cuts off this topic by asking
about medication.

Although the participants in this encounter do not again explicitly
discuss cancer and its frequent outcome, death, these issues hover at the

margins of the dialogue, never explored directly nor fully resolved. In some sense, the gob of matter then becomes a metaphor for larger concerns that comprise so much a part of living one's life at an advanced age. For instance, outside the patient's presence, as he prepares for the physical exam, his wife takes initiative in reiterating their mutual concern about the meaning of the gob of matter. In reply, the doctor raises the possibility of re-examination by a specialist and also expresses his own intention to examine the patient's throat:

W: Yeah. I wonder what that thing was that come out of his
    throat?   100
D: Probably . . sounds like a big chunk of mucus.
W: No, I don't think it was, was like flesh. 'Cause he called me
    to look at it.
                          [
D: Yeah, it could look
    like that.   105
P: Yeah. As big as a half a dollar.
D: Might be worthwhile to have him take another look at his throat
    you know.
                          [
W: Sprinkled with blood. Yeah,
    way down in here he said it was.   110
D: Have the ear, nose, and throat people look at his throat again?
    That won't, won't hurt. We'll go take a look at it.

Until this point, the doctor seems to rely on the patient's account of a prior negative specialty exam to assuage fears of cancer. Here, however, the patient's wife pushes farther, disagreeing with the doctor's hypothesis about mucus and implying that appearance of flesh, size as big as a large coin, and presence of blood all signify something worse; the unsaid something might well be cancer. Responding to the wife's initiative, the doctor begins to plan for another specialty referral.

This same cluster of symptoms returns to the dialogue after the doctor examines the patient and finds only a postnasal drip (line 132). Again, the doctor's attempts at reassurance prove not too successful. The doctor tries to provide a diagnosis of laryngitis but also discusses the need for another specialty evaluation:

D: Well, I think what we ought to do . . I think we ought to go back
    and take a look since you've been spitting up this stuff. But   150
    I think what you really had just is probably some laryngitis.
    Looks OK to me. I can't look way down with the light like he can.

In addition to laryngitis, the doctor then offers another benign diagnostic possibility, muscle spasms. In reply, the patient disagrees and again alludes indirectly to cancer and its relation to smoking, as he mentions a previously abnormal test, possibly a cytology exam. The patient also confirms that he has stopped smoking, a decision that the doctor reinforces positively:

D: This could also, just be muscle spasms which get tense and
    up tight at night but   160
        [
P: No I don't think it's been coming along from that,
    remember in the report you got from (words) for the dry throat.
D: Yeah, right.
P: I stopped smoking.
D: Yeah, you were wise to do that, but I think that you have   165
    nothing to lose by having him look again.

Toward the end of the encounter, the doctor extensively discusses the details of the follow-up referral to the specialist (lines 193–209, 218–24, and 238–40).

In short, these passages convey a picture of an aging couple very concerned about possible cancer and its implications for life expectancy. Through several maneuvers—an early cut-off that moves the dialogue from cancer to current medications, later attempts to offer less ominous diagnoses, and focusing on specialty referrals—the doctor directs the conversation away from the topics of aging, fatal illness, and death. In fact, the doctor embeds the entire discussion of aging per se within instructions about the physical exam:

D: Let's look here at your throat, if I can.
    How old are you?   125
P: I'll be 70 in December.
D: You that old really? Open real wide if you would. Say aah.
P: Aah.

As the patient, his wife, and the doctor direct their attention to technical details, the issues of aging and mortality drift to the margins of their conversation. A technical challenge of diagnosing the gob of matter thus concretizes and reifies broader concerns, including the physical deterioration of aging and the specter of approaching death.

Dragging and sagging. According to the diagnoses that the doctor lists in his questionnaire, the patient suffers from depression, a common problem for elderly people.[9] Despite the prominence that depression holds as the first diagnosis stated by the doctor, very little dialogue confronts the specifics of the patient's emotions. For instance, especially among men, depression frequently accompanies retirement from work, which for the patient presumably has begun within the past several years. In addition to work transitions, other losses can contribute to depression among the elderly. Further, the contextual problems of aging can exacerbate chronic depression, which if present may wax and wane over many years. Speculation about such precipitating causes, however, remains unsubstantiated in the present encounter, which deals mainly with technical questions of medication and the patient's response to it.

An initial reference to depression occurs early in the encounter, just as the doctor cuts off the discussion of cancer by asking about medication. In reply, the patient mentions amitriptyline (Elavil), an antidepressant drug that the doctor previously has prescribed, as well as penicillin, which a specialist has given him:

D: Are you taking any medication now?
P: Well, you gave me some little green pills, Elavil was it?   3
                                          [
D: Yeah, Elavil.
P: Elavil, yeah.
D: Yeah.
P: And —— gave me some, uh, penicillin pills.

The severity of depression then becomes clearer. Apparently, the patient had experienced not only sadness but also insomnia and diminished appetite—two of the so-called "vegetative signs" of serious depression. With the antidepressant medication, these problems have improved:

D: How about the green pill, uh, how how
                              [
P: What was that supposed to be?
D: That was for your nerves and your depression. You were really
    dragging and sagging last time I saw you.   5
P: They, they did the trick all right.
D: Did it help? Do you think it helped?
P: Of course it did.
D: Do you think it helped?
W: Yeah, I think so.   6
D: Yeah, yeah.
W: He used to go to bed a night and sleep; and that's something
    he wasn't doing.
D: You weren't eating, I suppose.
W: No. Oh, he's eating.   6
D: Now, yeah, the weight's come up.

All three participants here appear satisfied about the efficacy of a technologic approach to depression. No discussion occurs concerning the patient's emotional experience. Contextual sources of distress remain unexplored and thus become reified through the exclusive emphasis on pharmacologic treatment. It seems enough that the patient is sleeping better, gaining weight, and dragging and sagging not quite so much.

When the doctor then proceeds to ask a general question about how the patient has been feeling in other respects, a major functional deficit manifests itself, though only briefly. Apparently because of arteriosclerosis (the second diagnosis that the doctor cites in his questionnaire), the patient develops groin pain with limited exertion. His arterial insufficiency thus limits his ability to walk and to do household chores:

D: Otherwise how are you
   feeling, besides the throat?
P: I feel . . . not so bad, I got a little upset; I do get a pain
   once in a while down in here.
D: The groin.   70
P: That's my problem . . . on account of the artery.
D: Yeah. Right. Do you get it when you're resting or when
   you're walking around?
P: Walking and push . . when I push a lawn mower, something
   like that. I get it.   75
D: Yeah.
W: He has to sit down.
D: How long does it . . last when you sit down?
P: Well, when I feel it coming I can stop and in about three or
   four minutes all gone.   80
D: Well, that's pretty good.
   Let's take a look at you if I can Mr. ——.

Apparently, the doctor has decided to approach this problem conservatively, without surgery or medication. In describing his feelings about incapacity, the patient spares his words, as usual; he gets "a little upset," nothing more. Because rest for a few minutes relieves the pain, the doctor reassures him faintly before moving on to the physical exam. The patient thus bears his pain and functional limitation stoically, with minimal complaint.

In this part of the discourse, as well as elsewhere, the patient's wife figures prominently. She takes part actively in the dialogue, speaking about her husband's condition both in and outside his presence. The doctor turns to her frequently, asking her to confirm and to expand on the patient's comments. For instance, the doctor first asks the patient if he thinks the antidepressant medication helped but then requests the wife's confirmation (line 59 above). The patient himself gradually emerges as a rather passive character, who often defers to his wife while she speaks in his behalf.[10]

Within another brief and jovial discussion of the patient's weight, his wife mentions alcohol use. The doctor does not pick up on this cue but

instead cuts off the topic by asking about an administrative form needed
to schedule a new appointment:

D: Tell him I referred you, uh, let me see you in September if I
   can, Mr. ——. For a completer physical once a year sort
   of thing. Uh, just don't get too fat.   22
W: Heheh heh.
P: What was I the last time I saw you?
D: 154.
P: 154.
D: From 165.   23
W: Don't seem possible, all the whiskey going around.
D: It seems possible. Do you have your slip, the girls give you
   a slip?
P: Yes.
D: Uh, give this to them, they'll set you up.   23

When the wife mentions whiskey, it is already late in the encounter, and
the doctor is beginning to wind things down. Because he does not
respond at all, the elaboration required to understand the wife's rather
cryptic comment remains missing. From the phrase "all the whiskey
going around," chances seem at least fair that alcohol has become a
prominent part of the patient's and/or the wife's life experience. Although alcohol use is a correlate of depression among the elderly,[11] the
dialogue here marginalizes this problem, as the details of scheduling
follow-up appointments receive priority.

In short, depression assumes an evanescent quality in this encounter.
Contextual issues that precipitated or worsened the emotional difficulty
stay in the margins of the discourse, subject to speculation but not
confirmation. The doctor, the patient, and his wife take little initiative in
exploring the details of depression, except to note an apparent improvement that medication has achieved in the vegetative signs of insomnia
and reduced appetite. Although alcohol may contribute to the problem,
it attracts very tangential comment by the patient's wife before the doctor
changes the subject. Despite the doctor's listing depression as a major
diagnosis, the discourse excludes many elements of social context that, if
addressed, might prove pertinent. Meanwhile, the participants seem to
accept an assumption that depression comprises mainly a technical problem, amenable to a course of medication.

Ideology and structure. In contrast to Encounter 7A, the present encounter offers relatively scant information about the patient's contextual
experience as he ages. Perhaps because of the patient's laconic style, he
voices little commentary about what his life is like outside the medical
sphere. The patient and his wife fixate on some disconcerting throat and

airway symptoms. Such symptoms come to symbolize concerns about aging, fatal illness, and death. These larger issues then remain marginal, mentioned rarely and explored not at all. Further, the patient previously has retired from his work and has experienced a depressive reaction. What if any relation has existed between retirement and depression, what other losses may have occurred, and what contribution alcohol has made to this problem—the answers to these questions do not appear.

The encounter reinforces an ideology of coping with age, illness, mortality, and sadness through technical means and in relative isolation. Patient, wife, and doctor all value a specialist's further evaluation of frightening symptoms. The discourse does not encourage them to explore the specter of death that such symptoms convey. Similarly, the participants accept a reified, technical approach to emotional disturbance, relying solely on medication and leaving contextual concerns unstated. At no point in the conversation do they mention family, friends, or other sources of social support. Further, the limitations that the patient's arteriosclerosis imposes on his daily functional capacity are met with stoical acceptance.

Several structural elements become apparent in this encounter (figure 7.2). As in Encounter 7A, the principal contextual issue confronting this patient involves social conditions facing the elderly. These conditions include a functional incapacity to fulfill social responsibilities (such as yard maintenance), the impact of physical deterioration (including the perceived likelihood of serious illness portending death), loss of work identity associated with retirement, and isolation (A). Such issues lead to personal troubles involving depression and a deep concern about symptoms of the throat and airway that possibly are consistent with cancer (B). During the medical encounter (C), the patient and his wife discuss these symptoms on multiple occasions; their statements assume a partly metaphorical quality, reflecting larger questions about fatal disease, illness, and mortality. The doctor also elicits some brief comments about the patient's depression and about improvements noted with medication (D). Tensions related to contextual issues, however, arise at several points in the encounter. The doctor cuts off the patient's reference to cancer without discussing its emotional significance, the participants do not explore the problem of depression when the patient and his wife report some improvement, and the doctor changes the subject when the wife mentions alcohol use. Both in and outside the patient's presence, the doctor also holds side conversations with the wife, who seems to serve as an advocate or proxy for her husband (E). During the encounter, the doctor manages contextual problems associated with aging by emphasizing technical methods; these approaches include medication for depression and specialty referral for a symptom that might reflect fatal illness. Further, the doctor offers brief reassurances about depression and about pain

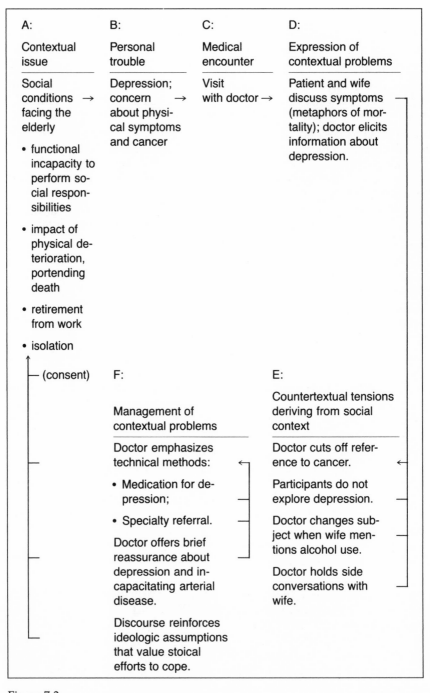

A:	B:	C:	D:
Contextual issue	Personal trouble	Medical encounter	Expression of contextual problems
Social conditions → facing the elderly	Depression; concern → about physical symptoms and cancer	Visit with doctor →	Patient and wife discuss symptoms (metaphors of mortality); doctor elicits information about depression.
• functional incapacity to perform social responsibilities			
• impact of physical deterioration, portending death			
• retirement from work			
• isolation			
— (consent)	F:		E:
	Management of contextual problems		Countertextual tensions deriving from social context
	Doctor emphasizes technical methods: ←		Doctor cuts off reference to cancer. ←
	• Medication for depression;		Participants do not explore depression.
	• Specialty referral.		Doctor changes subject when wife mentions alcohol use.
	Doctor offers brief reassurance about depression and incapacitating arterial disease.		Doctor holds side conversations with wife.
	Discourse reinforces ideologic assumptions that value stoical efforts to cope.		

Figure 7.2
Structural elements of a medical encounter with a retired man suffering from arterial disease, throat and airway symptoms, and depression

from incapacitating arterial disease. The discourse reinforces ideologic assumptions that value stoical efforts to cope with physical and emotional problems, through technical means and with little social support (F). After the encounter, the patient and his wife return to the same contextual conditions to which they previously have consented.

This encounter differs in several ways from the last one. Here the patient's terseness contrasts with the first patient's loquaciousness concerning contextual detail. In the second interaction, the patient complains little, if at all, as the doctor must elicit information more actively. Specific contextual elements also vary. For the first patient, difficulties of independence and loss figure more prominently, and the specifics involve activities centering on a woman's relation to home, family, and friends. In the second, contextual elements pertain to a man's retirement and his subsequent incapacity to perform day-to-day responsibilities in such areas as yard maintenance. Yet, such differences in style and substance between the two encounters do not diminish the similarities of structure that emerge. Contextual conditions of aging impinge on the participants in both encounters, creating difficulties that their discourse does not, and perhaps under present circumstances cannot, transcend.

ENCOUNTER 7C: DEATH OF A SPOUSE

SUMMARY

A man comes to his doctor for a routine semiannual appointment. During a short encounter, the patient reports that he is feeling good and has no problems. Doctor and patient review two psychotropic medications and the status of the patient's diabetes mellitus. They also discuss the patient's recent trip to Florida and his son's work activities but do not mention the patient's recent retirement or the death of his spouse.

In the questionnaires completed after the visit, patient and doctor provide some helpful information. The patient is a 66-year-old white male, who lists his occupation as "retired" and his marital status as "widowed." A high school graduate who also has taken some courses in college, the patient reports that his religious preference is Protestant and that his ethnic background is English. The doctor is the same one as in the last encounter;[12] to review, he is 38 years old, specializes in internal medicine and gastroenterology, and expresses a Protestant religious preference and an English ethnic background. Practicing in a Boston suburb, the doctor has known the patient for about three years and gives the following diagnostic impressions of the patient: "mature onset diabetes mellitus" and "mild depression secondary to death of wife from cancer."

An absence of problems. Why did the patient come? In his question-naire, the patient states that the reason for the visit is a routine, "semi-annual visit." During the encounter, which is distinguished from all others considered so far by its brevity, the patient indeed mentions no specific physical or psychosocial difficulties. As the encounter begins, in response to the doctor's general questions, the patient clearly says that, as far as problems are concerned, he experiences none. The doctor recon-firms this lack through sequential questioning:

D: How are you feeling?
P: Good, thank you.
D: Are you?
P: Yes.
D: No problems?
P: No.

The doctor's confirmatory questions seem a bit odd, unless he were expecting problems to be present. And well he might, based on changes that he knows have occurred in the patient's life.

Although the recorded dialogue does not at any time mention con-textual issues affecting this aging patient, information from the patient's and doctor's questionnaires indicates that at least two major life transi-tions have taken place. Since the patient is 66 years old and states his occupation as "retired," retirement from work likely has occurred in the not-too-distant past. Further, as the doctor notes in his diagnostic im-pression, the patient has become depressed since the recent death of his wife from cancer. Such transitions comprise substantial sources of stress. Yet in the discourse of this medical encounter, the contextual issues of retirement and loss of spouse remain conspicuously absent. An image of stoical and uncomplaining acceptance then emerges. If the patient en-counters difficulties with major life transitions, he does not discuss them openly. Nor does he give voice to sadness surrounding any losses that he has experienced.

Psychotropic medications and the achievement of normalcy. The lack of verbalized problems takes on a certain irony, when seen in light of the psychotropic medications that the patient is taking at the doctor's instruc-tion. These drugs include two pills, one of which is thioridazine (Mella-ril), a major tranquilizer used mainly for psychosis and sometimes in depression when a psychotic component presents itself. Although the other pill's name escapes mention, based on its description it probably is amitriptyline (Elavil), an antidepressant.

As the encounter begins, just after the patient denies active problems, the doctor reviews his medications and inquires about his "nerves":

D: What are you taking
  for medication now, Mr. ——?

P: Ah, Mellaril, Mellaril, those little green pills,
                [
D: Yeah
P: Doctor, and then the, uh, the large . . . white and blue pill.   25
D: The (word).
P: Yes, yeah.
D: How much, how much do you
       [
P: One a day. One of each a day
               [
D: How much of Mellaril—one of each, huh?   30
P: I find that the, uh, Mellaril, if that's the name of it, Doctor,
       [
D: yeah, uh mm
P: they make me a little bit loggy, so I just take one before I
    go to bed and it, uh, has me pretty well, you know
   [
D: Yeah. How're your nerves?   35
P: Well, they're (words), yeah, yeah. Uh, I
   [
D: (words) huh? How's the
    eyes doin'?

In this dialogue, several points become clear. The patient generally has
complied with his doctor's recommendations about these powerful psychotropic medications. However, he has experienced an uncomfortable
degree of sedation because of the Mellaril, a common side effect.[13] For this
reason, he has reduced the dose. On the other hand, he here expresses no
desire to terminate either the tranquilizer or the antidepressant. Further,
when the doctor asks the first direct question about "nerves," the patient
responds with a brief (and largely inaudible) account of psychologic
status. Then, when he asks about the patient's eyes, the doctor for the
moment cuts off the quick consideration of emotional life and moves to
other medical problems.

    In the midst of the physical exam, as he listens to the patient's lungs,
the doctor resumes the prior discussion of psychotropic medications, and
the patient responds by expressing a self-image of normalcy. The doctor
reinforces this self-image by brief conversational filler and then negotiates
with the patient about adjustments in one of these medications, before he
turns quickly to another technical observation concerning blood sugar:

D: Now breathe, breathe. In, breathe out, in. Take a real
    deep breath. OK. OK. OK. Uh, I think what you could do. Take   65
    your shirt off, but you could just take the Mellaril when you
    think you need it.
      [

P:　　　　Sure.

D: Don't take it on a regular basis. You know when you think you feel
off (words) OK.
[

P: At night time. See, I'm a (word) normal man, I don't
normally, nothing normally bothers me.
[

D: Yeah, right.

P: I could take one of those more or less
[

D: just as needed
　　　[

P:　　　　once in a while.

D: No, don't, don't bother during the day.

P: Oh, I see, I really don't need to, Doctor
　　　[　　　　　　　　　　[

D:　　　OK, yeah, now.　　　I'm with you there.
As I think the less we have you on the better.

P: Yeah, I'd rather not.
[

D: Your blood sugar is doin' fine.

Here the patient makes a claim about his emotional stability. Since "nothing normally bothers" him, he as a "normal" man usually would not need
medications like Mellaril. His comment about normalcy implies that his
present condition is abnormal in some way. Presumably, the patient is
alluding to his current emotional disturbance. In this as in all other parts
of the discourse, however, the contextual issues impinging on this patient remain absent, even though depression stemming from the wife's
death figures as one of the doctor's major diagnoses.

The positioning and emphasis of this discussion about psychotropic
medication do not provide much opportunity for exploring contextual
matters. Just after he asks the patient to take off his shirt within the
physical exam, the doctor suddenly returns to this topic. Further, the
doctor's advice here focuses exclusively on medication adjustments and
again cuts off the topic of emotional distress through the reassuring
comment about blood sugar. These features of the discourse serve to
marginalize the contextual issues that have proven most troubling for
this patient. Notwithstanding his claim to normalcy, the patient plans to
continue antidepressant medication regularly and also a major tranquilizer "once in a while." Medical discourse here lends itself to such
technical and reified interventions, while the social context remains absent.

Just before the encounter concludes, the doctor again returns to the theme of psychotropic medication and introduces an image of control. As he reviews the patient's prescriptions, he expresses satisfaction about the medications' impact:

D: Do you need new prescriptions, by the way?
P: No, I just had them both filled out.
D: Okay.
P: By the way, I did drop it down. They were giving me a
   hundred of the Mellaril, the little green pill   95
   [
D: Yeah, sure.
   [
P: And that would last me three months.
      [
D: Sure, I get fifty at a whack. I think as long as that's
   holding it, you look good and you say you feel good, so
P: Yeah, thank God.   100

Here both parties talk around the psychologic problem without mentioning specifics other than medication. By expressing hope that the concrete, technical intervention provided by medication will continue to "hold" the problem, the discourse values technical control of emotional reactions, in the face of stressful life transitions associated with aging. As doctor and patient negotiate about drug dosages, they leave these contextual issues in the margins of their talk.

Leisure and family. While much of this encounter focuses on the technical realm, a very brief portion of the dialogue deals directly with nontechnical matters. These passages mention the patient's recent vacation and his son's activities. Here, patient and doctor make the only attempts in the entire encounter to discuss the social context. Yet, in neither instance does the patient elaborate beyond a few short remarks, nor does the doctor pursue further details.

Just as the physical exam begins, the patient mentions a Florida vacation, which proved none too pleasant:

P: I came back two weeks ago today, I was in Miami. It was too hot,
   it was too late to go down there.   50
D: Yeah. I can't go anywhere for some sunshine.
P: Yeah, oh, I chase it (words) believe me.
D: I tell ya, I love the sun.

The patient does not indicate why he went to Florida and what kind of experience he had, other than facing excessive heat. The doctor pursues this topic only to emphasize his own craving for sunshine and the constraints that keep him from satisfying this need.[14]

Next, when the doctor initiates a brief discussion of the patient's son, the conversation focuses on the son's problems at work:

D: Is your boy out this way now?
P: Oh, yeah, he's,   yeah
   [[
D: You said he was comin' back
P: But he just, while I was away he went out to Detroit and had
   to fire a manager he hired, which was a kick in the fanny.
   So now, he's back in Detroit trying to find another man.
D: So he's, he's stationed here with, uh with (words)
                      [
P: oh, yeah, yeah, yeah.
D: Your pressure's good, 110 over 70.

That the son's job proves the main topic of interest for the patient reveals the patient's concern with work and its challenges, and he empathizes with his son's current occupational difficulties. Again, the degree to which the patient misses such challenges in work since his retirement receives no attention in the discourse. Further, the patient omits discussing any other aspects of his relationship with his son, including the degree to which the son serves as part of his own social support network.

A return to the technical again cuts off this quick dialogue about social context. Just as the patient confirms that his son continues to be "stationed" locally, the doctor mentions a favorable blood pressure reading. At no other time do they return to the contextual situation. Instead, the conversation stays grounded in the technical details of medications and additional brief references to the patient's satisfactory blood sugar readings (lines 82–86 and 104–10). In this way, the discourse again marginalizes the contextual issues facing this patient. During this encounter, social context thus devolves into stoical silence and medicine's technical maneuvers.

Ideology and structure. Certain similarities become apparent between these past two encounters. That the same doctor is involved, of course, engenders some of the likeness in discourse. Further, the two patients report similar ethnic backgrounds, although their different use of language leads one to suspect that the patient in Encounter 7B holds a more working-class background than the present patient. They both have retired during the past few years. The patients come across as men of few words, who initiate little if any discussion of the contextual issues that they are facing. Further, they face their troubles with a stoicism that leaves contextual problems for the most part absent from the dialogue. This absence becomes all the more striking, given that both patients suffer from depression and use substantial doses of psychotropic medications.

While the contextual issues affecting the present patient differ somewhat from those in the previous encounter (mainly concerning the loss of a spouse), the discourse manifests largely similar ideologic content. In the face of stressful life transitions associated with aging, stoical acceptance proves the most appropriate response. When the emotional reaction to such transitions becomes too difficult, the technical interventions that medicine offers, especially mood-altering medication, become useful options in re-achieving control. A vision of normalcy diminishes the degree to which personal problems are acknowledged or discussed. As a result, an individual copes with these problems mainly in isolation, with little apparent social support.

Some structural elements of the encounter appear as follows (figure 7.3). Again, social conditions facing the elderly comprise the chief contextual issue that affects this patient. Specifically, he has lost his wife through death and his career through retirement. Because his physical problems are limited to mild diabetes mellitus, his health has not deteriorated. On the other hand, he apparently leads his life in relative isolation, as he mentions only a son with whom he maintains regular contact (A). He suffers from depression, a personal trouble that his doctor attributes to the wife's death (B). In the medical visit (C), the patient denies the presence of any problems whatsoever. Instead, he alludes to his own normalcy, as he discusses adjustment of the psychotropic medications that he is taking (D). The absence of explicit reference to contextual issues, including retirement or the death of a spouse, introduces tensions in the discourse. Such tensions become evident as the doctor cuts off brief discussions of "nerves," the patient's feelings about medication dosage, and the patient's son. In each instance, the cut-off comprises a return to a technical matter—the patient's eyes, blood sugar, and blood pressure (E). Medical management mainly involves a continuation of psychotropic medications with an adjusted dosing schedule. In additional technical comments, the doctor also offers reassurance about diabetes mellitus. Partly through the absence of attention to social context, the discourse reinforces an ideology of stoicism and individual coping with the transitions of the aging process (F). With the aid of medication, the patient then continues to accept the contextual conditions that he faces.

In short, this patient and his doctor keep the social context mainly in the margins of their discourse. The death of a spouse and retirement comprise at least two transitions with which the patient must cope. According to the doctor's diagnoses, the patient has endured a rocky emotional response. Yet these contextual details remain virtually absent. In fact, one could not know their existence without additional information supplied in the questionnaires. Medicine's technical capabilities help doctor and patient exclude such details from their talk, and it is not clear that either party would have it otherwise.

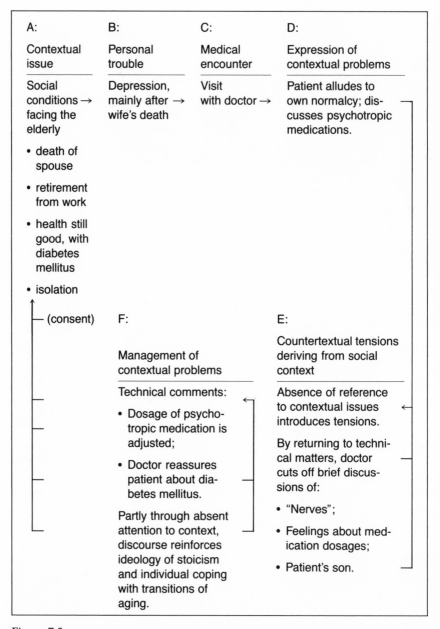

Figure 7.3
Structural elements of a medical encounter with a retired man who has diabetes mellitus and depression associated with the recent death of his spouse

THE DISCOURSE OF AGING

Three aging patients briefly enter and exit the medical realm. To varying degrees they voice the social issues that face them and many others as our society ages. In Encounter 7A, a feisty 80-year-old woman struggles to preserve independence in the face of physical decline, loss of home and community, and financial problems. As she expounds on her troubles, her doctor listens supportively, but the discourse does not lead to intervention or change in the contextual problems that trouble the patient. A retired man and his wife in Encounter 7B express concern about throat and airway symptoms that assume a metaphorical quality, representing the threat of fatal illness and death. Steering clear of exploration of contextual difficulties, the doctor adopts a technical approach to the specialty evaluation of these symptoms and the pharmacologic treatment of depression. The patient in Encounter 7C is passing through stressful life transitions, involving retirement from work and the death of a spouse, that typify the aging process. Yet the dialogue between patient and doctor leaves these issues entirely unsaid, as it focuses on technical adjustments to psychotropic medications.

All three encounters paint a picture of stoicism, acceptance, individualism, and isolation. The first patient tries to socialize and does not hesitate to talk with her physician about her problems. As the physical and social losses of aging take their toll, her cheerful attempts to maintain autonomy become more difficult, but she perseveres on her own. The last two patients scarcely refer to the contextual issues that they are confronting, as they obtain the psychotropic medication that their doctor offers. For these patients, medical discourse does not provide a forum for contextual discussion. Ideologic assumptions that pattern the life experience of elderly people receive no critical attention here. This silence implies that the patients will continue to walk as stoical individuals through the often troubled world of advanced age.[15]

A so-called "geriatrics revolution" currently confronts the practice of medicine in industrialized societies. As demographic patterns shift, the social issues exemplified in these three encounters will become more commonplace. Whether and in what ways medicine will deal with such contextual difficulties of aging then becomes a puzzle. Without doubt, the policy challenges raised by an aging society are beginning to attract some response. To what extent a critical vision will extend to the discourse of the medical encounter remains unclear. The answer depends partly on clarification of the practitioner's role, especially the degree to which intervention in the social context comes to be seen as appropriate and desirable. Medicalization of social problems, as noted previously, has its down side. How doctors should involve themselves in elderly patients' contextual difficulties therefore takes on a complexity (to be considered in the last chapter). Meanwhile, doctors and patients continue to face the context of aging, often indirectly, tensely, or silently.

CHAPTER 8

SELF-DESTRUCTIVE BEHAVIOR AND OTHER VICES

In medicine of the late twentieth century, prevention has become a guiding principle. The infections that once ravaged the populations of preindustrial societies now exert a relatively minor impact, although they persist in force within economically underdeveloped countries. Even in new infectious epidemics like acquired immunodeficiency syndrome (AIDS), the most devastating effects emerge in underdeveloped nations, and cogent medical approaches involve prevention of behaviors like drug abuse and certain sexual activities.[1] Because with economic development the principal health problems affecting populations shift to the chronic diseases, preventing such diseases becomes a challenge for the fields of medicine and public health. In the winds of health policy, the banners of prevention and health promotion then wave conspicuously.[2]

Self-destructive behavior causes trouble for those who espouse the lofty goals of prevention. One perverse irony of the human condition involves the pleasure that some people derive from activities that, over a long period of time, may destroy health and happiness. An example involves use of such substances as alcohol, tobacco, and a variety of mood-altering drugs. Some sexual activities also may lead to perceived adverse effects, through sexually transmitted diseases, instability of family and occupational roles, or interference with standards of common decency. These sad outcomes, of course, affect the person who indulges himself or herself in such ways. Even more disconcerting, such behaviors may spill over onto family, friends, professionals, and the community at large, thus creating widespread feelings of uneasiness and resentment.

Further, taking care of people who suffer physically and emotionally from self-destructive behavior costs a great deal of money.³ In societies like ours, this latter sin becomes the most unforgivable.

Medical encounters frequently are occasions for dealing with, or at least conversing about, self-destructive behavior, and the following three interactions show how this happens. These sessions illustrate some variable ways in which professionals and clients approach activities that one or both parties see as damaging or even reprehensible. Because we recorded these interactions just before the AIDS era began, I expect that sampling done now would find an even deeper medical involvement in the processing of self-destruction. As in prior chapters, by looking for an underlying structure that may not be apparent from surface details, I emphasize elements of ideology and social control that present themselves as doctors and patients deal with self-destructive tendencies. While supporting the worthy purpose of prevention, I also point out, influenced especially by Foucault, some ambiguities of professional surveillance in the arenas of substance use and sexuality. Further, I explore the rather subtle ways that medical discourse reproduces dominant ideologies of society, while leaving intact important components of the social context that impede efforts to modify self-destructive behavior in more lasting and fundamental directions.⁴

ENCOUNTER 8A: SMOKING, DRINKING, AND SEX (PART 1)

SUMMARY

A man goes to his doctor for a premarital blood test. The doctor questions him closely about his drinking problem, his smoking, his job as a netmaker for fishermen, his family, and his plans for married life. Then the doctor encourages attendance at Alcoholics Anonymous and orders tests of liver function, in addition to the premarital blood test that the patient requested.⁵

From the questionnaires that patient and doctor completed after their interaction was recorded, the following information gives the encounter some perspective. The patient is a 39-year-old white Irish Catholic netmaker who has a high school education. He is about to be married. The doctor is a 47-year-old white male, who denies a religious preference and reports his ethnic background as Russian. He states that his area of specialization is general internal medicine. Patient and doctor have known each other about nine months. According to the doctor, the patient's diagnoses are "ethanolism [alcoholism] under control" and "excess cigarettes with asthmatic bronchitis." The interaction occurs in a private suburban practice outside Boston.

Inquisition. Apparently, the purpose of this visit, from the patient's point of view, is to obtain a blood test for syphilis, so that he can get a marriage license. At the outset, however, the doctor asserts that the blood test is not the only item on the agenda:

D: Now, you got the Hinton tests
   at the hospital.   15
     [
P: Right.
      [
D: So that that's all set . . .
   Your premarital slip is all signed.
P: Right.
D: I have to just examine you to make sure that you have   20
   no infectious diseases, which I'm sure you have not.
   I'm more interested in your liver. Now what has your
   situation been?

Instead of the premarital blood test, the doctor indeed is more interested in the patient's liver—and many other areas of the patient's life as well. What begins as a straightforward request for technical information required by the state becomes a wide-ranging inquiry into the patient's medical status, social relations, and personal habits. Eventually, a variety of moral judgments issue forth, all under the rubric of medical advice.

Aside from its content, the form of the encounter is noteworthy. The doctor dominates the interaction through a long series of questions. After the patient responds, apparently as honestly as possible, the doctor then asks more questions. The encounter takes on a staccato quality, largely because of the doctor's interrogatory behavior. A format of repetitive questioning, although to some extent required by medical history taking, establishes the doctor's dominance in the interaction with this working-class patient.[6]

This style distorts a lengthy parenthetical discussion about work, fatigue, and lobstering. An excerpt gives the flavor of this extended dialogue, which begins with the doctor's question about the patient's "situation":

D: Now what has your
   situation been?
     [
P: I . . .
D: How've you been?   25
     [
P: feel a little . . .
D: You look great
            [
P: tired.

D: Why? How much've you been working?
P: Not bad at all, running around the past week,
    fooling around, lobstering
                    [
D: What did you say?
P: Lobster pots.
D: What are lobster pots?
P: For catching lobsters.
D: What's that got to do with you?
P: I'm tired.
                    ((more details about lobstering))
D: No, I mean why are you allowed to and I'm not
    allowed to
    [
P: You're allowed to. You just have to
    file the permit.
                    ((more details about lobstering))
D: My Gosh! . . . My Gosh! I didn't realize that. Where
    are your pots?
                    ((more details about lobstering))

This part of the dialogue opens with the doctor's general questions about
the patient's status (lines 22–25). As the doctor immediately answers his
own question with a comment about how well the patient looks, the
patient simultaneously replies with the only symptom that he reports
during the entire encounter: he is "tired." The doctor hears this complaint twice in the lobstering conversation (lines 28, 37), and he briefly
asks about the patient's work (line 29), but he does not focus on the
patient's fatigue. Instead, the inquiry about the equipment, legalities,
timing, and location of lobstering continues. Even if the patient wished to
exert himself about his fatigue, it would be difficult to interrupt the flow
of interaction.

Work, family, and substance use. That the patient is tired, however,
does not escape the doctor entirely. The doctor connects fatigue to two
issues, both of which he considers later in the encounter: work and
family. Regarding work, the doctor asks about the patient's energy and
strength. When the patient responds, now for the third time, that he is
tired, the doctor immediately does some reality testing about the patient's work life and then congratulates the client for occupational reliability:

D: How's, uh, your general energy and strength?
P: I'm tired but
    [

D: but are you able to put out and work
                              [
P: Oh, yeah.   175
   [
D: and work a regular day?
P: Oh, yeah.
D: Wonderful.

Here the doctor reinforces his client's economic role and appears to take fatigue less seriously than if it interfered with productive labor.
    In addition to professional surveillance of the patient's role in economic production, the doctor also inquires about family life. For instance, the doctor asks about the patient's sisters and father, particularly regarding changes that will occur after the patient's upcoming marriage. The dialogue reveals some problematic family dynamics:

D: Oh! I didn't know that . . . And how's —— [fiancée]?
P: Good. Now.   80
D: And how are your sisters?
P: They're just . . . well . . . I don't get along with them . . .
D: Maybe you don't, but . . .
P: After next week it's all over.
D: Why?   85
P: I get married.
D: And then?
        [
P: Sunday
          [
D: And then?
P: Well, I'll move.   90
D: Where?
P: Where? Where'm I going to live? ——, maybe.
D: And where do your sisters? . . .
P: Oh, they live at home.
D: Why do you think they'll then get off your back?   95
P: I dunno . . . I think . . . I'll just do my work.
D: What about your father?
P: Well, he's . . . good, I guess.
D: Who's going to live with him?
P: No one.   100
D: Going to live alone.
P: Right.
D: OK, fine. So then . . . who's going to watch over him?
P: Well . . . well, I guess my sisters . . . probably. I imagine
   I will . . . 'bout the usual.   105

D: You'll share it.
P: Yeah.
D: Instead of you doing it all.
P: Right.

In this passage, the doctor leads off by asking about the patient's fiancée. With characteristic understatement, the patient replies, "Good. Now." He thus implies that she was not good previously but provides no further details. Then, in response to the doctor's questions, the patient recounts conflict with his sisters, uncertainty about his own future living arrangements after marriage, and lack of clarity about caretaking responsibilities for his father. Perhaps because of concern about the patient's stress, the doctor strongly encourages division of labor between the patient and his sisters.

Throughout the encounter, marriage and family become intertwined with fatigue, alcohol use, liver disease, and smoking. The doctor himself juxtaposes cigarettes, fatigue, and marriage:

D: And your cigarettes . . . And you're tired . . . You're getting   ₁
   married next . . . Sunday?

At the encounter's beginning, as noted earlier, the doctor indicates that he is more interested in the patient's liver than in the medical requirements of the marriage license. Just before the session ends, the doctor connects bronchitis, marriage, and the liver:

D: Open your mouth. Say ah.
P: Ah.
D: Good. Now don't smoke that much. You're   ₂
                      [
P: I won't.
D: You're all loaded with junk and wheezes. You're doing
   great. I signed the slip. You're all set for your
   wedding. Uh, your liver's down to normal.
P: Whew!   ₂
D: Yeah, heh heh. We're starting anew, just anew.

Although the patient is "doing great," the doctor nonetheless wants additional liver tests and notes that, because of heavy smoking:

D: you've got your lungs
   shot. It's, it's, I've never heard it this bad.   ₂

On the other hand, apparently because of the patient's upcoming wedding, the doctor advises a reduction in smoking rather than a complete stop:

D: I'm not saying stop smoking, 'cause I can't, uh,
     because right now you're in a tense situation, but, uh,
     cut it down, please. Good luck. Best wishes.

P: Thank you, doctor.
D: Have a happy life.   280
    [
P: Uh huh.
    [
D: Give my best to —— [fiancée].

The patient thus receives mixed messages about self-destructive habits and family, voiced with the authority of scientific medicine.

Seeking to bring the patient's behavior under tighter control, the doctor attaches symbolic values to the problems of smoking and alcohol. Smoking is "the 32 dollar question." When the patient gives a therapeutically incorrect answer, the doctor advises a straightforward act of will:

D: OK. Uh, the 32 dollar question: How's your cigarettes?   110
P: Bad.
D: How bad?
P: . . . I haven't cut down. Well, I mean, I started cutting
   down, but I went back up again.
D: Why?   115
P: I don't know. I have a cigarette in my mouth
   (words).
D: Whenever you find that happening, put the cigarette out.

For a person hooked on cigarettes, such willpower may prove less than fully successful; the feasibility of this approach, however, does not receive further attention.

Without specific suggestions about smoking cessation, the doctor moves on to alcohol, "the 64 dollar question," which draws greater emphasis. The patient also gives a wrong answer to this question. At his prenuptial stag party, the patient has broken the vow of abstinence required by Alcoholics Anonymous (AA). AA claims that, for an alcoholic, any drink creates a risk of full-scale re-addiction. The doctor affirms this principle:

D: And then the 64 dollar question, of course, is how's the
   booze?   120
P: I'll tell you, I've had a few beers, that's all.
D: Now . . .
P: At the stag party
   [
D: Now . . .
P: I swear   125
   [
D: You're skating on thin ice.

In minute detail, the doctor then questions the patient about alcohol consumption before, during, and after the stag party:

P: I went to that
   stag party last night; I didn't have a drink.
D: Really? For you
          [
P: Right.   1
          [
D: Terrific.
P: Right.
D: How many guys?
P: Um . . . I have no idea . . . Biggest one I've seen. ((chuckles))
                                    * * *
D: You didn't, you had how much?
P: ((chuckles)) Cold Duck and beer
          [
D: and no beer?   1
P: No. I'll tell you I had a beer afterwards, though.
   I went to ——'s house afterwards, and I had one beer,
   and we split that. That's all.
D: Now, that's great. That is . . .

In this passage, the patient switches his story several times as the doctor
tries to pin him down. First, the patient says he drank only a few beers, at
the stag party. Then, in the midst of other details about the party that the
doctor elicits, the patient mentions that he had Cold Duck and beer.
When the doctor perhaps mishears this statement and asks, "and no
beer?" the patient now replies, "No," but then confesses to one beer at a
friend's house after the party. The doctor's interrogatory format, at least
in this passage, becomes more understandable in light of the patient's
slipperiness.

Soon the patient makes it clear that he does not fully accept AA's
principle of complete abstinence. Based on the pleasure that he takes in
the goings on at his stag party, the patient apparently enjoys drinking
quite a bit, and he also likes to be present at scenes where other people
drink. He questions whether a lower level of alcohol consumption would
prove acceptable. Yet he does not push very hard. When the doctor
expresses doubt about one's ability to hold the line, the patient makes a
rather radical promise, to which the doctor responds enthusiastically:

P: Now will that one beer bother me? I'll never go back
   on booze again.
       [
D: Look. It won't bother you if you can
   stay there, you know.
              [

P: I can stay there.
            [
D: The thing that   155
   bugs me, you said that the last time.
                        [
P: Yeah, well I'm . . .
   I'm a little smarter this time.
                        * * *

P: I'll go without it.   165
D: Huh?
P: I'll go without it. There won't even be beer in the,
   uh, refrigerator up there.
D: Just terrific! Just terrific! Just terrific!

Staying on the wagon, based on previous experience, may prove easier
said than done. Yet it cannot hurt for the patient to promise or for the
doctor to reinforce him. In this way, both parties acknowledge a standard
of ideal behavior, motivation to do better, and forgiveness for past foibles.

The patient's promise, however, is not enough. To prevent relapse, he
also needs social support. After mentioning again the patient's impending marriage, the doctor stresses the importance of continuing participation in AA, and the patient reveals his irregular attendance:

D: Shew! Have you gone to any AA at all?   185
P: Uh, just in the last three months, I missed the last
   three ones. I, uh, got reminded of your appointment
   today, and I remembered that I missed the one last
   week and, the last two weeks . . .

The doctor then outlines a rather comprehensive approach to the patient's alcoholism. Rather than relying on the patient's motivation, which
has proven spotty in the past, the doctor tries to orchestrate a support
network that will serve as an "alcoholic base." Specifically, he offers three
such supports: himself, the alcohol counselor, and AA as an organization:

D: Yes, I'd like to give you some sort of, uh, alcoholic
   base, uh, that is, when things get bad, you know you
   can always come here.
P: Right, right.
D: You know that. You know that —— [counselor] will kick   205
   your ass, and you know that you can always depend on me, too.
   And then you also know that you'll have the AA who are
   used to dealing with people like you. So that I think
   that it's very important, not that you'll ever use it,

but if you do   21|

    [
P: I would go to him. I'll tell you if I
goofed again. I . . .
D: But we need contingency plans.

"People like you," the doctor implies, need a great deal of surveillance to
stay away from booze. While he may not go as far as the alcohol counselor in "kicking your ass," the doctor states his willingness to be depended
upon. By coordinating a variety of resources, the doctor presumably can
assist the patient in controlling, if not kicking entirely, a troublesome
habit. In this way, doctor and patient presumably can cooperate in mini-
mizing the risk of further "goofs."

    Moral control and medical technique. Aside from such practicalities,
the discourse that follows also reveals a moral element. From Foucault's
perspective, professional surveillance seeks to enhance a patient's welfare, as a medical practitioner coordinates resources to help modify behavior. Along with professional surveillance, the subsequent dialogue
conveys an ideologic message that, when temptation beckons, self-
control is paramount. The image of control extends not only to the
physical impact of such activities as smoking and drinking, but also to
their moral implications. Although social supports are desirable, ultimately a person must resist decline through the force of will, and alone.
Final responsibility for a healthy life, physically and morally, rests with
the individual.

    Medically phrased moralism occurs at several points in the encounter,
but especially during the physical exam, when doctor and patient discuss
what to do when social pressures encourage a deterioration into bad
habits. The doctor paints a picture of personal fortitude in suppressing
one's inclination to indulge in booze, tobacco, or—now mentioned for
the first time—sex:

D: Deep breath . . . You hear that? Boy, your
lungs are loaded with uh wheezes . . . Boy, you're smoking
up a storm.
P: I did last night something awful. 'Cause everybody was
on my back about . . .   22(
D: Yeah, well when people get on your back, you can't go
to booze or cigarettes or . . or sex
                    [
P: Oh, no
                    [
D: you've got to
think of something where you can hang out by yourself   22!

and control
[

P: What are you gonna do when you're sitting
        up at the table and the guys go after you?
D: Then you have to . . . here, take a deep breath, a real
   deep breath, now, does this hurt at all?   230

The doctor's reason for bringing up sexuality remains mysterious, unless
he views sex as simply one other form of deviant and possibly self-
destructive behavior, along with smoking and drinking. Perhaps the
earlier discussion about a stag party raised the specter of sexual diversion,
since that is what traditionally happens at such gatherings. The patient
seems to begin a denial of sexual misconduct ("Oh, no," line 223), but the
doctor interrupts him with statement of ascetic philosophy: "you've got
to think of something where you can hang out by yourself and control."
Unsure about his ability to achieve such rectitude, the patient pushes
harder by asking what to do when others tempt him ("the guys go after
you"). The doctor then retreats into the physical exam but gives a physical
instruction that ironically answers the patient's question through a double meaning: "Then you have to . . . here, take a deep breath, a real deep
breath." This instruction conveys an image of a man alone, breathing
deeply to restrain himself from sensuous, self-destructive distraction.
    The doctor's concern about these issues, of course, is understandable.
The patient's habits apparently are turning him into a physical wreck.
Yet, while laden with value judgments, this encounter remains nearly
devoid of information concerning the patient's physical condition. The
doctor provides no details about the impact of alcohol on the liver or the
effect of smoking on the lungs. Physical observations remain brief and
uninformative, such as, "You hear that? Boy, your lungs are loaded with
uh wheezes . . . Boy, you're smoking up a storm" (lines 216–18), or
". . . you've got your lungs shot" (lines 274–75). In this interaction, the
symbolic aura of medicine gives credence to ideologic messages that aim
to control major facets of the patient's life experience. By such mechanisms the medicalization of self-destructive behavior takes place.
    Toward the end of the encounter, the doctor depicts himself as an
arbiter of good and presumably of evil. Here, just after commenting that
the patient's liver has returned to normal size and just before requesting
tests of liver function, he expresses a preference about when a return visit
should occur:

D: ——, if you do good, that's it. If you don't do
   good, I want to see you.
P: I won't.
D: Now I want to just . . . when was the last time we did a   260
   liver test on you?

Again, a double meaning appears. By "doing good," the doctor may refer to how well the patient feels symptomatically. Based on his immediate return to the liver and the liver's relation to alcohol intake, however, the doctor also probably is alluding to the patient's drinking behavior. Further, the term *doing good* conveys moral overtones. Bad behavior, in the sphere of alcohol use or other less clearly defined areas of life, warrants medical surveillance. If the patient does badly, the doctor wants to intervene.

Although such efforts in social control outweigh the technical content of this encounter, the doctor employs technical material at several points to cut off discussion of contextual issues. For instance, the doctor's question about smoking terminates, without resolution, a dialogue about problematic family relations:

D: Instead of you doing it all [caring for the patient's father].
P: Right.
D: OK. Uh, the 32 dollar question: How's your cigarettes?

Similarly, questions about appetite, energy, and strength cut off conversation about the stag party before the patient's forthcoming wedding and the social pressures that encourage alcohol intake:

P: I'll go without it. There won't even be beer in the,
   uh, refrigerator up there.
D: Just terrific! Just terrific! Just terrific! How's
   your appetite?
P: Same.
D: How's, uh, your general energy and strength?

In the same vein, the doctor's instructions about the physical exam interrupt the give and take concerning the patient's alcohol support network:

D: But we need contingency plans, and this is for, uh, sit
   up on here ((long pause)) and come on down here a minute,
   and let's poke a little and see. Let me listen to your
   heart first . . .

Further, as noted earlier, the doctor's instruction to take a deep breath terminates with a double meaning the discussion of what to do when "the guys go after you" (lines 227–30 above). While this doctor goes to great lengths in exploring the contextual factors that may worsen or improve the patient's self-destructive habits, he also uses technical cutoffs in returning to the somewhat surer terrain of the medical history and physical exam.

   Ideology and structure. To summarize, this encounter manifests ideologic assumptions that emerge in not particularly subtle ways. The practitioner dominates the discourse through an inquisitory style that extends to minute details of the patient's occupational life, leisure-time activities, family relations, and personal habits. Consistent with his working-class background, the patient asks very few questions himself and usually provides laconic responses to the doctor's numerous questions.[7] The doctor tries to assure that the patient's participation in work is continuing reliably, and he offers advice intended to produce smoother relationships with family members. Contextual problems regarding irregular work and family dynamics affect the patient. The conversation focuses intermittently on such contextual difficulties but ultimately marginalizes them by highlighting the patient's self-destructive actions as an individual problem.

In discussions of smoking and drinking, the doctor tries to reduce the patient's tendency toward self-destruction, partly by orchestrating an alcohol support network. Except in a brief reference to social pressures from male friends, the dialogue does not explore the connections between social context (for instance, work and family life) and alcohol. A support network that the doctor advocates aims toward professional surveillance of the patient's deviant behavior. The doctor also mentions the importance of impulse regulation. Through the medicalization of self-destruction, the discourse conveys an ideology that emphasizes moral rectitude and individual control.

By reinforcing such virtues, medical ideology here hails (to use Althusser's term)[8] the patient as a subject, who assumes concrete responsibilities in defined social roles. His self-destructive behaviors become important not just as they injure his body. Rather, these vices also threaten a web of relationships that depend on his performing reliably. The doctor's language hails the patient not only as a wheezing man with a liver swollen by alcohol, but also as a worker, a son, a brother, and a future husband. In all these roles, the patient's behaviors, especially those related to drinking, interfere with what he is expected to do. On behalf of medicine as a social institution, the doctor here speaks the language of ideologic reproduction, prevailing on the patient to march down a more straight and narrow path.

As already noted in chapter 3, several structural elements come to the surface (figure 3.3). The contextual issue facing this patient involves the patterning of a man's role expectations (A). To support himself and his family (thus earning the "means of subsistence"), the patient must hold a job steadily. In relations with family members, including his sisters, father, and wife-to-be, his performance should be more or less stable. Because the patient is a heavy drinker, his ability to meet these role expectations about work and the family is not straightforward. Actual or potential conflicts due to alcoholism then comprise a personal trouble that the patient experiences (B). In a medical visit (C), the doctor initiates detailed discussion and suggestions about alcohol; he also inquires and advises the patient about heavy smoking, work, family relations, and forthcoming marriage (D). At several points when tensions arise in the discussion of contextual issues, the doctor cuts off the dialogue and returns to technical matters of the medical history and physical exam; his technical comments prove brief and not too informative (E). In managing the patient's contextual difficulties, the doctor emphasizes participation in AA and tries to coordinate an alcohol support network. By his request for tests of liver function, he also advocates a technical maneuver pertinent to alcoholism. Regarding the patient's self-destructive behavior, the doctor conveys ideologic assumptions that support individual control and moral uprightness under medical surveillance. Such messages encourage stable function at work and in the family, as the patient consents to "doing good" (F).

In an encounter that confronts the difficult scenario of self-destruction, medical discourse manifests mainstream ideology and by doing so introduces an element of control to an out-of-control situation. Unsavory behaviors involving substances like tobacco and alcohol apparently bring a certain pleasure to this patient's life, fraught as it is with troublesome contextual issues. With an interrogatory style, the doctor enters the patient's social world and tries to rearrange it in a more orderly fashion. The doctor manifests a keen motivation to aid his patient to turn back from a road leading toward physical and moral degeneracy. There are no heroes or villains here. It is doubtful that the ideologic content of the discourse reaches conscious awareness. Such processes occur in a caring relationship, where the professional's concern for his client's well-being is beyond dispute.

ENCOUNTER 8B: SMOKING, DRINKING, AND SEX (PART 2)

SUMMARY

A man who is on vacation visits a doctor because of a cold. Answering a question about allergies, the patient mentions Antabuse (a medication that provokes an unpleasant physical reaction when taken with alcohol) and describes how he stopped drinking. After congratulating him for sobriety, the doctor diagnoses bronchitis, gives him a penicillin shot, and prescribes oral penicillin as well. In view of the patient's success in giving up alcohol, the doctor advises him *not* to stop smoking. The doctor also instructs him about physical activity during his vacation.

Some pertinent data about patient and doctor come from the questionnaires that they filled out after their interaction was recorded. The patient is a 52-year-old white man who works as a "setter" in a large industrial factory. He received a high school education, reports a Protestant religious preference, is married, and has three children, ages 27, 18, and 14. Regarding his ethnic background, he provides no information. A practitioner of general internal medicine and endocrinology, the doctor is a 43-year-old white male. He reports a Mormon religious preference and a "Danish Scottish English German" ethnic background. During this encounter, patient and doctor meet each other for the first time, in a private practice on Cape Cod. The doctor describes the patient's diagnoses as "bronchitis" and "alcoholism in remission."

Instrumentalism and a theory of hiccups. As the encounter begins, doctor and patient get down to business right away. They introduce themselves, the patient states his complaint—"a bad cold" (line 8)—very briefly, and the doctor immediately instructs him to get undressed. In the passage that follows, after the doctor asks a series of brief questions about fever, cough, phlegm, sore throat, and earaches, he quickly examines the lungs and takes the patient's temperature (lines 17–41). Although he does not say so, time seems to be of the essence, since the doctor then requests that the patient answer further questions while the thermometer is still in his mouth:

D: I'll ask you some yes and no questions that you can answer
   with your mouth . . . occupied. Do you smoke?
   Do you get hiccups very often?   45
P: Nope.

Such instrumentalism, which emphasizes technical procedures of the physical exam, inhibits storytelling, to say the least. These maneuvers not only create a physical obstacle to speech but also convey a message that verbal discourse is less pertinent than objective observation.

    While obstructing the patient's mouth, the doctor goes on to expound a theory of hiccups. The theory intrigues the doctor, and the patient expresses some interest as well, despite the explanation's irrelevance to the patient's present condition:

D: You have a long hair in your ear canal, and rarely that
   will irritate the
       [
P: Is that right?
D: canal and lead to hiccups. If you ever get a bad case of   50
   hiccups that won't stop, you tell the doctor to, uh, pull
   a hair out of your . . it's about an inch long inside the
   canal. I've always been waiting for someone with hiccups
   to cure them that way, but I guess I haven't found it even
   in you. Your ears are fine.   55

In the ear exam, the doctor apparently has found a long hair. This observation has reminded him of a relation that he recalls between hiccups and the ear. Such a connection seems little appreciated, since it does not appear in the pertinent medical literature.[9] Expounding his possibly idiosyncratic theory, the doctor expresses disappointment that it does not apply to the patient's case. His ease here in propounding a nonmainstream notion also foreshadows another unusual theory that proves more pertinent later.

Before voicing his next theory, however, the doctor continues in an instrumental mode, eliciting information through questions presumably to be answered yes or no while the patient still holds a thermometer in his mouth. The doctor also cracks a joke and obtains contextual information about the patient's work, from which he now is vacationing:

D: Do you take any medicines   5
everyday? Do you have any chronic diseases, diabetes,
high blood pressure, meanness? No meanness. What kind
of work do you do?
P: Ah unh, I work in, uh, —— ((name of factory)). I'm a setter.
D: Been working there a long time, haven't you?   60
P: Oh, eleven . .

When the doctor asks an ambiguously humorous question about meanness, he sets a jocular tone, although the humor remains rather dark.[10] The joke leads into two brief questions about the patient's work, the answers to which establish that the patient has participated reliably in industrial production over a period of many years. Even on his vacation, the patient proves eager to perform work-oriented activities, as he states toward the end of the encounter, "I have half an acre of land to clear" (line 183).

Meanwhile, after several other question-answer couplets, the doctor briefly explains his diagnostic impression, which includes an interruption concerning another patient. Worthy of note, the interruption again illustrates the doctor's instrumental approach, since he refers to the other patient as a symptom rather than a person:

D: Your chest is clear in the sense that there's no deep pneumonia,   70
no signs of asthma. ((To woman)) Where's the earache?
WOMAN: In your office.
D: ((To woman)) We'll fix him up. ((To patient)) OK. Your
throat looks sore and boggy. There's no what we call exudate,
the sore that you get with strep throat.   75

For unclear reasons, in the midst of explaining his diagnosis, the doctor here engages in a side conversation about the next patient, to whom he refers as "the earache."[11] The doctor is about to continue an instrumental

approach to diagnosis and treatment, when contextual matters intervene.

Alcoholism, a disease under control. The patient, perhaps relieved to
get the thermometer out of his mouth, now begins an intimate description of a key part of his identity. When the doctor asks about drug
allergies, the patient mentions disulfiram (Antabuse), a medication that
produces a severe, noxious bodily response when taken with alcohol. For
this reason, Antabuse comprises a frequent part of alcohol detoxification
programs. Here are the details, which reveal the doctor's enthusiasm
about the patient's commitment to stay on the wagon:

D: Do you have any   75
   allergies to medicine?
P: No. The only thing I have an allergy to is . . . Antabuse.
D: Antabuse.
P: I'm an alcoholic.
D: Oh. Good for you, in the sense that you were a former   80
   alcoholic? Do you still drink?
P: No. Ten years.
D: Good for you. That's marvelous.

The doctor then clarifies if the patient's reaction to Antabuse constitutes a
true allergy, or simply the medication's intended effect:

D: But if you, do you have an allergy
   just to the Antabuse itself? I see.
P: No. But I can't take any medication with it.   90
D: I see.

In short, it is doubtful that the patient is allergic to Antabuse.

When the patient describes his alcohol detoxification program, the
doctor calls forth the image of a "disease under control." Patient and
doctor also refer to a beneficial impact of sobriety upon one's ability to
function in the social world:

P: But I only take it, Christmas time, you know . .
                    [
D: On the wet
   times of the year.
P: Right.   95
D: Well, I certainly respect you for it. Getting that disease
   under control.
P: I went to a . . We have in —— ((state name)) a —— —— Clinic
   in —— ((city name)).
D: I know that clinic.   100
P: And, uh. I was there for three weeks. And I had a little

Jewish social worker that got it across to me that the
world turns better without alcohol.

D: And it has turned better, hasn't it?

P: Beautiful, beautiful.   10

By referring to alcoholism as a disease, the doctor is reiterating an assumption promulgated by AA and accepted by a substantial part of the medical profession. That is, alcoholism is a physical disorder rooted in pathophysiology and requiring strict abstinence as a cure. From this view, although many contextual factors may precipitate alcohol binges or may contribute to chronic inebriation, they do not constitute the root cause.

When defined in this way, alcoholism becomes a reified, objective disorder that requires a profound degree of control, involving both personal will and professional surveillance.[12] In kicking his habit, the patient recounts that he has benefitted from both these forms of control—his own ability to modulate his inclinations during wet times of the year by self-dosing of Antabuse and input from other people like the "little Jewish social worker." The metaphor of the world's turning better conveys an image of smooth social relations, presumably at work and in the family. This passage tells a success story of prevention, as the patient vanquishes his disease and reliably performs his contextual responsibilities according to society's mainstream expectations.

Despite his praise, the doctor cuts off both this and a later discussion of alcoholism by returning to the technical matter of penicillin. The first instance occurs when he again reverts to the matter of drug allergy:

D: And it has turned better, hasn't it?

P: Beautiful, beautiful.   10

D: No allergies to penicillin specifically?

P: No.

A second cut-off arises toward the encounter's end, when the doctor repeats his congratulations for sobriety and terminates the patient's response—concerning an alcoholic family member—with a shot in the buttock:

D: and you're to be greatly
respected for stopping alcohol.

P: Wasn't easy. And I have a sister-in-law who laughed at me.

D: Why?   15

P: Because I was going up . .

D: Is she a drunk?

P: Six or seven years later she was up there herself. And
afterwards she apologized and said that she wished she had
gone when I had.   16

D: Stand up and lean over. I'll give you this in the butt.

Contextual discussion thus seems fine up to a point. As scarce time passes or relevance declines, however, cut-offs that return the discourse to a technical plane become useful devices.

Smoking and a libidinal economy. Just as the doctor begins to describe his treatment of the patient's upper respiratory infection, however, a second self-destructive behavior rears its ugly head. Although the patient's alcohol use is "under control," his smoking is not. Continuing to smoke, the doctor notes, may exacerbate the patient's current respiratory infection and may interfere with treatment. At first, while offering an explanation of bronchitis, the doctor notes only that smoking may cause some irritation:

D: You're not dying, but you're miserable. This
  is the story of a
          [
P: Yeah   110
          [
D: bronchitis.

* * *

Not everyone dies of these things obviously, before we
invented antibiotics. But I think having a two or three day   115
history of it now, having productive phlegm coming up
now, you'd be better off and get better faster, especially
since you're smoking which tends to irritate it a little
bit, um, if you, uh, if we gave you penicillin.

Beyond the possibly reassuring allusions to death, smoking becomes part of the doctor's rationale for prescribing an antibiotic.

At this point, the doctor voices another of his rather idiosyncratic theories of clinical medicine, but one with more pertinence to this patient than the hair-in-the-ear theory of hiccups. Despite his acknowledgment that smoking worsens the patient's bronchitis, the doctor advises the patient *not* to stop smoking. Immediately, the patient recognizes the doctor's rationale, and both parties confirm that they see eye-to-eye on this matter. The rationale involves a perception that, regarding alcohol and smoking, abstinence is an either-or phenomenon. For a patient on the wagon, smoking cessation on top of sobriety may prove too much to handle:

D: Incidentally, doctors will probably tell you to stop smoking
    all the time. I'm . . I'm not sure you should. Let me tell   125
    you why.
P: I'm going to tell you why.
D: Well, you tell me.
P: I quit drinking, and I got . .
D: That's enough.   130

P: That's enough.

D: That's exactly my thinking. Now tobacco isn't the best
thing in the world for you, but you don't have emphysema,
and you don't have any serious complications of it.

P: But I, uh, have cut down.   13

D: It's just a little too much of a burden on you to stop
alcohol and tobacco. So let me be one doctor to tell you
that you probably ought to keep smoking.

In this way, the doctor theorizes that conquering one self-destructive habit is honorable, but that trying to vanquish two such habits may prove unfeasible. Further, the passage implies that clamping down too tightly on tobacco may lead to slippage in sobriety.

Here the dialogue conveys an image of a libidinal economy, in which only so much energy is available for self-control. When one faces a choice about the expenditure of such energy, the decision should favor the retention of whatever destructive habit is least socially disruptive. The underlying ideologic assumption of this passage then becomes apparent. Being a drunk threatens one's performance at work, in the family, on the highway, and so forth, much more than smoking cigarettes. Many clinicians and laypeople recognize some difficulty in tapering a second dependency after controlling a first.[13] Because of the differing social impacts of the two dependencies, the selection of which one to prioritize also seems somehow appropriate. For instance, the dialogue would become quite surprising if the doctor counseled the patient to start drinking again so that he could give up smoking. Although smoking's deleterious effects on health and longevity rival or surpass those of drinking, the consequences for reliable participation in social life according to mainstream expectations differ substantially. If limited libidinal resources require selectivity, the choice of which noxious habit to suppress thus becomes fairly obvious.[14]

The libidinal economy that governs self-destruction also takes on a moral dimension. Elaborating on the choice among adverse alternatives, the patient introduces the topic of sex, a third element associated metaphorically with dependency on harmful substances. Smoking, drinking, and sex—this triad becomes an almost inescapable image for indulgence and the difficulties of moral control. The emergence of sex in the discourse, without any other information about actual sexual behavior, reinforces the subtle imagery of an economy governing human drives, an economy that is ultimately libidinal.

In a variation on Encounter 8A (where, as noted earlier, the doctor cautions the patient, "Yeah, well when people get on your back, you can't go to booze or cigarettes or . . or sex"), the patient here compares giving up cigarettes, on top of alcohol, to the absurd option of giving up sex:

P: Well, my dad said, "Gee," this is about a year, year and a
   half after I
       [
D: Tell me.

   [
P: stopped drinking, he was in his late eighties, he said, "Now   145
   you've stopped drink-
               [
D: Yeah

   [
P: -ing, why don't you stop smoking?" And I says, "Well, Christ,
   next year you'll want me to stop having sex." ((laughs))

The moral weight attached to noxious habits manifests itself by two
further elements. First, the patient refers to an elderly father as he introduces the metaphorical triad. He counterposes his own defensiveness to
the father's quest for clean living. Secondly, he introjects a religious
allusion. Presumably Christ would forgive a less perfect outcome than
the father, who figures here as both external authority and superego,
might prefer. The patient's laughter at the end communicates that for him
the libidinal economy governing human vices has become no laughing
matter.

   While the doctor then reiterates his concurrence with the theory of
libidinal economy, he also begins to cut off the topic by returning to the
technical mode of treatment, and painful treatment at that. Here the
doctor juxtaposes the patient's mention of sexual deprivation to the
image of a syringe:

D: OK. Fair enough. I think it's important . . . Give me the . . .   150
   syringe . . Uh, I think that's . . I think your logic is correct,
   and, uh, I'm with you on that, and you're to be *greatly*
   respected for stopping alcohol.

In this transition back to the realm of the technical, the doctor readies a
tool of his trade, whose penetration into the patient's persona carries a
meaning of punishment as well as cure.[15]

Ideology and structure. As in the last encounter, this one conveys
ideologic language that values impulse control under professional surveillance. Early in the interaction, the doctor assumes a dominant position, as he adopts an interrogatory format in history taking, moves quickly to the physical exam, and physically obstructs the patient's mouth.
After providing an idiosyncratic theory relating ear hair to hiccups, the
doctor reinforces the patient's success in controlling the "disease" of
alcoholism, with the help of social services that have assisted his reliable
performance at work and in the family. Yet an ideology of human weak-

ness in the face of temptation comes forth, as patient and doctor agree about the limits of personal will. A libidinal economy dictates that self-destruction can be addressed only one noxious habit at a time, and the failure to achieve a higher state of perfection can be forgiven. Meanwhile, socially disruptive behaviors receive priority for intervention, while other medically dangerous acts prove more tolerable.

Within the discourse, several structural elements emerge (figure 8.1). As in the last encounter, the chief contextual issue facing this patient involves role expectations governing a man's social roles at work and in the family. It is expected that such a person will continue to perform in these spheres as reliably as possible (A). Neither patient nor doctor refers explicitly to difficulties in these contextual spheres. Yet the context, and assumed expectations about reliable performance, comprise a backdrop for the personal troubles that emerge. Specifically, considerable attention gets paid to the self-destructive habits of alcoholism and smoking (B), within a routine visit for an upper respiratory infection (C). The patient takes initiative in characterizing himself as an alcoholic, describes his success in eliminating alcohol intake, and mentions the professional help that he has received (D). Tensions manifest themselves when the doctor twice cuts off the patient's descriptions of alcohol detoxification programs by returning to technical matters of antibiotic treatment for bronchitis. As might be expected within a brief encounter for a limited physical problem, the dialogue does not explore relationships between the social context, for instance involving work or family, and self-destructive habits such as alcoholism or smoking. Yet this absence in the discourse tends to marginalize whatever contextual issues the patient may be facing, no matter how pertinent to the personal problems at hand. Further, when the adverse effects of smoking on the patient's present condition of bronchitis become apparent, a theory of libidinal economy allows doctor and patient to produce a trade-off between smoking and sobriety (E). The doctor helps manage contextual issues by concurring with a technical definition of alcoholism as a disease under professional surveillance. He also reinforces the patient's control of the disease through willpower and self-dosing of a medication, Antabuse. Finally he discourages cessation of smoking, another noxious but socially less disruptive habit. The discourse conveys ideologic messages of human weakness in the face of temptation, and impulse control under professional regulation (F). Afterward, the patient returns to a work-oriented vacation and presumably later to his usual social roles, having won professional approval of his balanced approach to dealing with self-destructive tendencies.

Encounters 8A and 8B show some of the variability in medical processing of human vices. Although the first patient continues to destroy his body through booze and tobacco as he approaches the major life transition of marriage, the second patient has regulated his behavior more

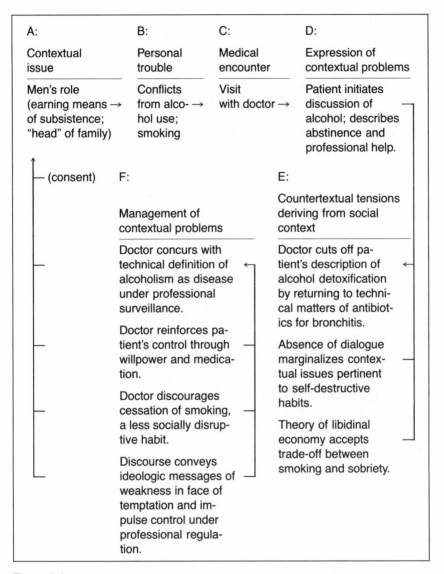

Figure 8.1
Structural elements of a medical encounter with a man who has ceased alcohol use but whose smoking exacerbates his bronchitis

successfully, at least in relation to alcohol. According to the first doctor, his patient needs all the help he can get to stop drinking, as well as moral instruction about impulse control in the areas of smoking and sex. While the second doctor congratulates his patient for sobriety, the metaphorical triad again arises, as the patient jokes that giving up smoking might prove as difficult as sexual abstinence, and the doctor concurs that suppressing more than one pernicious habit at a time would prove too burdensome. In these encounters, doctors comfortably reinforce the importance of professional surveillance and control in dealing with their patients' self-destructive tendencies. Meanwhile, specific contextual problems that these patients face go largely unexplored, as doctors and patients focus on technical matters and medical management. Narrowing their attention to the vices at hand, all parties seem to take pride in whatever small victories they win in the battle against self-destruction.

ENCOUNTER 8C: DRUGS AND OTHER RECREATIONAL ACTIVITIES

SUMMARY

A young man comes to a doctor because of possible high blood pressure. The doctor takes an extensive medical history, which includes repeated questions about drug use. Patient and doctor also discuss some mild respiratory symptoms. After the physical exam, the doctor reassures the patient that his blood pressure currently is normal. The doctor also recommends lab tests, a follow-up visit, and an antihistamine for nasal congestion, but no antihypertensive medication.

In their questionnaires, the participants give the following information about themselves and their encounter. The patient is a 19-year-old white male who states that he is entering his second year of college and who mentions no other occupation. He reports his religion as Jewish and his ethnic background as American. A 54-year-old white Jewish male, the doctor reports his specialty as "internal medicine, primary physician." Although patient and doctor are meeting each other for the first time in this encounter, the doctor has cared for other members of the patient's family for about fifteen years. Based on this encounter, which takes place in a suburban practice outside Boston, the doctor diagnoses the patient's problem as "hypertension etiology unknown prob[ably] labile."

A workup of hypertension. Much verbiage in this encounter involves the details of medical history taking. In particular, the doctor devotes extensive effort to the "review of systems," that part of the history which searches for symptoms in each of the patient's various organ systems.[16] With the exception of some material about colds, sneezing, and nasal congestion, the medical history yields little new data. Interrogatory couplets again dominate the discourse, as the doctor poses short, factual questions and the patient enunciates brief answers. Notably, the patient does not ask a single question during the entire encounter.

Regarding etiology and precipitating factors in hypertension, the pa-

tient gives a very brief clue, which neither he nor the doctor later pursues. The clue appears early in the encounter, when the doctor asks an
open-ended question about what is "bothering" the patient:

D: Well, supposing I let you tell me the things that might be
bothering you at this point.
P: Mostly, (words) my arm (words).
[
D: Uh huh.
[
P: About a month or so ago, and . . . . . my blood pressure was high.   40
D: That's good.
P: I don't know if it was just from being nervous or what so I
[
D: Have you lie down, and try it again or they just said fine?
P: No, I went back, uh, three days.

Here the patient reveals more about his internal life than he does at any
other point in the entire transcript. He speculates that "being nervous"
may have contributed to the abnormal blood pressure readings at school.

In the encounter, further discussion of emotional problems, or about
contextual issues that may trouble the patient, remains absent, despite
the widely recognized impact of stress and other psychologic factors in
hypertension.[17] The doctor again quickly alludes to emotional "strain"
during an explanation of hypertension:

D: Many people who have that, has no (words)
significant, just says, that when they get (words) under the
strain (words). Uh, your upper level blood pressure, the one   205
that tends to bounce more and is less significant

After mentioning a differential diagnosis that includes endocrine diseases, kidney problems, and hereditary conditions, and after describing
a diagnostic workup and treatment that he may recommend if hypertension persists, the doctor again refers to the patient's feeling "upset":

D: Right
now I can do nothing. It's just, you know, a thing that's got   245
you upset a little bit, and, I think I'm going to wait. So, for
now I do nothing about that.

The doctor states his intention to follow the patient's blood pressure with
a limited technical evaluation and without treatment. Here, explicit comment about emotions ceases, and assessment of pertinent contextual
factors does not begin.

Quest for drugs. Although the doctor explores neither the patient's
feelings nor the possibly troubling details of social context, he enters into
professional surveillance of recreational drugs. At first, the doctor im-

plies that mind-altering drugs may have affected the patient's blood pressure:[18]

D: Repeated it three times, and stated it was still high. And so far, (words) you did nothing to make it go up that you know of.
P: (words)
D: Take (words), did you take pill, amphetamines or anything else?
P: (words)
D: OK, because that would eliminate a lot of other things that we would have (words)
P: Once I took a couple of caffeine pills.

When the patient provides no confirmation, the conversation returns to the review of systems. During this sequence of question-answer couplets, the patient briefly refers to a girlfriend and her cat. Besides mentioning that he sneezes more at the girlfriend's house, the patient also notes his frequent presence there:

D: You may be right about the cat, cats are very common offenders (words).
P: My girlfriend has a cat, and I'm over at her house a lot.
D: Cats are common offenders for people who are allergic.
P: It seems when I'm outside I don't sneeze that much.

This news begins to paint a picture of a rather loose and carefree young-adult life-style, albeit hampered somewhat by nasal congestion. (Despite his surveillance of recreational drug use, the doctor does not pick up here on the symptoms of sneezing and nasal congestion—hallmarks of the cocaine era.)

Shortly afterward, the doctor inquires more directly into the paraphernalia associated in the popular imagination with such a life-style. The inquiry starts in the midst of the review of systems concerning the head, as the doctor asks about headaches, dizziness, and vision. Suddenly the doctor uses a question about double vision to renew the inquiry about pharmacologic "aids" to mind expansion:

D: Need glasses? Have them, but don't use them? You never see double or instead of one person you see two or any unusual visual things?
P: No.
D: Even with any kinds of aids like alcohol, grass, or anything?
P: No.
D: You use some of those?
P: I used to for a while.
D: Was it grass or other means, not amphetamines or (words). Speed or acid?

P: No.
D: Nothing stronger?
P: Alcohol.
D: But you don't drink a pint of booze a day?
P: No, I couldn't afford it. I stopped smoking last June,   130
cigarettes, I haven't had any since last June.
D: Your ears giving you any trouble, with this cold or allergy?

In his questions, the doctor shows, or tries to show, sophistication about the subject matter. Using vernacular terms, he substitutes grass for marijuana, speed for amphetamines, and acid for LSD. While the doctor employs concrete questions that are not open-ended, he gives the patient an opportunity to elaborate. At this point, however, the patient does not do so. The patient's response that he is drinking at a low level and has stopped smoking seems to bring relief, since the doctor cuts off this phase of the dialogue by returning to technical matters, in this case concerning the ears.

From the patient's side, a series of laconic answers to the doctor's closed-ended questions leaves the dialogue redolent with understatement. Among the ambiguities in this passage are the following. First, by using the past tense, the patient indicates that he has used mild hallucinogens previously but leaves vague his present usage. Secondly, economic constraints have proven the main inhibition limiting alcohol consumption. That is, regardless of whether he would like to drink "a pint of booze a day," financially the patient cannot afford to consume this much. By keeping his answers quite short and by not expanding on these themes in any way, the patient subtly truncates a discourse on substance use and abuse that could otherwise grow much lengthier and more detailed. If the doctor wished to engage in further professional surveillance of the patient's possibly self-destructive adventures in mind expansion, the patient himself provides little room for maneuvering.

Not superboy. At several points, the doctor's questions and statements suggest a standard of customary and expected behavior, against which the patient measures up not too well. Generally, such behavior involves athletic prowess. In the first instance, again as part of the review of systems, the doctor introduces this theme as he asks about exercise tolerance pertinent to the heart. Because of responses that indicate a rather slothful activity level, the doctor semihumorously notes that the patient is "not superboy":

D: OK. You get any chest pains? You physically active? You do things?
P: Not a whole lot.
D: What kinds of things do you do?
P: Uh, ... I do some rough house physically (words).   150

D: You don't go to the gym, play ball, you don't play hockey.
P: Sometimes; I play football.
D: You're not superboy. (words)
P: Yeah.
D: Have you been ice skating lately, for example? Some activity.   1

The doctor's characterization implies that somehow this youth has gotten on the wrong track in life, indulging as he does in drugs, alcohol, tobacco, and sex instead of good, clean sports.

Just as the encounter ends, the doctor tries one more time to get the kid into shape. After reassuring the patient about his medical status, the doctor encourages more exercise. Again, the patient remains undemonstrative and noncommittal:

D: I don't think it is anything to
worry about. It won't restrict you in any way. You can do any   2
damn thing you want. You can play ball or, I think it's good
for you to keep in general physical condition and shape. Lift
weights if you want. I don't know how much weightlifting
you do?
P: None.   2
D: I thought you said something, oh no, no, what were you going
to, oh, situps, pushup, oh yeah, all right, you can do those.
So, you do that, and let me look forward to seeing you sometime in the springtime.

In encouraging physical conditioning, the doctor seems to strive toward several ends. First, he apparently espouses exercise as a general principle of preventive medicine, with a view that physical conditioning proves beneficial for health. Further, although he does not say so, the doctor may feel that exercise would tend to lower the patient's blood pressure somewhat, a method that some specialists advocate for patients with borderline or mild hypertension.[19] Finally, in continuity with other parts of the encounter, the doctor may want to encourage exercise as a form of sublimation for this patient, who shows signs of slipping along a path of degeneracy. While he need not become superboy, at least the patient might stay out of trouble if he lifted weights and did calisthenics. By doing so, the patient would find his way through a winter of temptation, before the doctor checks up on him again next spring.

In loco parentis. Throughout the encounter, the doctor assumes a partly parental role. As the patient enters adulthood, he, of course, encounters the usual contextual issues associated with leaving the parental nest. Although he continues to depend on his parents in various ways, he also is beginning to live more independently. Both the patient and the

doctor mention, in their questionnaires, the doctor's long-standing relationship with the patient's parents, for whom the doctor has cared during
the previous fifteen years. In the dialogue, traces of the doctor's allegiance
to the parents create tensions affecting the relationship that begins to
emerge with the son. These tensions center on professional surveillance
of the patient's family and also on the doctor's probing about life-style.
Further, the doctor does not assure the patient that information transmitted between them will remain confidential from the parents, nor does
the patient ask about this matter. In the end, the doctor continues to ally
himself in large part with the parents, and his allegiance to the son
remains ambiguous.

These themes appear shortly after the encounter begins, as the doctor
moves quickly into a brief family history. The doctor himself manifests
some tension in his initial reference to the patient's parents:

D: Family history. Hardly need to belabor (words) to worry
    about, uh, your mother, father.   20

Here the terms that the doctor uses to refer to the parents become flags of
strain and anxiety, as he says there is no need to "belabor" or "worry
about" them. Such terms reveal a negative undercurrent which then
extends into a brief discussion of the patient's siblings:

D: And you have what, one   20
    brother, one sister. How old is your brother now?
P: I think he's 22.
D: What's he doing?
P: He works for ((corporation name)). He works in a warehouse.
D: Sister is now how old?   25
P: I think she's 11 or 12. Think 11.
D: And she's OK. Is she at home or away?
P: She's away.
D: Where is she?
P: She's in New Hampshire.   30
D: As far as you know, she's well?
P: Yeah.
D: Do you see her?
P: Yeah.
D: Good.   35

This perfunctory exchange carries several messages. First, the patient's
relationships with his brother and sister prove not particularly close. For
instance, he reports their ages only as approximations. Second, the patient's very brief responses to the doctor's questions manifest emotional
distance. The patient's bland statements convey facts but not feelings, as

he provides no elaboration about his siblings. Further, the doctor's questions remain very general and concern social more than health matters. Thus, the doctor asks only about the brother's work, not about any aspect of the brother's health; as depicted by the patient, the brother's job appears none too challenging or rewarding. Regarding the sister, the doctor concerns himself mainly with her whereabouts and the patient's relationship with her, while he leaves the medical inquiry at the vaguest level ("As far as you know, she's well?" line 31). This passage elicits no technical information at all; it mainly portrays a social constellation of family relations. The picture that emerges conveys tension and distance. Through his queries, the doctor engages in surveillance of the patient's familial role and (for instance, when he labels as "good" the patient's seeing his sister, line 35) approves those elements that reflect mainstream expectations of closeness and stability.

A final reference to family comes up at the end of the encounter. Here, in his farewell to the patient, the doctor reinforces the value of a close-knit "home":

D: When will you be back? Around June?
P: May.   2
D: May. All right, when you come back, we'll check that. If you
   want, in the interim, you might pop in to the nurse at school
   when you feel real relaxed and have her take your blood pressure
   and make note of it. She'll give it (words). Good luck and
   give my best to the home.   2
P: OK.

By asking the patient to check his blood pressure when he feels "real relaxed," the doctor again implies that emotional tension may artificially raise the pressure while he is at school. Rather than pursuing the theme of tension and relaxation, and its relation to the patient's social context, the doctor here swings the dialogue back to family, but in an impersonal manner—mentioning "home" instead of specific individuals. In this way the doctor tips his hat to the mainstream value of home, which he asks the patient to greet without reference to any of the (possibly unrelaxed) individuals who live there.

Ideology and structure. In an encounter intended to evaluate hypertension in a young man, a number of ideologic elements come to the fore. As he enters adulthood, the patient faces issues of dependency and independence. While at school and perhaps at home, he has experienced nervousness as he has gotten involved with a girlfriend, has experimented with drugs, has smoked and drunk within the limits of his pocketbook, and has led a generally sedentary life-style. Presenting himself as an ally of both the patient and his parents, the doctor engages in professional surveillance of these somewhat unsavory conditions. The doctor does not inquire about contextual sources of nervousness, nor does the patient volunteer information. On the other hand, the doctor paints a picture of clean living. This more desirable life-style includes control or at least moderation of self-destructive habits, especially those involving recreational substances. Body and soul also benefit from participation in the sublimated activities of the gymnasium. Moreover, the quest for autonomy should not infringe upon the values of hearth and home.

The encounter reveals several structural components (figure 8.2). The chief contextual issue facing this patient involves the transition from adolescence to adulthood. En route to achieving autonomy, he is dealing with the expectations of the educational system and family members, upon whom he is still dependent (A). As he confronts these issues, he has become troubled by nervousness and also has experimented with a number of substances whose continued use could become self-destructive (B). In a medical visit intended to evaluate hypertension (C), the patient briefly mentions his nervousness but does not elaborate. Through an extensive inquiry, the doctor extracts information about the patient's substance use, sedentary habits, and love life (D). Within the dialogue, tensions manifest themselves in several ways: the patient's laconic style of answering questions, references to the patient's family in which the doctor's allegiances remain ambiguous, and the doctor's cut-off of a discussion about substance use and family through return to technical matters (questions about the ears). Meanwhile, both patient and doctor stay silent about the specific contextual problems that contribute to the patient's nervousness (E). The doctor manages contextual difficulties by monitoring substance use and other potentially damaging components of the patient's life-style. In addition to encouraging clean living through athletics, the discourse communicates mainstream values that support familial closeness and educational advancement. Critical attention to the contextual sources of distress that face youths such as this one remains absent from the dialogue (F). Leaving the encounter, the patient consents to giving his "best" to the home, and to coping in a more relaxed way with pressures at school.

As in the previous two encounters, the doctor benignly observes self-destructive behavior and encourages prevention. Although the contextual issue here involves the transition to adulthood, professional surveillance exerts itself within a broadly similar structure of discourse. Whether this patient concurs with the doctor's vision of clean living and closely knit family relations remains hidden beneath an unrevealing terseness of expression. Regardless of the patient's compliance, at least the doctor has tried to help him get back on a healthy track.

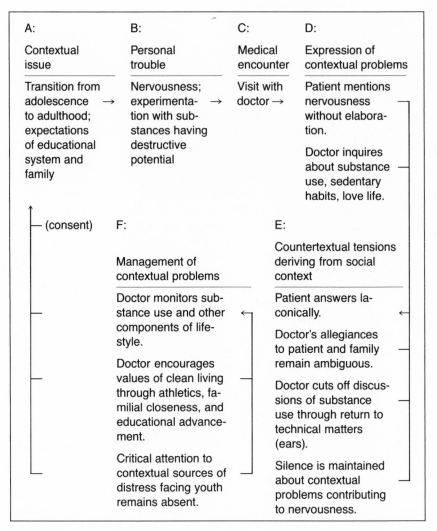

Figure 8.2
Structural elements of a medical encounter with a youth undergoing evaluation for hypertension

SURVEILLANCE OF SELF-DESTRUCTION

In the present period of the history of medicine, who could argue against prevention? The greatest challenges that health professionals and the general public now face involve problems that respond to preventive intervention. In economically advanced countries, chronic diseases have become the main causes of morbidity and death. Prevention and health promotion aimed toward reducing self-destructive behaviors, as many (including myself)[20] have argued, then seem worthwhile goals. Even in infectious epidemics, like AIDS, prevention of certain behaviors involving substance use and sexuality becomes desirable. From this perspective, the day-to-day routine of the competent and caring physician comes to include preventive activities. Within doctor-patient encounters, such activities frequently include discourse concerning personal behavior that appears dangerous to self, intimates, or the wider community.

One down side of prevention, however, involves the policing component of the medical role. That policing functions are involved in effective prevention comes as no surprise, since leaders in public health have recognized this fact for more than a century.[21] Surveillance of unsavory personal behavior, after all, becomes essential, if preventive medicine is to be effective. Social control then emerges as one part of the medical task, as does the propounding of ideologies that encourage patients' conformity to a safe, straight, and narrow path. That the quest for prevention involves social control and ideologic assumptions, at least to some degree, remains dimly if at all perceived by many doctors and patients who speak with each other about healthier life-styles.

The three encounters examined here show some of the variability in the medical processing of human vices. On the road to self-destruction, the patients have arrived at different milestones. At a rather young age, the first patient is wrecking his liver and lungs with booze and tobacco. Alternatively, although the second patient has partly cleaned up his act as far as alcohol is concerned, cessation of smoking remains beyond his reach. Just entering adulthood, the third patient is experimenting with mind-altering drugs, alcohol, and tobacco; whether he will return to cleaner living remains unclear.

While all three doctors staunchly advocate prevention, they differ somewhat in style. The first doctor adopts a take-charge approach, as he initiates a wide-ranging inquiry into the patient's habits and tries to intervene actively in an alcohol support network. When he encourages self-control in the face of temptation, the doctor "hails" the patient ideologically as a subject whose performance within a web of social roles ought to become more reliable. In the second encounter, the doctor also invokes imagery of control, as he congratulates the patient for controlling the "disease" of alcoholism. However, a theory of libidinal economy leads him to encourage the patient to continue smoking; energy devoted to smoking cessation thus might allow the patient to slip off the wagon of sobriety. In the third encounter, the doctor quests for mind-altering substances, which by implication would prove dangerous for health and happiness. Further, he paints a picture of a more sublimated life-style, involving athletics and a closely knit family. While the efficacy of these tactics cannot be known, they at least convey some range of current realities in the routine practice of preventive medicine and health promotion.

Critical attention to contextual issues, despite their pertinence to the goals of prevention, remains marginal or absent in these encounters. In Encounter 8A, the doctor and patient do discuss some social situations that encourage drinking, and the doctor tries to orchestrate a support network. Neither here nor in the other encounters, however, do patient and doctor explore the social context in any detail, even though all three patients confront contextual issues that may heighten their inclination to indulge in the noxious habits that they have adopted. Pressures associated with work, family, and life transitions such as marriage and leaving the parental home affect the patients to varying degrees. Although medical discourse encourages individual control of human vices, it assumes that such contextual constraints will persist in more or less unalterable form.

To sum up: In seeking diversion and gratification amid the difficulties of social life, some people choose activities that might be seen as potentially disruptive or at least self-destructive. Because such activities sometimes cause ill health and functional incapacities, they can become the subject of conversations between patients and doctors. While professional norms foster a certain tolerance of personal foibles, medical discourse also conveys fairly precise ideologic expectations about appropriate behavior. Through explicit pronouncements and implicit discouragements communicated in part by an absence of criticism of context, medical discourse reinforces safe, nondisruptive, and usually austere forms of gratification. Such is the day-to-day practice of prevention in a society enlightened about the adverse impact of self-destructive habits.

CHAPTER 9

TROUBLESOME
EMOTIONS

Troublesome emotions creep into conversations between patients and doctors, even in some of the most technically oriented encounters. While psychiatry remains an option for some people, physicians who are not psychiatrists often find themselves dealing with patients' emotional distress. Most doctors who see patients on a regular basis expect to face such problems, as a routine part of the medical role. Although some primary-care physicians take pride in their own socioemotional skills, others approach such difficulties with dread or at least apprehension.[1]

A time-worn criticism leveled against traditional psychiatry involves its inability, or unwillingness, to change the social conditions involved in psychiatric disorders. From this viewpoint, clients' emotional disturbances frequently derive at least in part from oppressive circumstances in work, the family, or other parts of the social context. Although psychiatrists can help people adjust to these circumstances, such limited approaches leave intact the contextual roots of personal distress. "Radical" visions of psychiatric intervention involve some attempt to improve these contextual conditions—through reforms of the work process, changes in family roles, community-based support networks, and so forth.[2] Although such alternative visions have achieved results in certain localities, they have remained very much a minority position in psychiatry and have not influenced routine psychiatric practice to any great extent.

If traditional psychiatry has encouraged individual adjustment rather than social change, what happens as primary-care physicians deal with their patients' emotional difficulties? The primary-care fields have re-

211

ceived much less critical attention in this respect, despite the high proportion of encounters (usually estimated between 25 and 50 percent) that involve substantial psychiatric disturbance or emotional distress.[3] Yet, in contrast to the psychiatric visit, primary-care practitioners and their patients seldom see emotional problems as a major reason for the medical encounter. Emotional content thus tends to enter medical talk indirectly. Further, contextual sources of psychologic distress often appear at the margins of the dialogue, whose customary purpose remains the diagnosis and treatment of physical disease. In the primary-care setting, an attempt to change the social context then might seem incongruous, awkward, or at least unusual. On the other hand, helping the patient to cope with emotional distress usually calls for some kind of medical action.

The scope of professional responses to troublesome emotions has become apparent in prior chapters. To recapitulate, here are only a few examples. Emotional concerns also manifest themselves in other encounters as well, though less centrally.

- For a man who suffers from depression after a heart attack and who faces financial insecurity if he returns to work during a strike, a doctor prescribes psychotropic medications and emphasizes the psychologic benefits of working (Encounter 5A).
- With a depressed woman going through a divorce, a doctor explores options for psychotherapy, which the patient doubts she can afford, and tries to deal with her suicide potential by mentioning several emergency contacts. Her occupational frustrations, childrearing responsibilities, and social isolation receive little attention, although the doctor does suggest renewed efforts to date other men (Encounter 6A).
- When a woman complains of multiple somatic symptoms, a doctor diagnoses "suburban syndrome" and encourages rest, although the patient has not found vacation trips helpful previously. After several requests by the patient, the doctor reluctantly prescribes a tranquilizer. Aside from social obligations that the patient finds burdensome, the sources of her emotional distress remain unexplored (Encounter 6B).
- An elderly woman mentions to her doctor a series of upsetting experiences, including visual symptoms that she fears may interfere with independent living, the loss of her home and community, and the inevitable approach of death. While making no specific suggestions, the doctor supportively listens to her concerns (Encounter 7A).
- A man in his late sixties and his wife focus with their doctor on upper airway symptoms. In response to the doctor's questions, they mention briefly that the patient's depression has improved with psychotropic medications. What contextual circumstances might have contributed

to the depression, such as the patient's retirement from work, remain unclear (Encounter 7B).

■ A man in his mid-sixties recently has retired and has lost his wife to cancer. His doctor reviews the patient's psychotropic medications, but neither party mentions the depression that the patient has experienced nor its sources (Encounter 7C).

■ For a man whose alcoholism has created liver disease, a doctor orchestrates a support network intended to help him stop drinking. Facing uncertain employment, family tensions, and a forthcoming marriage, the patient reports fatigue. The doctor responds with comments that encourage self-control and responsibility in social relationships (Encounter 8A).

These encounters show several reactions to emotional distress. In some instances, technical intervention with psychotropic medication becomes the main response. In others, doctors offer counseling, referral to other professionals, or supportive listening. At times, doctors utter explicit ideologic pronouncements about desirable behavior. At other times, these assumptions remain background understandings about what patients must continue to do in their lives, although the social conditions that they face may prove quite troubling. The possibility of contextual change as a route to happier living generally remains unexpressed. In these encounters, suggested modifications in life-style usually aim toward more satisfactory compliance with mainstream expectations.

Although previous chapters explore such troublesome emotions, here I want to focus on the processing of another common difficulty—psychologic disturbance that seems directly related to physical disease and its treatment. Certain illnesses cause psychologic symptoms, through effects on the central nervous system. Such problems can become quite challenging, especially since they sometimes exist with other socioemotional difficulties that do not derive from the disease in question.[4] Sorting out the physical and nonphysical components of the psychologic disorder then may emerge as a central theme during a medical encounter.

Patients who experience physical causes of psychologic upset, of course, carry out their lives within a broader social context, some elements of which also may affect the emotional disturbance. In such instances, patient and doctor may enter a verbal labyrinth, as they recount the interplay of physical, psychologic, and social factors in the etiology and treatment of emotional distress. Although such difficulties may present themselves less frequently than the nonphysical disturbances considered earlier, the single encounter that follows illustrates that ideology and context may figure just as prominently in the "management" of such patients.

ENCOUNTER 9A: EMOTIONAL MANIFESTATIONS OF PHYSICAL DISEASE

SUMMARY

A woman with a chronic inflammatory disease affecting her muscles comes to her doctor for a routine follow-up appointment. Complaining of fatigue and emotional distress, the patient asks for higher doses of corticosteroids (for her muscle disease) and antidepressants. Patient and doctor discuss the impact of muscle disease, adrenal dysfunction, and medication on her symptoms. The patient mentions concerns about ability to do housework and about her mentally retarded son. The doctor modifies the corticosteroid therapy and suggests a subsequent appointment.

In the questionnaires that they completed after the encounter, patient and doctor sketched some information about their own backgrounds. The patient, 62 years old, is a graduate of high school and secretarial school who reports her occupation as "housewife." She is married and the mother of three children, aged 33, 30, and 26. Although she does not answer the question about her ethnic background, she reports her race as "white" and her religion as Catholic. The doctor, who practices internal medicine, is a 44-year-old white male, of German and English descent, who denies a religious preference. Patient and doctor have known each other for about one year. The encounter takes place in a suburb of Boston. According to the doctor, the patient's diagnoses are polymyositis (a chronic inflammatory disease of muscle) and "cortisone reaction" (side effects of corticosteroid medication).

The big debate. Throughout much of this lengthy encounter, patient and doctor argue about many components of diagnosis and treatment. The patient consistently questions and refutes the doctor's judgments, while the doctor tries to justify his opinions. An undercurrent of hostility emerges, as patient and doctor bicker about one topic after another. Still, in the end, patient and doctor reaffirm their intention to continue their relationship, and the patient expresses satisfaction with the encounter. The doctor's interpretation of the patient's psychologic disturbance as largely a manifestation of drug toxicity, as well as the patient's incapacitating illness, may strengthen their perseverance, despite the verbal jousting that transpires.

Right at the outset, the patient pushes the doctor for an increased dosage of dexamethasone (Decadron), a corticosteroid:

D: All right.
P: Just give me permission to take two Decadron a day. I can't

go on with one.

[

D: I'll,

[

P: I'm half dead most of the time.   5

Because the patient feels "half dead," she wants more corticosteroid
medication. However, to the doctor this symptom may mean several
things. It may reflect worsening of the patient's muscle disease, a side
effect of medication, or depression. Further, the doctor has been trying to
limit the corticosteroid dosage, in view of potential toxicity. He has
tapered the medication and has used an every-other-day dosing schedule. This approach has received wide advocacy in clinical medicine, as a
way to prevent suppression of the adrenal gland and other side effects
that corticosteroids predictably produce.[5] When the doctor again advises
maintaining alternate-day dosage, the patient objects, claiming that she
would prefer symptomatic relief to the presumed long-term advantages
of less frequent dosing:

D: When, when we're, uhm, while we're talking about the Decadron   25
let me ask you one other thing and that is, you remember you
were taking two tablets every other day.
P: And you changed it to one a day.
D: Right. Now, are you just as bad? Worse? Better? Does

                                                        [

P: I'm   30
worse, it's getting worse the longer time (words)
D: So it's worse on one tablet a day.
P: Because it's like more length of time, you see, it's two and
a half months since I was on two a day.
D: You mean two every other day.   35
P: No.
D: Oh, you mean back when you were taking two a day? Yeah.

[

P: when I was back when I was taking two a day.
That seems to be it, now, whether it shortens the lifespan
or not, I'm going to take a chance.   40
D: Ha ha ha ha.
P: This is not living.
D: Yeah.
P: I can't just do anything.
D: Well, uhm, you know there's another possibility and that is,   45
uh, rather than taking two every day, you can try three
every other day.
P: What would be the point of that?

Here the patient begins the challenges that continue throughout the encounter. First, she corrects the doctor's account of her prior medication schedule and indicates that she is willing to accept the risks of increasing the corticosteroids. Nonetheless, he persists in advising alternate-day dosing, but the patient doubts his purpose.

Beyond her skepticism about medication schedule, the patient next questions the doctor's interpretation of her adrenal glands. Apparently, the doctor previously has explained to her that corticosteroid treatment suppresses the function of these glands and that tapering the treatment will lead to a resumption of normal adrenal function. Although she complains about muscle weakness, the patient interrupts the doctor to state her preference that he attend to the adrenal suppression rather than the muscle inflammation:

P: Yeah, you were trying to get them- but do you- I don't think
   that gland's going to come back. We've tried what, three
   times now.
D: Oh, it'll come back. Sure. No, your gland, your adrenal
   gland does
          [
P: I don't
          [
D: function.
P: A little bit.

* * *

P: What are you treating, the inflammation?
D: Yeah.
P: Why don't we skip that and just stick to the gland? Let's get
   that straightened out.

Despite the doctor's reassurances to the contrary, the patient does not accept his claim that her adrenal function would return to normal if the corticosteroids were discontinued. Instead, she pursues her concern about the adrenal glands and their impact on her symptoms. In the ensuing dialogue, she challenges the doctor further, expressing doubt that muscle disease, rather than adrenal dysfunction, is her main problem:

D: You see, no, it's not a question of that [adrenal dysfunction].
   You trouble is your muscle disease, right?
P: I don't think so.
D: Well, it has been.
P: You should know, of course. But
   [
D: Well, you haven't had a- nobody was treating adrenal disease
   in you, ever.
P: No, it started treating the muscles, of course-
D: Fine.

P: But the adrenal then works on, I mean the Decadron then works
    on the adrenal, which stops that from functioning.

The patient's faint praise of the doctor's knowledge (line 82) does little to
reduce her implied criticism of his diagnostic acumen. Perhaps as a
result, he continues his attempts to convince her that his perception of
physiologic truth is correct, but he enjoys little success.

What is the patient driving at here? She may well have reason to
question the doctor's clinical assessment, but more seems to be going on
than that. Psychologic distress, to be discussed later, has become at least
as great a problem for her as physical weakness. Higher doses of corticosteroids often produce euphoria, which improves a patient's subjective
perception of emotional well-being.[6] From the patient's perspective, up-
ping the dose now might be desirable, to produce a "steroid high." From
the doctor's perspective, inducing such a side effect would prove coun-
terproductive.

As patient and doctor focus on muscle inflammation versus the adrenal gland, the discourse concretizes and (to use Lukács' term) reifies a
complex socioemotional reality.[7] By focusing solely on physiologic details, the participants temporarily skirt the psychologic disturbance that
both parties realize is occurring. Further, the debating stance that they
assume deflects attention from the patient's grief. Meanwhile, the patient
vents her frustration and probably some anger as well through quibbling
about physiology.

The debating style and undercurrent of hostility persist until the end
of the encounter. At times, the doctor's patience seems to wear thin, for
instance as he responds to a challenging question, "Well, uh:::h, that's a
good question, but it's been answered" (line 124). Later, when the doctor
reiterates that the patient's adrenal function was "quite good" when she
was not taking corticosteroids, the patient replies, "Well, I didn't give a
hoot" (line 144). The patient also disagrees with the doctor's claim that
her blood pressure is normal:

D: Well, your blood pressure's always been fine.   260
P: You call that fine, a hundred forty was it over eighty six?
D: Yeah, that's normal pressure.
        [
P: I call it high.

Finally, doctor and patient argue about the meaning of the patient's
visual symptoms:

P: I've got spots in front of this eye, now,
    I've got to have my glasses changed, I read too much.   305
                        * * *
D: OK. Uh, uh, they're uh, actually those so-called floaters are
    not uncommon, they usually don't mean anything, uh.   315

P: Means I'm reading too much.
D: Well, even that, not necessarily.
P: Oh really?
D: No.

If she reads too much, perhaps the patient knows too much, or at least enough to present herself as an articulate, skeptical, challenging person, who holds high regard for her own knowledge and doubt if not disdain for the doctor's. Yet the banter goes beyond the usual bounds of doctor-patient repartee. Throughout this debate, a tense emotional undercurrent flows just beneath the surface.

A mental state. To reiterate, as the encounter opens, the patient requests more Decadron and claims, "I'm half dead most of the time." What does this mean? Here is how the topic of emotional distress initially enters and leaves the dialogue:

D: But the main problem now is the weakness?
P: Yes, just no ambition. Nothing. I started on the, uhm, the antidepressants. Have you got a stronger one, they're no good.
D: Uh huh, well, uh,
P: I'm really in a state, I'm in a mental state, there's no doubt about it.
D: When, when we're, uhm, while we're talking about the Decadron, let me ask you one other thing and that is, you remember you were taking two tablets every other day.

Apparently, then, when she says that she is "half dead," the patient's metaphorical language refers mainly to depression. Although she alludes to depression only indirectly by mentioning the antidepressant medication, her lack of ambition and disturbed mental state signify a depressed mood. While she answers affirmatively to the doctor's question of whether the main problem is weakness, her account reveals that weakness has become a subjective disturbance, linked to emotional upset and going beyond whatever objective muscle weakness may be present. Moreover, the image of being half dead raises the question of when the patient will be fully dead. The extent to which death preoccupies her, as one element of depression, remains unclear in this particular passage, since neither patient nor doctor pursues the theme until nearly the end of the encounter. Here the doctor cuts off this theme by returning to technical questions about Decadron dosage.

Later, within their lengthy debate, patient and doctor return to the problem of no ambition. Here they each interpret this symptom quite differently. The patient doubts that lack of ambition comes from her muscle disease; she implies that something else is causing this difficulty, either adrenal dysfunction or, more likely, her "mental state" itself. However, the doctor reinforces his view that muscle disease remains the main explanation:

D: Yeah. But that is uh:::h not. Uh, really, your adrenal,
that's not because you have adrenal disease. You don't.
You have muscle disease. If you, if you didn't have
muscle disease then we'd stop your Decadron.   105
P: And we'd have, still have no ambition, and stuff. That has
nothing to do with your muscles, your ambition, and your desire
to do something, your ability to do it.
D: Sure it does. You have muscular weakness. You tell me you
cannot walk really very much-

Thus the patient pinpoints the difficulty in an experience of absence: a lack of "ambition," a lack of "desire." For her, such a lack mainly constitutes a psychologic phenomenon, part of her distressing "mental state." This interpretation of her own experience emerges as an essentially psychoanalytic one. The doctor's interpretation, however, remains quite at odds from the patient's. For him, lack of ambition does indeed reflect an organic process of some kind.[8] Here he claims that muscle disease itself can explain the patient's mood disorder, since it limits her physical mobility.

In the discussion of adrenal dysfunction, he adds a further organic interpretation, concerning the impact of corticosteroids on emotions. Predictably, he notes, the adverse emotional response to this medication improves when the drug is stopped:

D: and the, uh, emotional response takes
a long time to get back to normal too. That's why we fought
so hard to keep you off the steroids.
P: Seven weeks and I'm mmmh back in bed.   150

Based on clinical experience and the medical literature, the doctor believes that the patient's emotional lability likely would improve after discontinuation of corticosteroids.[9] Still, the patient remains unconvinced, as she again describes how lack of ambition keeps her in bed.

Despite its rationale, the doctor's reified, organic interpretation of psychologic disturbance does not encourage dialogue about socioemotional difficulties that the patient experiences. For instance, the organic theory leaves unexplored those contextual issues that may be troubling the patient, beyond her physical disease and its pharmacologic treatment. No doubt, the organic factors that the doctor is postulating may well be involved. The doctor's rather tenacious attempt to persuade the patient on this score, however, moves the discussion away from other matters that may prove even more pertinent to the patient's emotional upset, as eventually becomes clear.

The patient herself later returns to the theme of emotional distress, as she raises the option of seeing a psychiatrist. Although she longs to consult a psychiatrist, she states that she cannot afford to do so:

P: I can't, if someday I get
  to the point that I can have a psychiatrist to help me, he
  won't solve them, but he might help me in, and like for
  instance, I have worries like fury and that takes so much out
  of you, you, you just don't go to sleep just thinking about it.
D: Have you thought of seeing a psychiatrist?
P: I can't afford one.
D: ((laughs))
P: That lets that out.

Here the patient takes the initiative in pointing out some limited goals for psychiatric help. She believes that her "worries" and resulting insomnia might become less burdensome through psychotherapy. Despite such potential advantages, financial limitations stand in the way. The doctor's laughter after the patient mentions this constraint may convey his own discomfort in facing the contextual impediment.

Although the doctor then makes a suggestion about less expensive alternatives for mental health services, the patient replies that these options have failed in the past. Specifically, she complains that less than fully trained psychiatrists have accomplished little in her case. Further, she concludes on a pessimistic note, claiming that she sees no hope for solving her emotional problems:

D: Yeah, uh, although there, there's an outpatient clinic with
  the, uh
P: Yeah, and they send you to a social service psychiatric girl
  that's a waste of your time.
                    * * *
D: Is Dr. —— a psychiatrist?
P: He sent me on to one of these girls, what do they call them,
  psychiatric workers, or something, and she was as good as
  nothing, and I went to her a few times.
D: ((laughs)) Well, it's difficult. Well, we'll put that in the
  back of our mind at the moment.
P: You know there's nobody's gonna solve these problems, 's gonna
  help me to live with them, that's about the size of it. And
  when you're sittin' there looking at nothing, why you, you just
  don't solve them. I've got spots in front of this eye, now,
  I've got to have my glasses changed, I read too much.

Seeing no psychiatric alternative, the patient reverts to an image of solitude and suffering, in which a person stares into empty space. In the pain of the moment, the picture of looking at nothing slides into the process of vision itself. Thus, the patient changes the topic slightly to a concrete visual symptom—a potentially more manageable problem than looking for help and finding only a lack.

Later, the theme of death crops up again, together with an innuendo of suicide. As the doctor recommends a change in brand of cortico-steroid, the patient asks for a stronger antidepressant medication. The ensuing dialogue reveals that the patient has not used the previous antidepressant for a long enough time to judge its therapeutic impact. Further, she talks of death and hints at self-destruction:

P: Have you got a stronger antidepressant?
D: Well, how much of the amitriptyline are you taking?
P: Well, I just started over again the other night, taking one at
    night and one in the morning.   355
D: Ah, you know that is not going to work for weeks, it's a
    strong antidepressant, but it won't work till you build up a
    level.
P: ((in a whisper)) Dear God. ((back to normal)) I'll take
    two of something else beforehand, I'm afraid. ((laughs))   360
    Go off, someday, I, really, some days are murder.
D: Yeah, I, I think really the best thing is to stick to that and
    don't stop it. You see, if you stop it, you're back at point
    zero again. And it generally works, but it does take a while.
P: Oh, all right. But really, I'm very preoccupied with death.   365
    I know there's an awful lot of mental stuff mixed up with that.
D: I know, uh, what we got to do is get you feeling better, and
    then you won't be.
P: Maybe that is the answer, I hope . . . . .

When the doctor asks her to wait "weeks" for the original antidepressant, amitriptyline, to take effect, the patient whispers a religious introjection and then laughingly refers to taking "something else beforehand." What does this dark humor mean? The patient does not say, and the doctor does not ask. However, the patient immediately gives a hint, when she says that "some days are murder" and adds that she is preoccupied with death. If she thinks about dying in the midst of depression, has she contemplated killing herself? The doctor does not inquire about any concrete plans that she might have, nor does he assess her suicide potential in other ways. Rather, he offers a reassuring statement that portends an improvement in the patient's physical health through tech-nical manipulation of her medications. Wistfully, the patient concurs that this approach may help, although (as she indicates through the words "maybe" and "I hope," line 369) substantial doubt remains. Without the economic wherewithal for psychiatric assistance, and with a technical change in corticosteroid brands recommended by her internist, she thus returns to the day-to-day vicissitudes of her "mental state."

Housewife and mother. The patient's responsibilities in the home weigh heavily upon her. Although she graduated from secretarial school, she defines her occupation as "housewife" and has maintained the family's household for quite a long time, apparently without much assistance. She defines the functional effects of her muscle disease and psychic distress largely in terms of impact on housework and family relationships, especially children.

The lack of "ambition" that characterizes her depressed "mental state" limits her ability and desire to perform simple household tasks. At several points in the encounter, she alludes to this deficit, for instance when she notes that the disinclination to dust has become more important to her than difficulty in walking:

P: I can't walk, but that's not bothering me, I can't even dust,
   is more important.
D: Hm.
P: But I don't want to dust. That's the main thing. It's a,
   bumped into a mental attitude.
D: Sure. But don't you see that the only way to get around that
   is to get off Decadron or get on a dosage of Decadron that isn't,
   uh, too large.

Physical weakness because of muscle disease thus has not emerged as the principal factor restricting performance of her customary social role. Rather, her "mental attitude" has become the main impediment. The doctor does not explore her psychic distress at this point but instead switches back to the reified, technical realm, as he reiterates his preference to reduce corticosteroid medication. This return to the technical cuts off discussion about emotional components of functional incapacity, as the patient not only fails to meet the usual expectations of her social context, but increasingly does not even want to meet them.

As she relates her perceptions, however, the patient's problem of "mental attitude" applies not only to housework but also to her children. About midway through the encounter, within the debate about adrenal disease and alternate-day corticosteroid treatment, the patient mentions a theory that her muscle disorder may have a hereditary basis:

P: Have you ever thought, did you, that possibly I was born
   with that, problem.
D: Which problem?
P: The muscle one, the adrenal.
D: Well, I don't think you have an adrenal problem.

With characteristic initiative, however, the patient does not let the matter drop. Even if the adrenal gland is not pertinent, she hypothesizes, the muscle disorder may be congenital. In response, the doctor equivocates in saying that the disease could be either congenital or acquired:

P: Well then maybe it was the muscle stuff I was born with,
    because I had this
        [
D: We::ll,   220
  [
P: same reaction only not so often in my younger days.
D: Yeah, uh, that's harder to say because we don't know a great
    deal about the causes of this sort of, uh, muscle problem
    anyhow. It's, uh, an inflammatory disease of muscle, it is not,
    you know, usually you, felt not to be born with it, but, uh, I   225
    don't think we can prove that one way or another.

Why does the patient express such interest in the congenital versus acquired causality of her disease? In some respect, her style here resembles that elsewhere; the intellectualized, argumentative format seems to defend against the troubled emotional undercurrent.

In the passage that follows, however, the patient finally reveals a more substantive and rather guilt-ridden concern: that a hereditary tendency somehow may have affected both herself and her two retarded children. She has given birth to three children, of whom two were born retarded. Of the latter, one has died, and the other presents a series of problems that the patient describes through much of the remaining encounter. At first, as she interrupts the doctor to introduce the topic of congenital retardation, nervous laughter accompanies both her remarks and the doctor's subsequent response:

D: So I don't think it's anything you did or didn't do,
    at least as far as we know.
    [
P: Y'know, I'm always in the back of my mind trying to
    find out why the two retarded, ((laughs)) (words) conniptions.
D: ((laughs)) I know, ah, if you find out let me know. Uh, yeah.   235
P: They found a lot of them, but not mine.
D: Pardon?
P: They find out a lot of them, but not mine.

Searching for clues from medical researchers (to whom the patient must be referring with the pronoun "they"), she has found none pertinent to her own offspring. After the doctor expresses doubts about the relation between muscle disease and mental retardation, the patient reveals that her concern about adrenal disease stems at least partly from a possible hereditary connection between herself and her children:

D: Yeah, I think in that case, well, offhand, at least, there's
   no relation I ever heard of between your muscle disease and
   mental retardation in the children, uh.
P: No, well, I was thinking glands, you see.
D: Oh, I see. Well, no, even, even if we thought there was adrenal
   disease, uh, uh, it would be any
   [
P: Well, they seem to be finding out more about glands now in
   connection with it,
D: Oh, sure, that's true.
P: but, uh, even so. Now, well, that's why I ask some of these
   questions. That's always in the back of my mind.

With this revelation, the patient's contentiousness about the adrenal gland becomes more comprehensible. Her adrenal dysfunction holds more than academic interest for her; nor is her concern about the adrenals simply a matter of her own physical and psychic distress. The adrenals also may hold a secret that would give meaning to the awful burden of producing defective offspring. Again, the doctor gives an equivocal rejoinder to the theory of hereditary connection, as the patient continues to ruminate about this explanation.

Besides retardation, her son suffers from hypertension and obesity, which the patient next laments. Just before patient and doctor begin to argue about blood pressure, the patient mentions the son's condition:

P: The retarded that's left has got high blood pressure now, that's
   enough to let mine up worrying about it.
D: Yeah.
P: We got his down, but they (words)
D: He has high blood pressure?
P: He eats like there's no tomorrow. He weighs two hundred
   and ten pounds.
D: Well, your blood pressure's always been fine.

Although the patient may want to discuss or at least emote about her son further at this point, the doctor's reassuring comment about her own normal pressure cuts off the contextual dialogue.

Later, the topic of antidepressant medication jogs the patient to return to the theme of the retarded son. The conversation here involves a series of steps, including references first to the antidepressant, then to the patient's own blood pressure, and then to the son's blood pressure:

D: Stick to the amitriptyline at the moment.
P: Okay. Oh, I think that was all I had in mind.
D: Okay.
P: Long as the blood pressure stays down there.   390

* * *

P: —— [son]'s down, but I worry about his.   400
D: Really? Is he doing all right?
P: Oh, he's down to 140 over 82.
D: Well, that's pretty good pressure.

Again, the doctor's attempt to reassure apparently produces little effect, since the patient then expresses concern about the son's weight and the lack of an effective diet for him:

P: Yeah, but you see, they don't put him on any diet, or they, he's
    on that pill, and (word) or something like that, (words), or   405
    something like that.
D: For his pressure.
P: For his pressure. They brought it right down. But what good's
    a pill if you're gonna be eatin' like that,

In this way, the patient continues to worry about the treatment of her re-tarded child, who now has reached adulthood. During the dialogue, the doctor offers brief reassurances, without eliciting further details about the home situation or the patient's caretaking responsibilities.

Just before the encounter concludes, the patient conjures a fantasy of the son's death. Her imagery conveys a presumption that death would become a more charitable outcome than the suffering that life offers:

P: If the Lord would take him in a massive stroke, that I could
    take. But being, God, just crippled, a half cripple, why,
    that's worse.
D: Let's hope that doesn't happen either, right.
P: No, that's what I think. But's those high blood pressure's   420
    that go. All right, thank you.
D: OK. I'll see.
P: I'll make an appointment for a month, anyway,
D: Yeah, if you would.
P: and then I'll call you first of the week.   425
D: Sure.

The patient's allusion to her son's death contains ambiguously mixed messages. While death might prove more humane for him, his demise also might bring emotional relief for the patient. Further, these words recall her own death wish, conveyed by the subtly suicidal preoccupations that she expresses earlier. In the end, patient and doctor together consent to cutting off the theme of death, as their words move to the more routine matter of scheduling a follow-up appointment.

In those parts of the dialogue that involve the patient's role as housewife and mother, pertinent elements remain absent. For instance, at no time does the patient's husband enter the conversation. Although in her questionnaire the patient gives "housewife" as her occupation, the man whose wife she is stays invisible. If the husband has left the household, because of death or other reasons, the patient mentions nothing about it, nor does the doctor ask. If the husband still lives with the patient, his relation to the patient's physical and psychic problems receives no attention. Further, alternative arrangements to ease the burdens of the housewife role go unexplored. The patient clearly feels these burdens, as she mentions how her lack of ambition and possibly her muscle weakness interfere with such activities as dusting (lines 111–14 above). Extra resources to help the patient perform these chores (such as homemaking services), or changes in role expectations within the family that would take these responsibilities off the patient's hands, do not arise as feasible possibilities. Similarly, caretaking options for the patient's adult, retarded son do not present themselves.

Such missing elements treat the patient's family context as given and essentially unchangeable. On the other hand, interventions to modify family roles might help the patient deal with her functional limitation. Alternatives to the contextual status quo would seem not particularly radical nor necessarily upsetting for the patient and her family. Yet the discourse accepts an assumption that the patient will continue to cope as best she can in a burdensome situation, with whatever assistance a switch in her medications can provide.

Ideology and structure. Through much of the encounter, as socioemotional matters give way to technical ones, the discourse reinforces an ideology of reified, scientific technique. Medical science explains the patient's experience mainly as a psychologic manifestation of physical disease and medication toxicity. Despite the debate that the patient's skepticism generates, the doctor makes diagnostic judgments about what causes what. The doctor's expertise, for instance, leads him to conclude that adrenal disease is not significantly involved and that the patient's psychic distress should improve through adjustment of corticosteroid medication. From this view, muscle disease requires just enough corticosteroids to suppress inflammation, without creating unpleasant emotional responses or other undesirable side effects. The doctor also assumes responsibility for making such technical decisions about treatment, although the patient challenges him at many points. While suggesting antidepressant medication, he accedes to the patient's complaint that psychiatric therapy is beyond her financial reach and that less expensive options would not be helpful. As highly charged contextual issues present themselves—financial insecurity, the stress of family responsibilities, the associated preoccupation with death, and so forth—the dialogue returns in each instance to the technical content of diagnosis and treatment. That, after all, is the medical task.

Here an emphasis on scientific technique also conveys another ideologic assumption, regarding individual acceptance of contextual difficulties. The discourse does allow the patient to express at some length the sadness and stress that she experiences, largely in relation to the responsibilities of her role as housewife and mother. Yet, change in context does not arise as an option. Instead, the discourse assumes that the patient will continue to shoulder her customary burdens, albeit with some help from adjustments in medication. The ethos of individualism guides the patient along her lonely path. Ultimately, the dialogue leads her to continue a stoical course, as she sees that no one will solve her contextual problems and that she simply will have to "live with them" (lines 301–02).[10]

From this encounter, several structural elements become apparent (figure 9.1). In her role as housewife and mother, the patient faces a difficult contextual issue of maintaining role responsibilities in the face of incapacitating physical disease. The family constellation includes a demanding, mentally retarded, adult son; another mentally retarded child who has died; and a husband whose whereabouts and impact remain uncertain. Financial limitations have restricted her ability to obtain assistance, for instance from a psychiatrist. Although she received training as a secretary, recently she has not worked outside the home (A). These issues have generated personal troubles that include depression, preoccupation with death, and distress about the inability to perform her customary duties. An emotional reaction to corticosteroids also may worsen these sorrows (B). During an appointment with her doctor (C), she complains at length about her current "mental state," the burdensome details of her family obligations, financial problems, and unsuccessful attempts to get professional help (D). Throughout the encounter, tensions arise as doctor and patient debate with each other about elements of diagnosis and treatment. In response to the patient's concerns about depression and functional incapacity to perform household duties, the doctor restricts the focus to technical manipulation of corticosteroid medication. Further, patient and doctor cut off a discussion of death by turning to the administrative procedure of scheduling a follow-up appointment (E). In managing the patient's contextual difficulties, the doctor relies on techniques of scientific medicine, which in this case involve a recapitulation of past diagnostic maneuvers and an adjustment of future medications. The reified focus on technical matters reinforces an ideol-

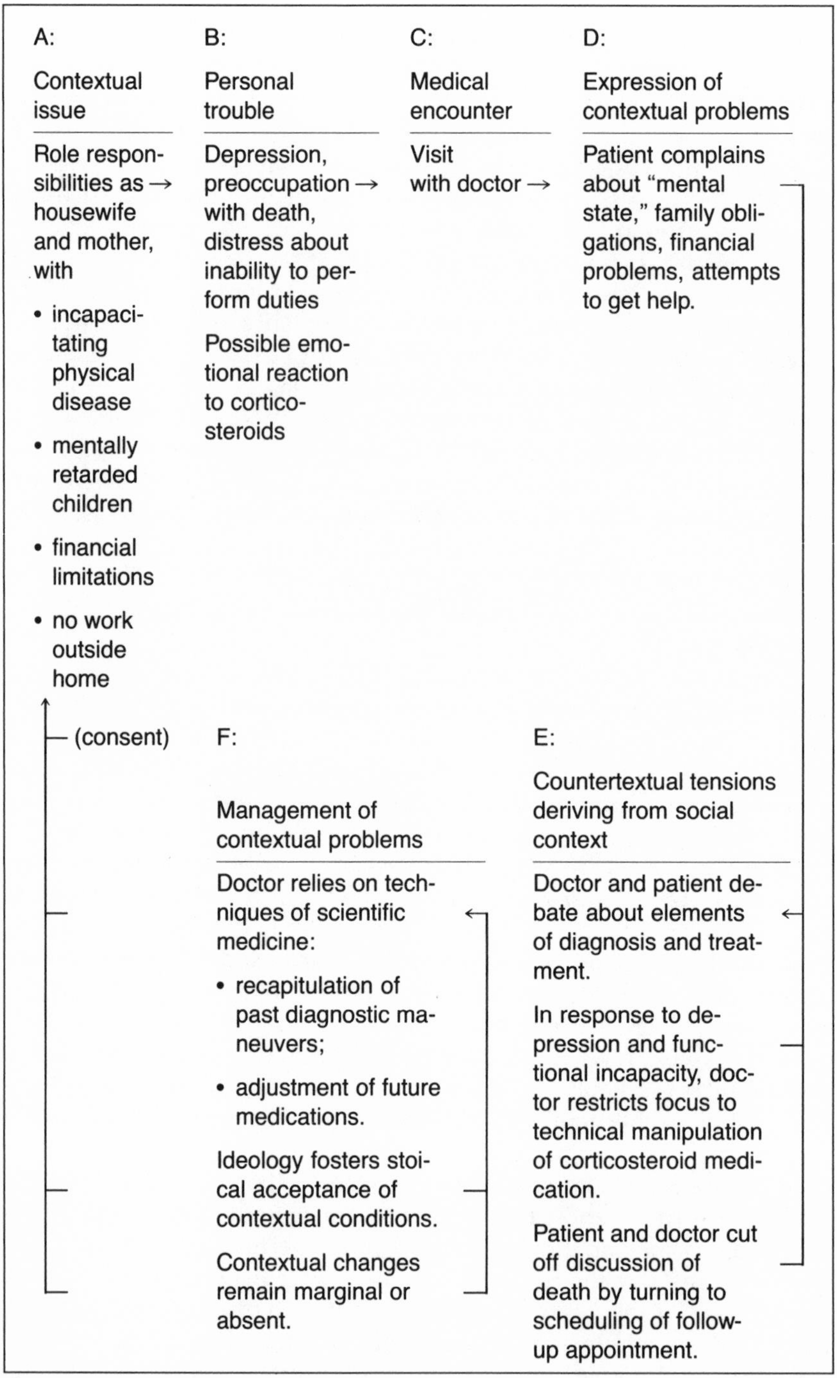

A: Contextual issue	B: Personal trouble	C: Medical encounter	D: Expression of contextual problems
Role responsibilities as → housewife and mother, with • incapacitating physical disease • mentally retarded children • financial limitations • no work outside home	Depression, preoccupation → with death, distress about inability to perform duties Possible emotional reaction to corticosteroids	Visit with doctor →	Patient complains about "mental state," family obligations, financial problems, attempts to get help.

— (consent)

F: Management of contextual problems	E: Countertextual tensions deriving from social context
Doctor relies on techniques of scientific medicine: ← • recapitulation of past diagnostic maneuvers; • adjustment of future medications. Ideology fosters stoical acceptance of contextual conditions. Contextual changes remain marginal or absent.	Doctor and patient debate about elements ← of diagnosis and treatment. In response to depression and functional incapacity, doctor restricts focus to technical manipulation of corticosteroid medication. Patient and doctor cut off discussion of death by turning to scheduling of follow-up appointment.

Figure 9.1
Structural elements of a medical encounter with a woman whose emotional distress may reflect toxicity from corticosteroid treatment of inflammatory muscle disease

ogy that fosters stoical, individual acceptance of troubling contextual conditions. Consideration of simple contextual changes that might ease the patient's role responsibilities remains marginal or absent from the dialogue (F). Afterward, the patient returns to her previous situation, presumably aided by a modified corticosteroid regimen and a continuing dose of antidepressant medication.

Patient and doctor here work a puzzle containing physical and socioemotional pieces. Both subjects try to put together the pieces in good faith, despite differences in position and motive. In doing so, they use an implicit set of ideologic instructions, which lead them to focus on technical components first and foremost.[11] Because nontechnical, contextual pieces do not fit very well in this scheme, they move to the margin. Emphasis on the technical then produces a picture with missing parts, jagged edges, and a sense of incompletion, yet not for want of trying.

PROCESSING TROUBLESOME EMOTIONS

While it is no surprise that troublesome emotions appear in medical encounters, their frequency goes beyond what one might expect. The interactions considered in this and earlier chapters come from a random sample of internists and clients.[12] For this reason, what transpires here would seem fairly typical of such encounters. Although statistical claims based on this sample probably are not warranted, the processing of troublesome emotional content within "primary care" doubtless occurs frequently enough to comprise a substantial part of what doctors and patients do when they meet.

Contextual issues figure prominently in the emotions that patients and doctors discuss. These issues typically involve work and associated economic insecurity, men's and women's roles in the family, aging, and substance use. Medical encounters provide one forum for the expression of such issues and the personal troubles that they generate. These concerns, however, usually differ from what is viewed as the task at hand. As a result, tensions arise, and contextual issues tend to gravitate toward the margins of the dialogue. Conversational devices that accomplish this marginalization include interruptions, other cut-offs, de-emphasis, absence of attention, and similar maneuvers.

Sometimes, as in Encounter 9A, troublesome emotions emerge, at least in part, as manifestations of physical disease or drug toxicity. Even here, however, contextual issues enter. Such problems can present special challenges, which involve sorting out physical and socioemotional causes. In the sorting process, however, the technical gaze of medicine tends to reify contextual matters while focusing on physical factors and their manipulation. Although such factors may play a relatively small part in a patient's experience of psychic distress, they prove relatively amenable to technical comprehension and management.

As doctors and patients process troublesome emotions, they turn to several characteristic alternatives. In many cases, they adopt the technical option of psychotropic medication. In other instances, doctors provide counseling, referral to other professionals, or simply a sympathetic ear. At some point in the encounter, the dialogue usually moves away from contextual issues that generate personal troubles. To whatever extent possible, doctors and patients avail themselves of medicine's technical and humanistic armamentarium, which does not generally include a critique of social context or advocacy of contextual change. As the medical encounter calms emotional distress, it conveys an assumption that patients will somehow continue to cope with the often distressing routine of their day-to-day lives. The absence of contextual options casts a shadow over what doctors and patients can hope to accomplish in each other's presence.

THE NEGATIVE
CASE
NONPROBLEMATIC
ENCOUNTERS

Until now, the encounters have more or less confirmed a single theoretical point of view. Or, at least, the transcripts, which illustrate the variability in sampled doctor-patient interactions, have not contradicted the theory too much.

To recap briefly, the theory argues that medical discourse contains an underlying structure, rarely recognized consciously by doctors and patients who speak with each other. In the social contexts of patients' lives, issues arise that create personal troubles. Such issues include difficulties with work, economic insecurity, family life and gender roles, the process of aging, the patterning of substance use and other "vices," and resources to deal with emotional distress. To varying degrees during the medical encounter, patients express these troubles. Although some humanistically inclined doctors supportively listen to such concerns, the traditional format of the interview does not facilitate their expression. Countertextual tensions then arise, sometimes manifested at the margins of discourse, or through dominance gestures like interruptions, cutoffs, and de-emphases that move the dialogue back to a technical track. The management of contextual problems involves reified, technical solutions (such as medication) or counseling, but also subtler verbal processes that maintain professional surveillance of individual action and that reproduce mainstream ideologic assumptions about appropriate behavior. Medical management also reproduces ideology through crucial absences—for instance, a lack of criticism focusing on social context

231

and an exclusion of such unspoken alternatives as collective action leading to social change. In the process, medical discourse contributes to social control by reinforcing individual accommodation to a generally unchanged context. With the technical help and emotional gratification that they have received, patients perhaps become better equipped to cope, as they continue their consent to the social conditions that troubled them in the first place.

Yet, to argue that *all* medical encounters manifest this underlying structure would be a mistake. In fact, many do not. How many? Based on the random sampling procedures that we used in this study,[1] I estimate that a substantial minority—between one-fourth and one-third of sessions involving similar doctors and patients—do not show many or most of the characteristics described here. This statistical inference obviously remains rough, based as it is on a sample of 50, selected randomly from a larger random sample of 336 encounters. Among the 50 fully transcribed encounters, we found 15 that showed little or no evidence of contextual issues, personal nontechnical troubles, ideologic reproduction, social control, or the other key elements of our theory. If the study were repeated, I cautiously predict that the nonoccurrence of these patterns would approximate the proportion that we found.

The existence of the "negative case" leads to certain trepidations. First of all, it limits the theoretical claims that one might make. Specifically, the theory as offered helps explain some, possibly most, but definitely not all medical encounters. Second, nonconfirmation in at least some instances raises a question about the theory's cogency overall. If the theory remains inapplicable to a substantial number of encounters, even a minority, how worthwhile a theory is it? Finally, the encounters that do not confirm the theory might share common characteristics. These features then may suggest a theoretical position different from the one developed here. For all these reasons concerning theory, one must get to know the negative case more intimately.

For methodologic reasons, as well, the negative case must be examined. Although this study tries to improve on some defects of prior research, the method adopted here calls for several compromises.[2] One compromise involves the search for variability of content. Our research team expected in advance that a random selection process would lead to a range of findings, only some of which would support our theoretical leanings. We therefore planned to pay attention to those encounters that lacked the substantive themes that most interested us. Becoming acquainted with the negative case then becomes a methodologic requirement, notwithstanding its humbling potential.

The following interactions convey a spectrum of encounters that lack the underlying structure described previously. Specifically, contextual issues and personal nontechnical troubles do not enter the discourses.

Although the encounters vary considerably, they share certain commonalities. Understanding the common features sheds a new light on the theory that the encounters superficially seem not to confirm. Further, the characteristics of these negative findings reveal some reasons why contextual issues sometimes do not appear in medical encounters.[3]

ENCOUNTER 10A: A CAMP PHYSICAL

SUMMARY

A teenager visits her doctor because the camp that she wants to attend requires a medical checkup. The doctor takes a medical history, performs a physical exam, and completes the necessary paperwork for camp.

Here is some information about the participants in the encounter, as revealed by the questionnaires that they filled out afterward. The patient is a 13-year-old white junior high school student who reports her religion as Eastern Orthodox and her ethnic background as Russian-Swedish-Danish. A general internist, the doctor is a 44-year-old white man, who expresses no religious preference and gives his ethnic background as German-English. Patient and doctor meet for the first time in the present encounter, which takes place in a Boston suburb. According to the doctor, the patient has no active medical problems.

Bureaucratic goals. This encounter belongs to a genre of medical visits whose purpose is to meet bureaucratic requirements, rather than the felt needs of a patient or doctor. Typically, a patient wants to do something in affiliation with an organization that requests medical authorization before accepting the applicant. By demanding medical clearance, an organizational third party presumably wants to avoid unpleasant surprises about physical disorders after the applicant begins activities for which the organization might be held responsible. In addition to camp physicals, such evaluations become commonplace before entering some schools, starting certain jobs, obtaining specific types of drivers' licenses, purchasing some kinds of insurance policies, gaining permission to immigrate to another country, and so forth. These settings usually involve an application procedure, one part of which comprises a physician's certification of good, or at least adequate, health.

Since in a sense the doctor becomes a gatekeeper for a third party, such encounters often take on unpleasant attributes. First, for physicians, visits with bureaucratic goals tend to become boring. Patients seeking routine medical clearance seldom manifest technically challenging problems, nor would they likely seek medical attention at the particular time if bureaucracy did not so require. Second, the definition of the situation calls for the doctor to assume a role of double agent. That is, the doctor must represent the interests of the organizational third party, as well as those of the patient. Even if the patient presents no pertinent pathology, the standardized and rather dull information usually requested in the paperwork of medical clearance can prove irritating. From the patient's perspective, the need to spend time and money on a medical evaluation desired not by oneself but by an organizational entity can raise hackles as well. Third, a patient on occasion may actually manifest a physical disorder that the doctor knows would adversely affect the likelihood of success. In that case, a doctor may feel obligated to bear bad tidings to both the patient and the organization in question. Alternatively, patient and doctor may enter a negotiation about "doctoring" a report to strengthen the patient's chances. For all these reasons, a medical encounter whose chief goal is bureaucratic may not exactly make one's day.

In this light, the participants in a bureaucratically oriented encounter reasonably would narrow their dialogue. Predictably, they would discuss information sought by an administrative third party, but without much elaboration. Although comprehensiveness proves beneficial in other settings, extra revelations here might muddy the water. When the purpose is to fill in the blanks on a standardized form, as efficiently and with as many correct answers as possible, there is no point in exploring potential problems in either the physical or social realm.

The bureaucratic focus accounts for the perfunctory and task-oriented content of the present encounter, a cordial first meeting between a teenager and an internist. Their exchange remains friendly and almost entirely factual, without any evidence of contextual difficulty, ideology, social control, or marginalization of concerns—despite several opportunities that would foster the appearance of these structural elements under other circumstances. Doctor and patient frame the encounter by affirming its administrative character. They begin:

D: You got a form to fill out?
P: Yeah.
D: Sit down a minute, won'tcha?

The same form, successfully signed, signals their departure:

D: Yeah . . . . Okay, I guess, uh, you want this back?
P: Yeah. We want to be able to send it to it to the camp.
D: I have my signature on it.
P: Yeah, okay.
D: Yeah.

Doctor and patient seem content to leave their future options open, since they do not mention any follow-up. In satisfying the camp's administrative requirements, they have met their goal.

Smoking mari-. During this encounter, the doctor interrupts very little, but one cut-off quickly seals Pandora's box. The passage in question occurs in response to the doctor's question about smoking, as the patient begins to provide information that is probably the last thing her camp counselor wants to hear:

D: Do you smoke at all?
P: Mari-   60
      [
D: Never smoke cigarettes?
P: No.
D: No. Good. Okay. Maybe we could bring you
   in here and take a look at you.

At 13, the patient apparently still believes that honesty is the best policy, even in dealing with bureaucracies. The doctor, however, knows better. If the patient smokes marijuana, the doctor does not want to hear about it. So he interrupts the patient, not even letting her finish the word. Qualifying his question about smoking, he immediately restricts the topic to cigarettes. Then the patient gives the correct, or at least more appropriate, answer. Subsequently, the doctor terminates the history entirely and begins the physical exam. The topic of illicit drug use then disappears from the conversation.

Under different circumstances, marijuana might not receive such a curt greeting. For instance, if the doctor were embarking on a longer term relationship with an adolescent patient, a person's volunteering information about recreational substances helps a physician gain a fuller picture of a patient's life-style. Further, monitoring and controlling drug use comprises a goal of prevention and health promotion, at least in some practitioners' view.[4] A doctor concerned about such matters might try to elicit further details about marijuana and maybe other substances that the patient uses. The social context—economic situation, family, school, friends, and so on—pertinent to drugs logically would warrant exploration. Finally, some pronouncement about life-style, conveying the society's more mainstream ideologic expectations, might come forth, as well as practical options for "detoxification." A bureaucratic rationale keeps the present conversation away from such themes, any one of which might keep this patient from going to camp.

Not exactly overweight. As adulthood flowers, this patient already has internalized an image of the healthy body. Specifically, like many other women in advanced industrial societies, she strives to be thin, even thinner than she already is.[5] Again, however, the encounter's narrow purpose truncates the discussion, as patient and doctor touch on this potentially problematic topic only in passing.

The theme emerges as the doctor asks a routine question about weight loss during the physical exam:

D: You haven't been
   losing weight?
P: Well, I've, I was trying to go on a diet, but it didn't do
   much for me.
D: You're not exactly overweight, you know.
P: I know, but,
   [
D: But you're on a diet anyhow.

According to the doctor, the patient shows no evidence of being over-weight. Nevertheless, she has been dieting, apparently trying to meet an unspecified standard that aims toward a weight a few pounds less than whatever it is at the moment.

Later the topic of weight returns, when patient and doctor negotiate about whether she should wear shoes on the scale; apparently, she would prefer to go shoeless, since this technique would yield a lower measurement.[6] The doctor's demeanor then takes on a touch of sarcasm:

D: We'll just see what your height and weight is here
                                    [
P: Okay, do you want me to peel off my sneakers?
D: No, okay, that'll do it with it on. If you weigh too much
   you can peel off those heavy sneakers.
P: Hheh hn.
D: With your clothes on, it's about 117.
P: I've gained two pounds.
D: Oh, yeah? Watch that.

Here the doctor implies that her scale anxiety about a few pounds more or less is somehow ridiculous. Yet such a concern lies beneath many an eating disorder among young women, who come to hold distorted body images because of a dominant cultural standard that values thinness.[7] Uncovering the social and psychodynamic bases of this problem, how-ever, would divert from the requirements of a camp physical. Perhaps reflecting the encounter's narrow goals, patient and doctor do not detour in that direction. In the end, the context of the patient's scale anxiety remains unexplored. The doctor's faint reassurance that the patient is "not exactly overweight" may or may not help her measure up to the culture's image of beauty.

Flubbing the softball throw. All in all, the patient's condition gives little reason for medical intrusion into the socioemotional context. She comes from a family well off enough to live pleasantly in an upper-middle-class suburb, to send her to camp, and to pay her medical bills.

True, she smokes a little dope and worries about her body a bit much. Yet she does well in school, enjoys social activities, reports no physical complaints, and passes the normal physical milestones of adolescent development (for instance, in the medical history, the doctor routinely confirms her onset of menses and normal menstrual periods, lines 50–58). In her comfortable situation, she can continue to experience the joys of youth, as her family provides the material means of subsistence.

Besides scale anxiety, the only other worry that the patient expresses involves athletics. Just after the doctor signs off on the camp physical, the patient describes some physical fitness tests that she has been taking at school. Although she does fine in running events, the arm hang, and the broad jump, the softball throw frustrates her ambition:

P: But I know I'm gonna flub it up when it comes to the softball throw. I can't throw a ball.
D: Oh really?
P: I can throw 'em, but not very far. I'm supposed to throw them ninety feet.   130
D: Really?
P: Maybe I can do it.
D: You'll have to practice that, I think.

As opposed to marijuana use and weight reduction, the doctor reinforces successes in athletics. If one has to worry about something, flubbing the softball throw seems not too bad.

Although the patient may not be mentioning other problems, a more likely explanation is that such problems simply have not arisen to any major extent. The patient is living her life in the realm of normalcy, fulfilling a set of expectations about what a normal person at her age ought to be doing. Even her indulgence in marijuana probably has become a normal part of upper-middle-class young adulthood.[8] Further, the bureaucratic goals of the encounter impose a framework that discourages contextual meanderings. There is no need for messages of ideology and social control here; the patient is meeting the society's ideologic expectations well enough at this point, and adequate controls already are in place.

ENCOUNTER 10B: PAIN AND DISCHARGE FROM THE PENIS

SUMMARY

A young man comes to his doctor because of pain during urination and a discharge from his penis. Doctor and patient discuss possible diagnoses, including venereal diseases like gonorrhea. After a brief physical exam focusing on the genitals, the doctor swabs the penis for microscopic examination, requests a urinalysis, cautions against sexual intercourse, and asks the patient to return for treatment the next day, after the lab results are ready.

Information about the participants is available from the transcript and the questionnaires that they completed. Although some demographic data are missing from the patient's questionnaire, it is apparent from the transcript that he is a student in his twenties who has received at least some college education and who is not married. The doctor is the same one as in the last encounter—that is, a 44-year-old general internist. Patient and doctor have known each other for about six months, and they are meeting in a private suburban practice near Boston. The doctor describes the patient's diagnosis as "nonspecific urethritis."

Not a strep throat. The encounter starts with a joke, as the patient laughingly describes his genitourinary symptoms:

D: Sit down, Mr. ——, won't you?
P: It's not as if I have strep throat.
D: Uh huh.
P: .Hh, hheh.
D: What, what do you think you have, gonorrhea, or
P: I don't know, I just have a, you know, a sharp pain urinating.

For the patient, problems of the penis do not remain emotionally neutral, and they warrant a nervous laugh. The patient next describes severe pain during urination and a penile discharge:

D: ((cough, cough)) And I take it it is not severe, or is it?
P: Yeah, it's very severe.

* * *

P: There's been a fluid coming out, just coming out. A, I mean,
  I, it seems to me like it's trying to lubricate itself.

In short, the patient is experiencing a painful genitourinary disorder whose import, despite the clowning around, goes beyond a sore throat.

As patient and doctor well know, a common culprit in such matters proves to be an infected sexual partner. Therefore, information about sexual conduct becomes useful, or at least fills out the picture. When a diagnosis of venereal disease comes forth, public health standards also call for finding all such partners and treating them as appropriate. The doctor gingerly approaches the topic of sexual activity with an indirect question, which asks for the patient's opinion about possible sources for the hypothetical possibility of gonorrhea. In response, the patient shows sophistication about the pathophysiology of sexually transmitted disease:

D: Do you know, you know if you did contract gonorrhea, do you
  know when you would have contracted it?

P: I, well, I don't know, what, what's the incubation time?
D: Well, the incubation period for gonorrhea can be around a week.
P: I suppose I could, you know, within reason. Yeah.

Information about gonorrhea's incubation period helps place the patient's sexual activity within the realm of reasonable causation.

Here and elsewhere in the encounter, the participants deal with casual sex in a casual way. Some minimal level of data about sexual partners becomes useful, but the inquiry stays brief and to the point. Further, moral evaluation remains undetectable. If the patient dabbles, that seems to be his own business, and the doctor's chief responsibility involves clearing up the problem at hand. After the doctor completes the physical exam, he states his preference for deferring treatment for one day, until he clarifies the diagnosis from laboratory test results. Meanwhile, he cautions the patient to avoid sex:

D: Since it's possible that this is   105
    gonorrhea, I'm gonna urge you to avoid sexual intercourse
    tonight. And uhm,
P: .Hh heh, don't worry, .hh heh.
D: eh, until we establish what happens.

Although the patient responds with laughter, the doctor's advice remains nonjudgmental. Further, he does not refer to a specific partner or partners. His only concern, he implies, is that the patient avoid infecting or receiving infection from others in the interim before treatment begins.

Fitting the patient in. Aside from a single indirect question about sexual activity, no other element of social context enters the dialogue of this brief encounter. As patient and doctor discuss the emotionally charged experience of a diseased penis, they both express no concern whatsoever about the social origins or effects of the patient's behavior. The matter-of-fact discussion contains no inquisition, no moralism, no positive evaluation of mainstream expectations, no disparagement of deviance. Patient and doctor instead focus narrowly on the technical problem of the patient's genitals. Why is the discourse so spare?

In the first place, because he has fit the patient into his schedule, the doctor probably does not have much time. This situational constraint may motivate the participants as they limit the discussion to the bare essentials. Although the doctor himself does not call attention to the unscheduled nature of the visit, the patient does so, as he expresses gratitude just after he receives instructions about how to give a urine specimen:

D: Yeah, actually, one of these paper cups. (words) And we'll
    see if ah,
P: OK. Thanks for fitting me in.   150
D: It's OK.

From this perspective, neither party may want to burden the interaction with extraneous details. A characteristic of the situation then may have much to do with the absence of contextual concerns. This observation suggests that unscheduled appointments, which aim to resolve urgent symptoms promptly, do not lend themselves to exploration of the social context. The point in such an encounter is to get the patient in and out. If and when the patient returns for a lengthier visit, more time would be available to delve into such matters as compliance with norms of appropriate behavior.

The patient fits not only into the doctor's schedule, however; he also apparently fits fairly well into his other social roles. As an unmarried youth who has not yet settled down, the patient creates no major difficulties at work or in the family through sexual dalliance, despite its adverse penile consequences. He also appears able to pay his bills, including his medical bill. His sexual activity comprises an expected and relatively nondisruptive pastime for a person of his age and social position. For this reason, even in a more leisurely appointment, delving further into the social context would seem a rather square thing to do. Time and maturity will probably straighten the kid out. If he continues to catch sexually transmitted diseases in his thirties, or after he becomes a family man, or when he works in a prestigious job—that would become a more appropriate time for preventive intervention.

In sum, this brief visit illustrates two further reasons why contextual issues sometimes do not arise in medical encounters. First, certain visits comprise hurried responses to urgent symptoms. Here, time constraints and physical discomfort truncate the dialogue, eliminating or abbreviating whatever contextual discussion and messages of ideology or social control might otherwise appear. Second, some problems predictably exert disruptive social effects in certain circumstances but not in others. For instance, sexual involvements comprise "normal" behavior during the unattached exuberance of youth (despite standards of safe sex in the AIDS era). With the social and material encumbrances of middle age, however, the same behaviors become substantially less normal. As long as a patient's activities remain in the realm of expected normalcy, and as long as antibiotics cure any adverse physical effects, medical discourse can afford to leave well enough alone.

ENCOUNTER 10C: MIDDLE AGE WITHOUT STRESS

SUMMARY

A woman comes to her doctor for a routine checkup. Doctor and patient initially discuss their recent vacations. Later, the doctor takes a comprehensive medical history, including information about the patient's family, job, and stress. The doctor also performs a physical exam, cleans the patient's ears, and reassures her about her health.

In questionnaires completed after the encounters, patient and doctor provide the following data. The patient, who is 46 years old, works as a part-time secretary and dance teacher. Her education includes a master's degree in an unspecified field. A married woman with three children, whose ages are 15, 11, and 8, she reports her race as white and her religion as Jewish; she gives no further response about ethnic background. From her point of view, the visit's purpose is to obtain an annual checkup and to get her ears cleaned. The doctor is a 54-year-old white male who practices internal medicine as a "primary physician." He states that his religion and ethnic background are Jewish. Patient and doctor have known each other for about thirteen years. The encounter takes place in a Boston suburb. From the doctor's perspective, the patient's main diagnosis is "cystic mastitis," by which he refers to small cysts of both breasts.

Gray-haireds on the slopes. Throughout the first part of the encounter, patient and doctor discuss vacations. They talk about the pros and cons of Caribbean beaches versus New England mountains. Then they review downhill versus cross-country skiing, focusing on the relative advantages of each for middle-age conditioning.

The encounter begins with comments about the doctor's recent jaunt to the Virgin Islands. Perhaps noting his tan, the patient introduces this passage. When the doctor asks about the patient's Caribbean experiences, she mentions her honeymoon in Jamaica and her subsequent preference for the snow:

P: Been basking in the sun all week.
D: One week, and it was delightful.
P: Uh huh, you mean you sneaked away for school vacation.
D: Yeah, between Christmas and New Year. We went down to the
    Virgin Islands for a little while.   5
P: That's great.
D: Yeah, I recommend it highly. Only trouble was coming back.
    ((laughter)) Have you gone there at all?
P: Well, no, we went to Jamaica on our honeymoon, and I'm very much
    in favor of fleeing northward in the wintertime.   10

Whether the honeymoon was all she had hoped remains unclear. Without doubt, however, she and her husband now take pleasure in skiing, especially after a substantial financial investment in equipment for a growing family:

P: Well, my husband is always in favor of a lot of skiing, this
   year because we've spent so much money on equipment this year.
D: It gets expensive.
P: Oh well, the uh . . .
D: Not only the equipment, lifts (words)
P: Oh yeah. Well, we try to economize as much as we can here
   and there, like accommodations, and bringing our lunches and,
   but when it comes to the children's equipment, that does add
   up, believe me.

On hearing this scenario, the doctor makes another plug for the beach:

D: Yeah, well, you might as well go down to the islands as far
   [as] money is concerned. Probably about the same as taking
   the family skiing.

If so much money needs to be spent, the doctor seems to argue, why not
warm up in a more exotic place?

   The discussion then moves to cross-country skiing, which presents
both financial and physical advantages for vacationers as they age. In
continuing this dialogue, patient and doctor briefly confront their own
aging processes. Conditioning from cross-country skiing, it seems, provides gratification and safety, even under the specter of coronary artery
disease:

D: But when you get older, you (words) . . . .
P: No, we figure we're just switch to cross-country skiing it's
   [
D: That's what some of my colleagues are doing now (words) . . . .
   [
P: safer, it's wonderful, it's great exercise . . . .
D: (Words) They don't want to do it, they do downhill skiing (words).
P: That's another way we stretch our money out.
D: Yeah. My very best friends who were up in country (words) last week
                           * * *
P: It was last week we were skiing with a
   gentleman who confessed something (words) that he had already
   worked off his second coronary, and he does both downhill and
   cross-country, but he does more cross-country.
D: My brother-in-law is now what, 66 or something, and he still
   downhill skis.
P: There's nothing wrong with it, you see a lot of, uh,
   gray-haireds on the slopes.
D: Apparently so.
P: Pretty soon our own.

By taking to the slopes in a reasonable way, then, gray-haired people can keep in shape and save money, too.

In devoting the first one-sixth of the encounter to a discussion of vacations, what do the patient and doctor accomplish? The chit-chat first of all gets the visit off to a friendly start. As they share information about leisure-time pursuits, the participants show each other that their relationship goes beyond professional cordiality. Using time in this way also signifies that they have in a sense become friends. Introduction of such personal detail, most of which remains irrelevant to the formal purposes of the meeting, bridges the interpersonal distance that commonly characterizes the doctor-patient relationship.

A second effect of this long opening parenthesis, however, is to establish the similarity of the participants' social-class positions. Both individuals clearly have obtained the financial wherewithal to enjoy the good life. Although they both refer to techniques of cutting costs, clearly they feel comfortable having money and spending it to have a good time. With wealth comes the opportunity to prioritize leisure and to give themselves a bit of luxury.

Third, the vacation scenario conveys an image of stable family life and integrated social networks. By saying that "we" went down to the Virgin Islands (lines 4–5), the doctor almost certainly refers to himself and his wife. The doctor also refers to the skiing experiences of his "colleagues," "very best friends," and brother-in-law. Similarly, the patient talks about her cooperative skiing arrangements with her husband, children, and another "gentleman" friend. Through such words, patient and doctor reveal family relationships and friendship ties marked by presumed stability, propriety, and fulfillment.

In short, as they discuss vacations, the participants in this encounter come across as upstanding, upper-middle-class people who have accumulated financial resources and social graces. Through their accounts, they imply that their family lives bring them comfort and that their friendships enrich their experiences. Further, their circles of friends have come to include each other.

A father's merciful death; a mother you can't stop. During the next part of the encounter, the doctor begins a long and routine medical history. Because the patient comes for a checkup and ear cleaning, their scheduled appointment leaves a great deal of time to talk about nonurgent matters. As the doctor takes this opportunity to fill in many details of the clinical history, he updates his prior notes.

The first part of this excursion, involving the family history, reveals that the patient's father died three years earlier. Despite the length of time that has passed, the event apparently stays fresh for the patient,

since she mentions it immediately following a general question about her
family:

D: Uh, could you bring me up to
   date with what in your family?
P: Well, my father died.
D: Yeah. When did he die?
P: Gosh, three years ago.
D: How old was he then?
P: He was in his seventies.

Although the father suffered from several medical disorders leading to
weakness, he had remained relatively well until his death, which came
quickly and apparently painlessly during sleep. In describing her father's
demise, the patient seems to agree with the doctor that dying in this
manner comprises a merciful way to go:

P: But it was the wearing down effect (words) . . . . .
                                         [
D: Uh huh.
   [
P: of the emphysema. It really . . . . though that was not the
   direct cause. He had these (words) blood to his brain
   apparently, deteriorating, which caused the stroke in his sleep.
D: It's the merciful way.
P: Oh::h. He wasn't really sick, you know, he was, you know,
   just weakened, but not . . . .
D: I wish that on all people when they'll (words).
P: Oh::h. That was, it was really, my mother said, you know, she
   knew when it happened exactly, because he uttered a (words).

In this passage, the patient pauses three times without completing the
sentence that she has begun (lines 90, 92, and 97). Such breaks in her
speech occur rarely throughout the rest of the encounter. From the
pauses, she conveys a sense that the father's death remains somewhat
unresolved, and that grief may persist. Yet she does not elaborate on her
feelings, although the doctor gives her some opportunity to do so as he
leaves the silence of her pauses uninterrupted for substantial periods of
time. Verbally at least, the patient diminishes her father's suffering and
seems content to accept the doctor's consolation that he would wish such
a benign death for "all people."

   While the loss of a father has proven relatively unproblematic, an
elderly mother also creates no apparent burden. At 77, the mother remains alive and kicking:

P: She will be 77.
D: Right, and she's doing fine?

P: Oh! She's driving the car all over the place, you can't stop
   her. She's the family gatherer.   110
D: Wonderful.
P: Constant company. She has a big house, she keeps it filled all
   the time.

At an advanced age, the patient's mother still serves as a source of companionship and pleasure. She suffers no incapacitating physical problems and maintains her functional autonomy. Her car and big house indicate that money has not become a problem either. Further, the mother preserves her own social network, as she fills her home with friends and loved ones. With such accomplishments, the mother emerges as a paragon of senior citizenship.

The doctor's further questions about family history reveal no difficulties that affect the patient's well-being or equanimity. In this inquiry, he learns that a sister has developed an ulcer, a grandmother had cancer, and an aunt died from leukemia. But none of these events has impinged on the patient's own life-style. In particular, the burdens potentially imposed by elderly parents apparently have taken no toll for this particular woman. The family history reveals a stable set of relationships among individuals who enjoy relatively good health, financial security, and social amenities.

Pooped at work. As a result of the doctor's exhaustive questions during the review of systems, the patient's work enters the dialogue. Although the patient apparently would not have brought up these minor problems if the doctor had not asked, she has suffered some aches and pains as a result of exertion at work. Yet here again, the patient does not indicate any continuing conflict or stress. For her, work's physical requirements comprise an expected part of what she wants to do in the occupational side of her life.

One such difficulty involves a strain of the hand muscles, incurred as she moved a heavy drum while teaching dance. The patient injured herself slightly, but the problem subsequently has cleared up:

D: No (words) weakness in the hand?
P: Oh, that was severe at that point, but then it's gone   295
   now. I do take precautions to make sure (words).
D: How well, if I think I can remember correctly you were
   involved tom-toms or something?
P: Yes, I was holding a heavy drum, and I didn't realize it and
   again, that too went away.   300

Such a temporary limitation would seem a small price to pay for the pleasure that teaching dance evidently brings.

A more irritating challenge arises at her part-time job as a secretary.

Because her office has moved, she complains about fatigue from hauling heavy typewriters and notes:

P: I had to haul it up and down every day, but, boy oh boy, by the
   end of that week I was pooped.   3

Although the patient clearly does not appreciate the physical require-ments that the office move has imposed, she presents the difficulty as a minor problem. Certainly, it does not affect her overall view that her job is worth doing. In fact, she takes some pride in her ability to transcend the temporary chaos. Getting pooped then becomes a sign of doing the job well.

No stress. With thoroughness, the doctor undertakes a lengthy and largely unrevealing review of systems. The patient reports that a prior foot pain has improved with more judicious skiing. Subsequent ques-tions and answers deal with dizziness, eyes, ears (including a recurrent problem with earwax), throat, lungs, and heart.

A presumably routine query about stress then occurs, to which the patient gives a firm, negative reply. She also links stress to exercise:

D: You don't get
   palpitations, rapid heart action, irregular heart action?   2
P: No.
   [
D: Stress or other things?
   [
P: No, what if you exercise a lot naturally you're going to feel
   a little bit more, but that is part of normal adjustment.
D: Oh yeah, sure is. You get no chest pains however under   2
   those circumstances that we just mentioned?

Her zest for exercise brings pleasure:

D: You can walk up a
   hill in cold weather and not get chest discomfort?
   [
P: Oh, I love it. I like to get exercise every day.
   [
D: Uh huh, exercise. Anyway, you still dance and do those things?
P: Yeah. Not not quite as much, you know, I still ride my bike   2
   and walk and do other things.

She even has escaped overweight, the curse affecting so many modern women:

D: Great. Your appetite remains healthy?
P: Very good.

D: You don't look as if you gained any weight.
P: No. About the same.   240

To enjoy life without stress or excess fat—what more could one wish?

When the patient denies stress, it is difficult to read anything else between the lines. For the most part, worrisome conditions that affect others in contemporary society—economic insecurity, work demands, family pressures, and so forth—really do seem to have bypassed this particular individual. As fortune smiles upon her, the discourse of medicine finds few if any targets for either technical or social intervention. The patient is leading the good life, along a straight and narrow course. In middle age, she epitomizes a life-style that the dominant society values: stable family relations across several generations, rewarding (though sometimes tiring) work, financial well-being, pleasant recreational activities, lack of self-destructive habits, low stress, and even the ability to maintain a lean body. With all this going for her, the patient needs nothing more in the way of ideologic talk.

Sometimes the patient grows impatient even with medicine's non-ideologic surveillance. About halfway through the review of systems, she reminds the doctor that getting her ear cleaned is the main reason for the visit:

P: As I say, this ear isn't hearing right now. That's   206
        why I'm here.

At this point, the doctor promises that he will look at the ear later and explains why wax accumulates. Later, as the doctor reviews her joints, the patient gets a bit piqued:

P: Ah, you ask me all these crazy questions. Well, actually I don't   283
   think I have.

When the inquiry continues, the patient eventually protests good-naturedly one last time, although she accepts the doctor's rationale for a standardized methodology:

D: No bleeding?
P: Boy, you're going through everything, especially since I   335
   don't take (words).
D: (Words). The same questions every time.
P: That's right, you like to treat people . . . . . .

Experiencing so few problems and wanting only her ears cleaned, the patient may well wonder why the doctor is making a mountain out of a waxhill. Comprehensiveness in the clinical history and physical exam, however, remains the way this doctor does his job as it deserves to be done.

Forty more years. A lack of stress coheres with elements of context that appear elsewhere in the encounter. The patient's happy circumstances lead the doctor to prognosticate optimistically about the patient's future. Assuming that surprises do not occur, he jokingly estimates that this 46-year-old woman will live about forty more years:

D: And no new developments (words). If you can
   stay that way for next forty years or so; we'll settle for forty.
P: Forty! Oh, easily, sure, why not?

As the encounter concludes, the doctor also states that, aside from blood tests already in process, nothing more needs to be done:

D: I don't think there's anything we need to pursue further at this
   time. So, stay well, and have a good year.
P: Thank you. And the same to you.
D: We'll see you next year. We did draw blood for various things.
P: Yeah, if there're any problems (words).
D: Blood pressure is excellent, below normal.
P: That's fine, I like it to stay nice and low.
D: That's good.

In the end, blood pressure becomes a metaphor for the general pressure of life. For this patient, such pressure remains "nice and low," and she likes it that way.

While this encounter differs glaringly from those considered in earlier chapters, it is important to remember that such situations actually exist. Certain people do lead relatively stress-free lives. Somehow, they escape the troubles that social issues create for many others. At times, this pleasant condition reflects the benefits of social-class position, although wealth does not guarantee the inner peace seen here. At other times, a combination of physical health, comfortable upbringing, emotional tranquility, and personal achievement brings about a relatively unproblematic state of affairs. This patient's experiences conform in most ways to mainstream ideologies and expectations about what makes life worth living. Experiencing few difficulties herself, she apparently creates none for others either. Hers is a life of comfort without extravagance, social integration without loss of individuality, suburban advantages without the fast lane. In a context like this, medical advice would add very little.

ENCOUNTER 10D: GOOD NEWS AT AN ADVANCED AGE

SUMMARY

An elderly woman with hypertension and a prior urinary tract infection comes for a follow-up visit. Doctor and patient discuss x-rays and lab tests, which all have yielded normal results with the exception of mild emphysema. They also comment on the patient's recent bronchitis, diet, and exercise. The doctor performs a physical exam and does an electrocardiogram. In addition to asking frequent questions pertinent to her health, the patient mentions events in the lives of several friends and family members.

In their questionnaires, patient and doctor give some pertinent information about themselves. A 73-year-old white female, the patient has one child, a 45-year-old daughter. She is married and a high-school graduate, who reports her occupation as "housewife." Expressing a Protestant religious preference, the patient states that her ethnic background is "American." The doctor is a 44-year-old general internist of German-English ethnicity and without religious preference. Acquainted with each other for about one month, doctor and patient are meeting in a suburban practice near Boston. The patient's diagnoses, as the doctor reports, include hypertension and urinary tract infection.

Wonderful news. Throughout the encounter, despite various physical difficulties, the patient gives an upbeat account of her life and social activities. During the lengthy dialogue, the patient reveals a network of friends and relatives, who care for her and bring happiness. Through her social contacts, her life takes on a quality of orderliness and well-being.

Right after she sits down, the patient initiates this line of talk, without waiting for further instructions or questions. Her comments focus on another doctor, who also has become somewhat of a friend. Roughly the same age as herself, the other doctor has pulled through major cardiovascular surgery for an aortic aneurysm. After a one-month recuperation, he has started to drive his car again. For the patient, this outcome comprises "wonderful news":

P: I just had some wonderful news today.
D: Yeah.
P: My doctor, y'know, had the operation, with the bubble on
   the (word), and it's been just a month, and he's driving his   15
   car.

In the subsequent passage, patient and doctor discuss the other doctor's operation. As she mentions her elderly doctor-friend's youthful self-appraisal, the patient also refers to the pleasant impact of good news for a person her age:

P: He said, "while I'm young, I should have it [surgery] done."
   He's 72! ((laughs))
      [
D: Right! ((laughs))
P: Oh, dear. It's so nice to hear a few good things nowadays,
   you hear so many . . .   55
D: Now, where is his office?

Evidently, the patient's age often causes her to learn of illness and death among members of her own peer group; her pause (line 55) seems to convey this meaning. That her doctor-friend, one year younger than herself, refers to his own age as young makes her laugh; that he has thrived after major surgery makes her happier yet.

The present doctor, much younger than the patient and her medical friend, takes an unhurried approach to this kind of discussion, which reveals more about her social network than about her technical problems. Similar parenthetical excursions occur later in the encounter, for instance when the patient mentions her granddaughters' medical needs. One granddaughter is entering puberty and seems ready to switch from a pediatrician to an adult physician. After asking the doctor if he would be willing to see a teenager, the patient goes on to provide a witty and empathetic account of the granddaughter's dilemma:

P: Now, tell me Dr. ——, uhm,
    do you take girls in their teens?
D: Uh, I, ye::s, the, uhm, pediatricians sometimes take see
    patients up through their teens, and, at some point, patients
    usually decide to change (words)
                      [
P: Well, my,
    my granddaughter will be thirteen this month, and, uhm, her
    mother (words) and she said, "I am not going to Dr. ——
    again, (words) to sit there with all those little people
    running kiddy cars and," and then she said, "get a lollypop
    when I get through!"
D: ((laughs))
P: And I could see her point.

Later, the patient breaks the silence of the physical exam as she brings up the intimate detail of a second granddaughter's menstrual irregularity:

P: Mm, mm, ((words, rustling noises)) menstruating yet.
D: She's fifteen?
P: Mm hmm. She just, she won't be fifteen 'till (words)
D: That's, not unusual.

The patient then reveals her continuing interest in her family's development:

D: How old were you, do you remember?
P: I was fifteen, but I think my daughter was fifteen.
D: Yeah.
P: And she was very irregular for a long while. She'd go to
    camp and be there all summer and not have a period.

Despite her advancing age, the patient stays attuned to the developmental milestones of her children and their children as well. She even participates to the extent of seeking medical care for granddaughters during the awkward period of adolescence. Her integration in family life helps her fulfill an active and helpful old age.

Although the doctor retreats to the silence of the electrocardiogram, the patient returns to the theme of hearth and home. This time she asks about the doctor's marital status and confirms that the joys of family only increase as children grow older:

P: Are you a married man?   305
D: Oh, yes . . . . . I have four children.
P: (words)
D: Four, that's a lot, right?
P: Right, yes, it's a lot as one, can be a lot (words)
D: Right.   310
P: Oh, they're wonderful all the time, but, I mean as they
   get older.

Here the patient conveys how much she values family and her own continuing integration within it. As a spokeswoman for stable family life, the patient expresses mainstream ideology. While children, especially in large number, can create work (apparently the meaning of "that's a lot, right?"), these efforts prove worthwhile. Although the patient does not mention her husband during the encounter, in her questionnaire she indicates that he remains alive and presumably well. From the gratification of her own experience, she can tell the doctor a thing or two about what family life ought to be, in response to which he finds little to add.

Beyond familial integration, the patient maintains a circle of close friends, going beyond the doctor-friend whom she mentions at the beginning. Other parts of her social network appear tangentially, in the course of discussions about nutrition and allergies. While commenting on cholesterol and salt reduction, patient and doctor note the dietary restrictions that prevention warrants. Such nutritional requirements to some extent have cramped the patient's culinary style:

D: Yeah, your cholesterol is not
   bad. All right?   385
P: (words) I kind of hate to dine with somebody else, there's
   so many things I've tried to cut out.
D: For your blood pressure.
   [[
P: Yeah,   yeah.

Although these restrictions dampen her enthusiasm somewhat, she continues such social engagements. For instance, she refers to a specific "girlfriend." This reference occurs when she expresses satisfaction that she will avoid potential allergic reactions, since the doctor does not intend to add medications:

D: Yeah, I'm willing to stay with that at the moment.
P: Well, I'm awfully glad, my girlfriend, went on a trip;
   she got some new medicine, she broke all out in a rash all
   over, and she had a horrible time.
D: It can happen.

These comments, though fleeting, point to a network of friendships. Supplementing her strong family ties, these friends provide the give and take of social relations that help the patient avoid the common isolation and loneliness of advanced age.

Too sympathetic. While she maintains a closely knit social network, the patient also avails herself of keen mental and physical faculties that remain. Throughout the encounter, she takes the initiative frequently, asking pertinent questions and controlling much of the interaction. This active behavior paints a picture of an alert, capable senior citizen, who tries to increase knowledge that she can use to improve her health and life circumstances.

At the beginning of the encounter, after starting the discussion about her doctor-friend's successful bout with surgery, the patient changes the subject to her own medical evaluation. As a transition, she asks (line 67), "Well, what did you find out about me?" In response, the doctor explains the normal results of blood tests and mentions that the chest x-ray is not quite normal but not worrisome either:

D: And uhm, your chest film, oh, you know your
   lungs have a little emphysema, they're really not bad. And
   apart from that, your, ah, your chest x-ray looks normal.

The conversation later reveals that the patient has suffered from bronchitis and pneumonia in the past.

Concerning her respiratory disease, the patient shows a similar type of question-asking demeanor, which leads to a very full explanation by the doctor (lines 81–136). Just after the doctor describes her chest x-ray, the patient initiates a further question about prevention of exacerbations:

P: Well, is, is there anything I can do about this bronchitis, to
   avoid it? ((laughs)) I know that's a very silly question.

Despite a laughing denigration of the question's importance, the patient takes the lead in requesting information. While the doctor does not offer any preventive advice, he again emphasizes that the patient's symptoms are not unusual and that full recuperation takes a long time. During the explanation, the patient says that she is "glad to know" information about her respiratory disease. Her continuing success in requesting and receiving pertinent knowledge enhances her ability to manage her life in an autonomous style.

Throughout the encounter, similar patient-initiated comments about
prevention, nutrition, and exercise convey her positive attitude toward
self-care. For instance, she follows her cholesterol closely and wonders
how she can gain weight without worsening her lipid profile:

P: Now along with
   diets, I have, can you tell me anything that I can gain weight?
   Oh, uhm, how about the cholesterol? How much is that?   155
D: Oh, your cholesterol is not terribly high. It was 265.
P: It's gone up higher. It was 250 when I (words)

In the subsequent discussion of cholesterol, the patient reveals that,
despite her "love" for cheese, she avoids it, along with eggs and other
fatty foods. She also has tried to use lecithin as a cholesterol-lowering
dietary supplement. To these measures, the doctor responds with as-
surances that the cholesterol level is "not really high." When he states his
view that substances like lecithin are ineffective and a waste of money,
the patient expresses gratitude for this information.

   As a further attempt to improve her nutrition, the patient has been
taking a vitamin, and she questions the doctor about this medication also
(line 426). When the doctor advises that vitamins are unnecessary, the
patient laughingly notes her future financial savings:

D: I don't think you need 'em really, but, uh, it doesn't hurt you
   to take them, but I think it's, it's really wasted, that you   450
   don't need them at all.
P: Thank you very much. You've just saved me eight dollars a (word).
D: There you are. ((Both laugh.))

Throughout the extensive dialogue on diet and vitamin supplements, the
doctor respectfully follows the patient's lead, as she gains the data that
she needs for optimal self-care.

   Reassured about diet, the patient then turns to exercise. She indicates
that she has taken up walking as part of a self-inspired exercise program,
and the doctor expresses support:

P: I started walking though, I was   470
   round the block yesterday, and I went round the block this
   morning, and I (words) ((laughs))
D: So, you're all right. Well, keep it up, walking's good for you.
P: Well I'm tryin' to.

In this passage as elsewhere, the patient's laughter does not diminish the
seriousness of her efforts to care for herself at an advanced age. Self-care
and prevention emerge as clearly defined goals, which her keen wit and
social resources assist her in meeting.

   The quality of the patient's senior citizenship wins the doctor's respect. In particular, he praises her high spirits and concern for others. While he runs an electrocardiogram, for instance, he mentions depression as a common side-effect of reserpine, the patient's antihypertensive medication. Noting, however, that the patient does not seem sad at all, he comments on her emotional strengths:

D: Reserpine depresses some people, makes
   them feel really sad, and you don't strike me as being, ha!,
   sad at all. So I think
   [
P: My only problem is I'm too sympathetic.
D: Uh huh.
P: (words) and I feel so sorry for people.
D: Well, that's compassion, I think. We won't, uh, criticize
   you for that.

From the doctor's viewpoint, the patient's emotional equanimity and compassion for others warrant compliments.

Given the problems that seniors frequently face, this patient leads an exemplary life and expresses attitudes that prove difficult to criticize. She turns to her doctor for information, support, and technical assistance that she values, as she shows with her gratitude at the end:

P: You've made me feel a lot better.
D: Well, I think you're doing well.
P: Well, then, I can call you anyway.
D: Call me if there's any problem.

Her efforts to care for herself help preserve autonomy, and her social context has not brought discernible troubles. Such conditions are deserving of praise.

WHAT IS THE NEGATIVE CASE?

On first take, these four encounters do not confirm the theory developed earlier. Although this theory uncovers an underlying structure in a majority of the sampled interactions, a minority present negative findings. That is, even in passing, contextual issues do not appear, personal troubles remain absent, patients do not express and doctors do not elicit such concerns, tensions involving the marginalization of context do not arise, and the management of contextual difficulties—including messages of ideology or social control—proves unnecessary. That many or most encounters seem to manifest an underlying structure while others do not raises an obvious question—Why the difference? To answer, it helps to look closely at the characteristics of the negative case, at least some of which these examples illustrate.

As shown in the first example, some encounters occur for mainly bureaucratic reasons. The goal here often comprises certification of health for an organizational third party. In such instances, neither patient nor doctor usually wants to muddy the water with extraneous contextual details. When one or both participants note problems that might potentially interfere with a successful outcome, they feel pressure to exclude such difficulties from their attention (as when marijuana crops up in this encounter). In such encounters, expression and management of contextual concerns would not serve the mainly administrative purpose of the dialogue.

A second characteristic of the negative case, illustrated by Encounter 10B, consists of acute physical problems. Doctors often deal with these difficulties during brief, unscheduled visits. When a patient sees a doctor because of urgent symptoms, the focused and instrumental nature of the encounter does not lend itself to contextual matters. Time constraints also inhibit such dialogue. Especially when a patient is "worked into" a busy schedule, both participants may want to restrict their talk to the physical discomfort of the moment. If more time becomes available, as in a regular follow-up appointment, exploring and managing contextual difficulties may then become convenient.

Besides bureaucratically motivated encounters and those oriented to acute symptoms, a third characteristic of the negative case involves specific stages of the life cycle. Especially during youth, social role expectations demand less in the way of mainstream standards. As evident in Encounter 10A, adolescents who live at home, who receive material support from parents, and who develop according to normal milestones may experiment in various ways while staying within the realm of normalcy. Such behaviors do not disappoint nearly so much as they would if they included more extreme alternatives, which then might lead to medical intervention—hard drugs, pregnancy, and so forth. Similarly, for unattached youths living on their own, like the patient in Encounter 10B, certain foibles come to be not only accepted but also expected. If sexual escapades do not disrupt family life or work roles, medical expertise can provide technical help for unpleasant physical consequences, without going further into contextual matters. In this setting, notwithstanding advice about safe sexual techniques, moral messages would appear as rather unseemly baggage.

Advantages of social class create a fourth basis for the negative case. As Encounter 10C shows, wealth helps solve many a problem. Comfortable financial circumstances usually spring from stable work arrangements for oneself or one's spouse, or occasionally involve independent means. Such comfort lifts a contextual burden experienced by many others. Since doctors themselves usually have attained an advantaged financial position, they converse as equals with those of their patients who also are so fortunate. Under these circumstances, the difficulties of occupational instability or other sources of financial insecurity do not appear at the margins of medical discourse. Rather, some patients and their doctors can openly share the pleasures and opportunities that their common class positions bring.

A fifth feature of the negative case involves social integration and adherence to mainstream life-style. In Encounters 10C and 10D, patients speak of family and friends who provide integrated social networks. A middle-aged woman describes the leisure-time pursuits that she enjoys with her husband, children, and friends. She recounts the joy that she continues to receive from an active mother, describes work activities that prove rewarding though at times physically taxing, and mentions athletic activities that help keep stress low. An elderly woman gives an account of beloved friends and family members who apparently appreciate the vigorous role that she plays in their lives. Further, her keen intellectual faculties help her in self-care. These two patients lead model lives, the kinds of lives toward which societal standards cause others to aspire. Under such happy circumstances, medical discourse has little to add.

A proportion of medical encounters then, probably a minority, do not deal with contextual issues or the personal troubles that these issues often generate. During such encounters, patients do not express difficulties in their customary social roles, and the dialogue does not reveal evidence of ideology or social control. Certain instances of the negative case reflect characteristics of the encounter itself—for example, a bureaucratic rationale or an acute symptom requiring an unscheduled visit. At other times, patients' circumstances indicate that they are fully adjusted at work, in the family, and in their leisure activities, or so it seems. These persons have accepted the patterning of their lives according to the dominant framework of the society and have not yet experienced the personal troubles engendered by social conditions with which many other people must reckon. Medical discourse reinforces this "happy," though relatively uncommon, situation through absence. That is, by not addressing contextual issues, the dialogue supports patients' continuing satisfactory adjustment to the society's dominant ideologies and expectations. Such is the positive accomplishment of the negative case.

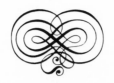

THREE

MEDICAL
MICROPOLITICS
AND
SOCIAL
CHANGE

CHAPTER 11

CHANGING
DISCOURSE,
CHANGING
CONTEXT

Before taking up the question of change, let me repeat a now familiar question: How do patients and doctors deal with social problems? If the encounters considered here are typical (and the random sampling procedures that led to their selection indicate that they probably are), such problems arise frequently in medical visits, perhaps in a majority of cases. The issues include work and economic insecurity, family life and gender roles, aging, sources of self-destructive behavior and other "vices," and resources for responding to emotional distress. Patients experience these contextual issues as personal troubles that they express, directly or in passing, during conversations with doctors. The structure of medical discourse tends to marginalize such troubles, despite tensions that remain as the dialogue returns to a technical track. Management of contextual difficulties takes place in several ways: through subtle ideologic messages that reinforce adherence to mainstream expectations, through the absence of criticism of context or exploration of collective action, through professional surveillance that enhances social control, and through therapeutic actions that provide personal gratification while reifying contextual issues and encouraging consent.

Some doctor-patient visits, however, do not reveal this underlying structure. These encounters, probably a minority overall, comprise what I have called the negative case. Here, social issues and the personal troubles that they generate do not present themselves. Several characteristics distinguish the negative case. Such interactions sometimes adopt bureaucratic goals, or they respond to acute symptoms during brief visits.

Alternatively, negative encounters involve patients at stages of the life cycle, especially youth, when potentially troublesome behaviors do not threaten customary roles in work and the family; or patients whose social-class position provides advantages that minimize contextual difficulties; or patients who integrate themselves satisfactorily into a social network and adhere to a mainstream life-style. Under such circumstances, the medical processing of social problems becomes unlikely, and this non-intervention reinforces an individual's already successful fit into societal norms.

Although this interpretation explains at least part of what does and does not happen in medical discourse, an obvious question involves change and how to accomplish it. The goal of improving medical dis-course implies that it is not enough to criticize. From this view, criticism also entails a responsibility to clarify directions of progressive change and even to work in those directions. That is, recognizing how the structure of medical discourse helps marginalize the social issues that create per-sonal troubles becomes only the first phase of a larger task. This task involves the creation, or at least the suggestion, of a new kind of medical discourse. To work toward this end also may require transformations of the social context within which medical encounters occur.

While the larger purpose of change goes beyond criticism's custom-ary bounds, such a call is not all that unusual. "The philosophers have only *interpreted* the world, in various ways; the point, however, is to *change* it," says Marx.[1] This weighty call has motivated generations of critical scholars, who have aimed to convert insight into action. In the current generation, this preference for criticism linked to action extends to Marxist-oriented literary critics who hope that their work contributes to progressive change. From this view, the critical analysis of both literary and nonliterary texts engages the social problems that those texts convey. For instance, such criticism seeks to demystify elements of culture that justify and help maintain patterns of social oppression. These patterns include domination based on social class, race, gender, age, and inter-national exploitation. Further, such criticism points to new forms of discourse that resist, challenge, and seek to transform the deeply embed-ded assumptions of not only literature but also everyday, nonliterary language.[2]

How might medical discourse change? While utopian visions have their place, there is no point in reaching for fantasies divorced from the reality of the here and now. It is easy to call for concrete modifications in the behavior of doctors and patients. But these individuals must continue to confront a social context where change often appears difficult or im-possible. It is also easy to argue for new social policies to reduce the contextual difficulties that clients and practitioners currently face. Recon-structing the social order, for instance, involves assurance of full employment, sexual and racial equality, security for senior citizens, and so forth. Such a reconstruction will require a future struggle that goes far beyond the boundaries of medicine.

Further, especially in the United States, the entire health-care system cries out for reform. The United States continues to lack a national health program that provides universal entitlement to basic services (the Republic of South Africa remains the only other economically developed nation without such a program). Those who justify the current situation point to individuals' freedom to choose from options that include the most technologically sophisticated measures available anywhere. Yet the ideology of free choice masks the fact that more than 40 million U.S. citizens cannot exercise this choice because they lack either public or private health insurance and otherwise often cannot afford to pay for services. The high costs and inefficiencies of present arrangements also have become well known. From this vantage point, the creation of a health-care system that assures access to needed care becomes another target for contextual change. Like the contextual transformations advocated earlier, the movement toward a national health program will require sustained activism during coming years.[3]

In this light, strategies for change in medical discourse ought to consider two periods of time. First, long-range strategies aim toward basic modifications in current patterns of power and finance in the larger society of which medicine is a part. Such strategies seek to change the contextual issues that create personal troubles on the individual level. For instance, long-term strategies try to reduce class-based economic insecurity by assuring regular employment and expanding public-sector health and welfare benefits. Creation of a responsive national health program comprises a key goal here. Other such strategies address unequal opportunities based on race, gender, and age. In the long range, contextual change involves nothing short of revolutionary restructuring of social institutions that now create suffering and unhappiness. By basic changes such as these, many of the most troublesome contextual patterns that patients and doctors currently face presumably would cease making themselves felt in medical discourse.

Short-range strategies involve modifications in medical discourse that could occur within the present social context. In the encounters considered here, the ways that patients and doctors deal with social problems reveal tensions and difficulties. For instance, the marginalization of contextual issues involves devices of interpersonal communication such as interruptions, cut-offs, de-emphases, or silences. Likewise, medical discourse often conveys ideologic assumptions consistent with those of mainstream expectations. While voicing little or no criticism of context, medical language generally encourages reified, technical responses. Such measures help patients adjust to troubling contextual conditions but generally do not modify these broader conditions. Even if contextual problems do not improve much in the short term, the structure of medical discourse need not remain what it is currently. En route to progressive change in the social context, now is the time to begin restructuring the manner in which patients and doctors communicate with each other.

All this is not to say that medicine is the only, or even the major, social institution that promotes society's current arrangements. The family, educational system, criminal justice system, mass media, and many other institutions achieve similar effects in service of the status quo, but their impacts have received wider recognition than those of medicine. Further, it is foolish to think that changing the doctor-patient relationship in itself would lead to wider social change. Although medical encounters may reinforce structural patterns of domination and oppression, a transition toward nondominating, nonoppressive doctor-patient relationships will not create social revolution (despite ardent claims by alternative health movements of various persuasions). Modification of doctor-patient relationships needs to accompany change in the larger contextual conditions that impede a decent and humane health-care system. Just as medical encounters are only part of the problem, their reform will comprise only part of the solution.

The following parts of this chapter aim to make some limited contributions to both long-range and short-range strategies for restructuring medical discourse. I will not spell out in detail the kinds of struggles that will be necessary to transform the social order of advanced capitalist countries. Such long-range strategizing, as crucial as I think it is to do, is best done in other settings and in more depth than is possible here. One modest contribution I want to make, however, is to describe changes that have occurred in medical discourse within some but not all postrevolutionary societies. The purpose is to point out improvements that are possible, after long-range strategies succeed in modifying the social context of medicine. Further, while recognizing the limitations of strategies that do not modify the social context, I also want to argue for certain ways that doctors and patients can alter their communication in the present. These suggestions assume that the medical processing of contextual issues can improve, even if contextual issues in the near future change little.

SOCIETAL CHANGE AND MEDICAL DISCOURSE: LONG-RANGE STRATEGY

Revolutionary change in social context does not in itself resolve the micro-level contradictions of doctor-patient communication. Although few observations of medical encounters in socialist countries are available, some very similar problems have persisted or arisen anew in post-revolutionary settings. On the other hand, marked changes in medical discourse have occurred in certain postrevolutionary countries; here, dialogue between patients and health professionals has come to deal differently with contextual issues.

The Soviet bloc. In the Soviet Union during the Stalinist period, the medical encounter became a tension-ridden experience, since individuals could obtain exemption from work only through medical certification.[4] If a person wanted a certificate of illness to miss work, he or she had to consult a physician authorized by the government to issue such certificates. To obtain certification from an authorized physician, a worker might simulate symptoms. As an alternative approach, an individual could consult a physician and simply request a medical certificate, without presenting any symptoms of illness. In this case one could offer the physician a story—most likely concerning a contextual difficulty, such as the necessity of missing work to attend to the needs of one's family—which would arouse pity or sympathy. A third possibility involved a person whose physical disorder was real and not simulated. A worker experiencing objective symptoms often sought the care of a physician who was known personally but who was unauthorized to issue medical certificates. Such a patient then might approach an authorized physician, requesting a medical certificate but no other attention.

Institutional cross-pressures also affected the medical processing of contextual difficulties during the Stalinist period. The physician's standing among political and professional superiors depended largely on how quickly his or her patients returned to their active responsibilities in the occupational system. Because production requirements did not permit an extended period of recovery, the physician limited medical certification to the shortest possible period of time; illness was to be certified every three days. On the other hand, the patient was free to denounce a physician by writing critical letters to the editors of newspapers. For these reasons, contact between physicians and patients was marked by mutual suspicion. Physicians were required to ascertain whether patients were faking their symptoms. Patients, some of whom actually experienced the symptoms they reported, had to convince physicians that their incapacity was real. With such cross-pressures, trust between patient and doctor broke down.

Although the constraints affecting medical discourse during the Stalinist regime represent an extreme, similar tensions also have arisen during other time periods and in different countries. For instance, even after the departure of Stalin, Soviet health professionals have participated in the psychiatric labeling of political dissidents. Through this process, psychiatrists have rechanneled and helped control individuals' criticism of exist-

ing social policies. Further, although the Soviet Union formally guaran-
tees universal entitlement to needed services, public dissatisfaction has
focused on bureaucratic inefficiencies and impersonal care within the
national health program. This dissatisfaction has generated proposals for
reform of Soviet medicine in general and the doctor-patient relationship
in particular. Analogous tensions and calls for change have arisen in other
Eastern European countries, where observations of medical encounters
(well before the momentous events of 1989 and 1990) have revealed
impersonality, lack of continuity, bureaucratization, and frequent requests for certified absence from work.[5]

China. The People's Republic of China has restructured doctor-patient
relationships substantially, although such modifications have varied in
different historical periods. Specifically, reform in medicine emerged as a
major goal during the Cultural Revolution, and sweeping change affected interpersonal communication, as well as many other features of
the health-care system.[6] At that time, hierarchies based on professional
authority received widespread criticism. Reflecting national policies and
political agitation, doctors had to share authority with nonprofessional
health workers, community activists, and patients themselves. As principles of criticism and self-criticism reached even clinical interactions, patients began to speak with doctors more as equals. Political struggle
extended to face-to-face medical encounters, where patients and advocates who accompanied them demanded full information and participation in decision making.

Further, health-care teams often included paraprofessionals like "barefoot doctors" and traditional healers, as well as representatives from
community organizations, unions, and political groupings. Although
local regions varied somewhat in their practices, health-care team members generally tried to address both the technical and nontechnical components of patients' problems. For instance, when contextual difficulties
involved work, economic factors, family relations, housing, or similar
matters, the team together would address these issues, along with the
physical disorder that the patient presented. Often the team initiated
multifaceted interventions, designed to improve both social and physical
conditions. In short, when contextual difficulties contributed to patients'
distress, members of the health-care team generally dealt directly with
the social context. Rather than marginalizing such concerns, the team
discussed contextual matters explicitly with patients and tried to modify
the broader social relations affecting an individual, beyond whatever
technical measures were needed.

After the death of Mao Zedong, some of these practices in medicine
have reversed, alongside parallel changes in other parts of Chinese society.[7] Local practices vary even more widely than previously. Generally,

physicians have regained much of their earlier authority, although some regions, especially rural ones, have retained a prominent role for paraprofessionals and the health-care team. With a re-emphasis on scientific medicine, especially in cities, practitioners and nonprofessional team members have become less likely to focus on contextual interventions. Because technical matters again receive priority, attempts to deal directly with contextual sources of personal distress have become less common. In the process, as much of Chinese medicine returns to a Western model, its discourse again moves context to the margin.

Cuba. In contrast to the Soviet bloc and China, the Cuban revolution has transformed both the context and the structure of medical encounters. Changes in medical discourse have occurred together with fundamental shifts in the health-care system and the society as a whole.[8] A brief summary of these shifts will put into perspective the modifications that have occurred in doctor-patient communication.

Before the revolution of 1959, Cuban medical services remained at a rudimentary level, except for a concentration of physicians and medical technology in Havana, the national capital. Although wealthy Cubans received care through the private sector, the majority of the population could not gain regular access to needed services. The people of Cuba suffered from malnutrition, widespread infectious diseases, and high rates of infant mortality. In short, a coordinated public health system was nonexistent, expensive fees and maldistribution left much of the population lacking care, and patterns of disease and early death that are characteristic of economic underdevelopment ravaged the poor.

The Cuban revolution permitted a rapid reconstruction of its health-care system. Although nearly half of the country's physicians emigrated by 1962, the new government initiated basic organizational reforms. Despite problems that remain, these changes have fostered the creation of a health-care system which, to a variety of even skeptical observers, appears the most responsive and effective in all of Latin America.[9]

In particular, the government placed a high priority on recruitment into medicine and initiated a policy of open enrollment in medical school for qualified students; additional schools opened in provinces outside Havana. Medical education was free, and previous barriers of social class, race, and sex no longer affected the number or composition of the profession. Students from working-class and peasant families, blacks, and women quickly entered the study and practice of medicine. As the class origins of the medical profession changed, the revolution provided mobility into a satisfying and relatively prestigious field of work. By the early 1970s, the ratio of doctors to population in Cuba resembled that of the United States and surpassed that of all other Latin American countries.

Government policies rectified geographical maldistribution. In exchange for free education, graduates have served a two-year period of compulsory practice in rural health centers and hospitals. Similar programs have provided for a redistribution of nurses and allied health workers. In addition to personnel, the government constructed hospitals and clinics in underserved areas. Within a decade, each of Cuba's provinces contained a regional hospital and an integrated series of clinics. More than half the new clinics were located in rural areas that previously had lacked such facilities altogether.

Despite these measures, the difficulties of practice led to a high turnover of physicians, who often returned to urban centers after compulsory service and undertook specialty training. To address the problem of continuity, in the mid-1970s the Ministry of Health began a program of "Medicine in the Community" (*Medicina en la Comunidad*). Among other initiatives, this program started teaching and research activities at decentralized clinics and required a rotation of professors between clinics and teaching hospitals. Beginning in 1984, a national residency training program in family medicine (*Medicina Familiar Integral*) led to the placement of primary-care teams involving a family practitioner and a nurse in every local neighborhood. The newly trained family practitioners, who commit themselves to at least five years of service within a single community, accept responsibility for the care of approximately 600–700 persons in a geographic area of two to three square blocks. Partly as a result of these policies, maldistribution and turnover have improved. A designated clinic and staff of health workers serve patients in each defined geographical location of the country.

The government also has sought to change prior patterns of class structure and racism that limited the accessibility of health care. Even when doctors were within traveling distance, the high fees of private practice before the revolution created barriers to access. Racism compounded the problem, since the number of doctors and clients who were white was disproportionate to the ratio of whites in the general population. In postrevolutionary Cuba, health care is free. Public financing assures that medical services, as well as most drugs and needed supplies, are available, regardless of income. Patients receive preventive, ambulatory, and hospitalization services without charge. Blacks have entered the profession of medicine in proportion to population, and racism does not hinder patients from seeking and obtaining care.

Mass organizations have taken an active role throughout the healthcare system. The Committees for the Defense of the Revolution (CDRs), based in neighborhoods and workplaces, initially concerned themselves with security and vigilance against counterrevolutionary activities. Later, the CDRs became the primary political structures for popular representation in policy decisions. In preventive medicine, the CDRs have coordinated immunization campaigns in neighborhoods and workplaces; they also have assisted people in obtaining early attention for medical problems. The Federation of Cuban Women has helped coordinate prenatal, maternal, and infant care. Regarding occupational health, the association of small farmers and the trade unions have monitored workplace safety and have organized educational campaigns about work hazards. From time to time, when national goals of high productivity have interfered with safe working conditions, the trade unions have intervened to protect workers. In local neighborhoods, senior citizens' associations (*círculos de abuelos*, "grandparents' circles") have organized activities for older people, emphasizing travel, exercise, nutrition, education, and social events. The grandparents' circles have assisted health-care workers with the growing challenges of geriatric medicine. Since the mid-1970s, elected representatives of municipal governments (*Poder Popular*, "People's Power") also have assumed responsibility for helping to coordinate local health and welfare programs. In short, central planning and activism by the mass organizations have fostered prevention, as well as accessible services.

These initiatives have led to remarkable improvements in morbidity and mortality, which demonstrate the impact of simple interventions in an underdeveloped country. The incidence and prevalence of infectious diseases have fallen drastically. Within fifteen years of the revolution, diphtheria, polio, tetanus, and malaria were eradicated in Cuba. Infant mortality fell from 52 to 27 per 1,000 within the same time period, and maternal mortality declined from 118 to 63 per 100,000. Subsequently, these important measures of health status continued to improve, as Cuba has achieved infant and maternal mortality rates equivalent to those of the United States and the countries of Western Europe. Since the 1970s, Cuba has resembled economically developed nations in illness and mortality patterns, as heart disease and cancer have become the leading causes of death. In occupations like sugar production, the chronic lung disease of bagassosis would be a predictable consequence of high productivity standards; measures to reduce bagasse dust in cane processing and regular tests of workers' pulmonary function have helped prevent this and similar occupational diseases. Such accomplishments would be hardly imaginable without the coordinated efforts of mass organizations and health workers.

In addition to these transformations of the health-care system, the Ministry of Public Health has devoted attention to the nuances of the doctor-patient relationship. As noted previously, staff turnover and an orientation toward specialty medicine have led to widespread dissatisfaction. Within the program of Medicine in the Community and the newer family medicine initiative, research and teaching efforts have emphasized the process of professional-client interaction. These educational approaches have focused attention on interpersonal communication.

Primary-care teams have played an even more important role than these centrally coordinated measures in improving doctor-patient relationships. Although multidisciplinary teams have emerged in many countries, their composition and activities in Cuba have differed from other models. Since the mid-1970s, primary-care teams have assumed responsibility for a designated panel of patients. On a day-to-day basis, team members include doctors, nurses, and allied health workers. Participation by psychologists, sanitary workers, epidemiologists, and social workers on these teams supports an integrated approach to each patient and family. In addition, representatives of mass organizations meet regularly with the team. For instance, team members are responsible for reporting to one or more representatives of the local CDR. These individuals provide suggestions and involve themselves in finding solutions when patients face contextual problems that go beyond the technical expertise of other team members. Many primary-care teams, especially those focusing on maternal and infant care, include representatives from the Federation of Cuban Women or other local women's organizations. Regarding problems in geriatric medicine, the teams receive input from the grandparents' circles. Further, when teams care for patients working in specific industries or agricultural enterprises, trade union representatives take part in the teams' deliberations.

Through the participation of nonphysician members, the primary-care team has altered the structure of medical discourse in a fundamental way. When technical problems of illness present themselves, the doctor, nurse, and allied health workers can respond with appropriate diagnostic studies and treatments. When contextual difficulties arise, however, team members try to facilitate changes in patients' living and working conditions that interfere with health and well-being. For instance, representatives from the CDR, People's Power, a women's organization, or a grandparents' circle may intervene to improve financial conditions, housing problems, and even family relations that become troublesome for individual patients. When job stress or other occupational difficulties create personal troubles, a labor union representative often collaborates with the primary-care team to seek modifications at the workplace. Educational campaigns in neighborhoods and workplaces also encourage citizens to express discontent and to suggest improvements, either to the primary-care team directly or through the mass organizations.

The primary-care team changes the structure of medical discourse by focusing on contextual issues, rather than marginalizing them. Further, team members deal with social problems through social intervention, rather than medicalization. When patients mention contextual problems, the team activates nonprofessional participants who can take action directly to alter contextual patterns. Instead of fostering consent to a troublesome status quo, the team seeks to diminish personal troubles by working toward change in social institutions.

Three case summaries illustrate how medical discourse in Cuba deals with social problems that patients and doctors confront on a day-to-day basis. I recorded interactions involving these patients, family members, and their primary-care physicians during visits to local family medicine clinics and to the patients' homes.[10]

■ A 40-year-old woman was hospitalized in 1984 because of methyl alcohol poisoning. Apparently, she had ingested the methyl alcohol during a celebration when she was offered home-brewed rum. Her acidosis and transient visual loss improved with intensive care. After discharge, the family physician assigned to her neighborhood (a woman in her late twenties) visited the patient at home.

Here the doctor uncovered a series of social problems. The patient's home was poorly constructed, with several safety hazards and inadequate sanitary facilities (an unmaintained latrine). Her husband had abandoned the family several years previously. The patient was not working outside the home, and there was no regular source of income. Her four children all showed signs of emotional disturbance and were not performing well in school. An adolescent daughter was becoming sexually active but had not received educational information about birth control and sexually transmitted disease.

In addition to supervising the patient's continuing convalescence, the doctor then initiated several interventions to improve these social conditions. At first, she involved a representative of People's Power, the municipal government, and also a local sanitary worker (*brigadista sanitaria*). These individuals coordinated reconstruction of the patient's home through voluntary labor by a group of community residents. This work group repaired safety hazards and built a toilet and piping that connected to the municipal sewer. In response to the doctor's initiative, the vice-president of the local chapter of the Federation of Cuban Women, who also serves as chief of the grandparents' circle, approached the patient and offered assistance. Largely through this effort, the patient obtained employment as an aide at a nearby hospital and began to participate in community organizations. Together with the nurse and psychologist members of the primary-care team, the doctor also began to work with each of the four children. One child's school problems improved after he started attending a "workshop school" (*escuela taller*), where students receive more individualized attention. After resolving difficulties with her studies, an adolescent daughter was able to finish secondary school and to begin working. A younger teenage daughter responded positively to birth control information and continued her studies in secondary school.

During a recorded encounter at home, the patient described the improvements in her life but noted that she still wanted to do further repairs in her home. When she complained that she had found mice recently, the doctor explained the rodent control measures that the patient could use. As the doctor departed, she pointed out trash in the patient's yard and stated that she would ask a sanitary worker to instruct the patient about trash removal.

■ In making her required rounds of homes in the neighborhood during 1985, the same doctor found problems involving an 11-year-old boy and his 70-year-old grandmother. The boy was experiencing difficulties in school and recently had failed to advance to the next grade. His teachers felt that he was mentally disturbed. After school, he seldom left the house and preferred to stay with his grandmother, who was very protective of him. On investigating further, the doctor learned that the boy was upset about a recent divorce of his parents. His father retained little contact with him, and his mother carried out extensive work responsibilities as a laboratory technician at a local hospital, where she often needed to work evening and night shifts. The grandmother suffered from anxiety, loneliness, and osteoarthritis of the hands and feet that limited her activity, as well as hypertension controlled adequately with two medications.

To deal with the boy's problems, the doctor initiated a series of meetings with his teachers, the coordinator of the neighborhood's youth center (*casa de juventud*), a representative of People's Power, and the leaders of the grandparents' circle. Teenagers active at the youth center visited the boy at home and asked him to get involved in the center's activities, including the construction of a new wing of the building. He responded positively and enjoyed learning construction skills. His school work began to improve. More recently, the doctor tried to arrange his participation in a residential "camp school" (*escuela del campo*), but he was hesitant to attend because of embarrassment about the perceived shortness of his penis and because of his recent experiments with masturbation. The doctor tried to respond to these concerns through counseling and reassurance.

For other family members, the doctor also took action to improve the social situation. She discussed the mother's work schedule both with her and her superiors at the hospital, but changes had not yet proven possible. For the grandmother, leaders of the local grandparents' circle visited the home and encouraged her participation in their activities. The grandmother then began to visit the grandparents' circle facility every day, where she socialized, watched television, and took part in a medically supervised exercise program.

During the recorded encounter at this family's home, the boy returned from taking a test at school and expressed gratitude to the doctor and to the leaders of the youth center. In response to the doctor's questions, he said that he was feeling better about his parents' divorce and that he hoped to attend camp school soon. Regarding the future, he said that he wanted to study for a career in auto mechanics, as he pointed to a car motor that he was repairing in a corner of the kitchen. In the same home visit, the grandmother reported that she was still very anxious about her grandson's behavior but that she was calmer and more satisfied since her arthritis seemed to be improving with daily exercise at the seniors' center.

■ A 38-year-old woman visited another family physician (a man in his late twenties) because of low back pain. According to the patient, who worked as a clerk in a retail store, the pain had been bothering her for about nine years. Because she had to stay on her feet at work for eight hours a day, she complained, her back symptoms gradually had grown worse. For this reason, she was requesting a formal medical evaluation of a problem that in her view represented an occupational disability.

In response to this request, the doctor took several actions. First, he issued a temporary medical certification that removed the patient from her usual work for a period of one to two months. During this time, she continued to receive 50 percent of her usual salary. The doctor ordered x-rays of the lumbosacral spine, which showed scoliosis and degenerative changes of osteoarthritis. He also referred the patient to an orthopedist for consultation. Further, to resolve the question of occupational disability, the family doctor convened a review board (*comisión de peritaje*). This independent panel of three physicians from different specialties was to consider the case and decide among three alternatives: that the patient should return to her previous job, that she should be assigned a new job (*puesto de trabajo*) with less taxing physical requirements, or that she should retire from work with a pension. Although the review board was to decide the case within one to two months, it had not yet reached a determination. Meanwhile, the doctor believed that the review board probably would recommend assignment to a new job.

These three cases all show how a new kind of medical discourse has emerged in Cuba. When social problems present themselves, they do not move to the margins of the dialogue. Instead, doctors can focus the conversation on the trouble at hand and can turn to a variety of community-based organizations or professional colleagues for help. With the first family, these resources included a representative of municipal government, a sanitary worker, an activist in a women's organization and senior citizens' group, school officials, and (as members of the primary-care team) a nurse and psychologist. For the second family, persons based in organizations outside medicine also helped resolve social components of the problems facing patients and their doctor; teachers and other school officials, leaders of a youth center, a representative of municipal government, and members of a seniors' group all made substantial contributions. In the third case, a patient who perceived that her job either created or worsened her physical symptoms initiated a standard process of medical evaluation, whose conclusion would not jeopardize her financial security. While none of these cases reached a completely satisfactory resolution, all participants agreed that major improvements either had been made or at least had been tried.

The social problems facing these patients and doctors are not particularly unusual. Similar difficulties arise routinely in the day-to-day practice of Cuban medicine, and they resemble those that occur in the United States and most other countries. Yet the social resources available to Cuban patients and doctors as they deal with such issues go beyond those available elsewhere. The transformation of Cuban society permits a broad-based approach to social components of medical problems. With great effort, patients and doctors in countries like the United States can mobilize similar kinds of assistance from community agencies, but no organized system helps accomplish this task. In Cuba, on the other hand, the participation of community organizations in dealing with such difficulties has become routine—enough so that the everyday discourse of medicine routinely finds ways to respond to social problems when they arise in individuals' lives.[11]

Deficiencies remain in the Cuban health-care system, as openly acknowledged within Cuba. In particular, difficulties imposed by underdevelopment limit further achievements. Yet Cuba has transformed its rudimentary and crisis-ridden medical services into a rationalized and accessible system whose accomplishments are startling even to the most skeptical observers. One of the most unusual of these accomplishments involves a change in the structure of medical discourse, which—with the help of nonphysician members of the primary-care team and representatives of other community organizations—has moved contextual issues from the margins to the center.

CHANGING MEDICAL DISCOURSE NOW: SHORT-RANGE STRATEGY

In the United States and other advanced capitalist countries, fundamental change in the social context of medicine will not happen today or tomorrow. Clearly, such contextual alterations do not assure that doctor-patient communication will necessarily improve anyway; observations in the Soviet Union, Eastern Europe, and China show that. Despite some shortcomings, however, the transformation of medical discourse in Cuba sets a standard of what proves possible when change in the social order coincides with attempts to restructure clinical encounters in a progressive direction.

Where does that leave us, living as we do in a social context whose resilience and resistance to change remain apparent to all who care to look? Although some other countries may provide models toward which long-range strategy can aim, medical encounters here continue to take place every day, under frequently adverse contextual conditions. While transformation of medicine's context seems far in the future, there are some ways that restructuring medical discourse may begin to occur in the short term. Lacking contextual supports, such a restructuring will prove neither easy nor popular. Further, a call for change contains an explicit ideologic assumption that change is desirable. Many practitioners and observers of medicine, who currently benefit from—or at least remain satisfied with—the status quo, predictably will see things differently; they will not appreciate suggestions to restructure medical discourse. But that is all the more reason to advocate these "reforms."

To begin on the most limited level, doctors and patients can alter their communication in simple ways. These alterations are not particularly radical, and the medical literature contains some similar suggestions.[12] Previous chapters have shown that many of the tensions in medical encounters derive from devices of language that maintain professional dominance. Such devices have become obsolete and should be replaced by new ways of talking. Specifically, doctors should let patients tell their stories, with many fewer interruptions, cut-offs, or returns to the technical. Especially at the beginnings of encounters, patients should have the chance to present their narratives in an open-ended way. Doctors should provide full explanations to patients, with information given in comprehensible terms without jargon. Patients also should take a more active role in questioning, challenging, and directing the flow of conversations. Such participation will benefit from efforts to educate and to support patients as they try to become more assertive "consumers" of health-care services.

When patients refer to personal troubles that derive from contextual issues, doctors should try not to marginalize these connections by reverting to a reified, technical track. Further, doctors' explanations and suggestions should avoid messages of ideology and social control, especially when these messages encourage patients' adherence to social expectations that cause them grief. Attempts to reduce ideologic and controlling language should occur particularly when contextual difficulties involve work, social class, and economic insecurity; gender roles and the family; the troubles of aging; personal behaviors outside the mainstream, including substance use and sexual preferences; and emotional distress deriving from social causes.

Even these limited alterations in medical discourse would require that doctors suspend, at least for a moment, the drive to reach a diagnosis that fits traditional diagnostic categories, as well as the drive to offer a technical solution. Transcending these motivations temporarily, to let patients tell their contextual stories, involves swimming against the stream of several generations of medical education. This observation means that doctors in training also should begin to learn from their mentors new ways of communicating. The high-control style that the traditional clinical history encourages should be eliminated from programs in medical education. Such changes will require a drastic rethinking and critical evaluation of what traditional history taking accomplishes. Without modifying the educational process by which trainees learn to communicate with patients, however, adverse patterns of medical discourse will remain entrenched.

It would be helpful if the conditions of clinical practice facilitated these changes in discourse, but current pressures point in the opposite direction. Multinational corporations have entered the health-care field and have assumed control over a greater number of hospitals and outpatient services. These enterprises have imposed more stringent productivity standards on physicians, with a frequent expectation that doctors see more patients per unit of paid time. Similar standards of productivity have become prevalent in health maintenance organizations and prepaid group practices. Such arrangements, especially as they aim to raise corporate profits, will put greater constraints on doctor-patient communication.

Changing the structure of medical discourse will take conscious attention and time—though not necessarily more time than doctors and patients now consume inefficiently in conversations that marginalize contextual issues. The process of change will not go well if doctors and patients are too busy or too rushed. Individual practitioners or the institutions for which they work may be willing to deprioritize interpersonal communication to increase the volume of patients and to maximize profits. But it is important to resist such policy decisions, which create almost inevitable ill effects in doctor-patient relationships. Especially from the standpoint of the society as a whole, the effort to deal more constructively with contextual issues would not necessarily increase costs or reduce efficiency overall. On the contrary, successful attempts to improve contextual problems would probably enhance the long-term economic productivity of individuals and would tend to reduce requirements for expensive medical and social services. While policy decisions in this arena should consider human values that go beyond cost and efficiency, a restructuring of medical discourse to deal with contextual issues might well prove "cost-effective" in the traditional sense as well.[13]

Aside from the limited changes described already, several others should prove feasible, although such alterations undoubtedly will generate controversy. These suggestions pertain directly to the boundary between contextual issues and medical discourse. While the qualities of

a "good" doctor-patient relationship are the topic of endless speculation, little of the available commentary deals with the ambiguities of
medical humanism. Sensitivity, compassion, nurturance—all these admirable traits may encourage a client's adjustment and acquiescence to
oppressive features of social and personal life. What kind of medical
discourse, then, heightens contextual understanding and motivates contextual change, rather than encouraging limited improvements that only
perpetuate current conditions? The empirical study presented here provided not a single example that met this criterion of a progressive discourse. Some preliminary thoughts about such a discourse, and about
how it might occur in a new kind of doctor-patient relationship, may be
appropriate in conclusion.

A vision of progressive medical discourse must include a conception of
how professional-client relationships either reinforce current social conditions or contribute to change in those conditions. This conception
should consider the specific ways that clinicians and clients, in the here
and now, can work together to overcome the historical contradictions of
their relationships. Such contradictions include medicine's tendencies to
reproduce oppressive social arrangements, despite the best intentions of
practitioners. In moving beyond the conservative dynamics of customary
discourse, however, new relationships should not encourage a further
medicalization of social problems.

Basic change in the social context requires long-term and difficult
efforts that increase democratization and popular control.[14] Typically,
these efforts take place in two spheres: the workplace and the local
community. In the workplace, organizing focuses on collective control
over the labor process, through workers' councils, progressive unions,
cooperatives, and similar organizations. In communities, democratic participation aims to achieve popular control of local institutions like schools,
transportation, hospitals, and clinics. The pace of such organizing is slow
and occupies decades.

In the short term, a progressive medical discourse should foster these
strategies of democratic participation. Obviously, there are limits to what
a clinician and client can hope to accomplish. Also, these considerations
clearly do not apply to all problems that patients present, or to all patients
and doctors.[15] On the other hand, when clients' distresses are socially
caused, it is important to expand the scope of medical discourse and to
address the linkage between personal suffering and social structure.
Some specific goals are worth considering.

First, in a progressive relationship, both participants try to overcome
the domination, mystification, and distorted communication that result
from asymmetric technical knowledge. Professionals try to communicate
thoroughly, honestly, and in comprehensible language both the content
and the limitations of their knowledge about physical problems. When

patients disagree or do not understand, they say so openly. Because differences of education, class, gender, ethnicity, and race make communication more difficult, doctors actively seek full discourse by encouraging patients' participation, skepticism, and disagreement. When the situation permits, the scope of medical discourse should be expanded to include a fuller, more explicit analysis of the connections between social structure and individual distress.

Second, doctors and patients should avoid the medicalization of nonmedical problems. This involves a conscious attempt to prevent medicine's symbolism from extending to nonmedical spheres. When such issues as work, family life, aging, substance use, and sexuality enter the conversation, both participants recognize that the doctor often has neither training nor authority to arbitrate these areas. Because such issues involve social problems, it is necessary to seek social solutions. Likewise, emotions such as anger, anxiety, unhappiness, depression, and loneliness frequently have social roots. A doctor's attempt to ease such emotions, either technically through medications or supportively through psychotherapeutic discussion, may deflect attention inappropriately from these underlying causes. Under such circumstances, reducing socially caused pain generally should not be the sole objective, however humanistic it may seem.

Instead, as a third goal, it is necessary to analyze the social origins of personal suffering. A doctor's participation in this analysis may or may not be appropriate. The health professional, for example, might refer a patient to a labor union, women's organization, cultural center, community group, or other organization for assistance. In making a referral, the purposes of the group taking the referral should be an important criterion. Organizations that aim toward outreach, advocacy, heightened democratic participation, and popular control should receive not only referrals but also other kinds of support from clinicians. In consulting such an organization, a client may decide that a change of social role is desirable, in work, the family, or another institutional setting. The client's integration into the organization and later participation in the group's efforts may become beneficial outcomes of the referral. In these decisions, the client's autonomy is essential, but so is the availability of a support system. From the start, decision making and control in such areas remain outside the boundaries of medical expertise and authority. In the United States, several community-based programs already have tried to grapple in a systematic way with the contextual issues that affect patients; such efforts deserve every support.[16]

Fourth, it is important to change the ideologic foundations of medical practice. Physical illness may demand technical intervention as therapy, but social problems require resistance, activism, and organizing. This distinction, often blurred by the undeniable impact of social conditions on physical health, is nonetheless essential to maintain if therapy is to include both physical and social elements. When occupational toxins, stress, or job insecurity produces symptoms, for instance, labor organizing is the preferred therapy, in addition to whatever physical treatment may prove appropriate. For the tension headaches and psychosomatic complaints of tedious housework, sexual politics aim directly at social causes. For alcoholism and other addictions that seek oblivion from the strains of social life, organizing at the level of local communities can begin to convert isolation to resistance. These rather facile examples oversimplify the clinical dilemma. The point, however, is that a progressive doctor-patient relationship fosters social change. Otherwise, the medical encounter dulls the pain of today, without hoping to extinguish it in the future.

NOTES

CHAPTER 1: INTRODUCTION

1. For some pertinent critiques, see Howard Waitzkin, *The Second Sickness: Contradictions of Capitalist Health Care* (New York: Free Press, 1983, 1986), pp. 3–43.

2. Examples of theorists arguing for the importance of noncoercive institutions in reproducing ideology and achieving social control include Antonio Gramsci, *Prison Notebooks* (New York: International, 1971), pp. 123–202, 375–77, 406–07; Louis Althusser, "Ideology and Ideological State Apparatuses," in *Lenin and Philosophy and Other Essays* (New York: Monthly Review Press, 1971), pp. 127–86; and Michael Burawoy, *Manufacturing Consent* (Chicago: University of Chicago Press, 1979), pp. 13–30, 193–203. These and other theorists will be considered in the next chapter.

3. A conspicuous exception to the lack of contextual criticism involves the "radical psychiatry" movement, which links individual therapy to social change. This movement, however, has exerted little impact on practitioners in the nonpsychiatric specialties and has remained a minority position in psychiatry as well. For pertinent examples, see R. D. Laing and A. Esterson, *Sanity, Madness and the Family* (Baltimore: Penguin, 1964); Hogie Wyckoff, *Solving Women's Problems* (New York: Grove, 1977); and Terry A. Kupers, *Public Therapy* (New York: Free Press, 1981).

CHAPTER 2: THEORETICAL APPROACHES TO MEDICAL ENCOUNTERS

1. C. Wright Mills, *The Sociological Imagination* (New York: Oxford University Press, 1959), pp. 3–24.

2. Useful overviews of this theoretical debate appear in K. Knorr-Cetina and A. V. Cicourel, eds., *Advances in Social Theory and Methodology: Toward an Integration of Micro- and Macro-Sociologies* (Boston: Routledge & Kegan Paul, 1981); and Jeffrey C. Alexander, Bernhard Giesen, Richard Munch, and Neil J. Smelser, eds., *The Micro-Macro Link* (Berkeley: University of California Press, 1987).

3. Although I have chosen a broad conception of ideology here, Althusser's famous definition has influenced the discussion that follows. According to Althusser, ideology is a " 'representation' of the imaginary relationship of individuals to their real conditions of existence." Ideology therefore represents individuals' imaginary relations with reality in their lived experience. "What is represented in ideology is therefore not the system of the

279

real relations which govern the existence of individuals, but the imaginary relation of those individuals to the real relations in which they live" (Althusser, "Ideology and Ideological State Apparatuses," pp. 162–65). Useful interpretations of Althusser's definition appear in Roisin McDonough and Rachel Harrison, "Patriarchy and Relations of Production," in Annette Kuhn and AnnMarie Wolpe, eds., *Feminism and Materialism* (Boston: Routledge & Kegan Paul, 1978), pp. 14–25; Gayle Greene and Coppelia Kahn, "Feminist Scholarship and the Social Construction of Woman," in Greene and Kahn, eds., *Making a Difference: Feminist Literary Criticism* (New York: Methuen, 1985), pp. 1–5; and Colin Sumner, *Reading Ideologies* (New York: Academic Press, 1979), pp. 10–56. I return to Althusser's work on ideology later in this chapter, when I also note some of the controversy that this work has generated; for a helpful review, see Ted Benton, *The Rise and Fall of Structural Marxism: Althusser and His Influence* (New York: St. Martin's, 1985). Among the vast literature on ideology, the following sources also have proven helpful: John B. Thompson, *Studies in the Theory of Ideology* (Berkeley: University of California Press, 1984); Martin Seliger, *The Marxist Conception of Ideology* (New York: Cambridge University Press, 1977); and Gunther Kress and Robert Hodge, *Language as Ideology* (London: Routledge & Kegan Paul, 1979).

4. Karl Marx, *Capital* (Moscow: Progress Publishers, 1971 [1894]), vol. 3, pp. 370–90, 790–94.

5. For an early and incompletely developed analysis, see Karl Marx and Friedrich Engels, *The German Ideology* (New York: International, 1939 [1846]), pp. 3–78. Economic determinacy and ideology are among the most difficult problems in Marxist theory. For example, although Marx mainly used the term ideology to refer to the false consciousness engendered by the capitalist class, later Marxist theorists have broadened the usage of the term. The relative impact of economic versus nonmaterial forces also has been a central focus of debate within Marxism. Although the complexities of the debate are beyond my purposes here, pertinent discussions include Richard Lichtman, "Marx's Theory of Ideology," *Socialist Review* 5, no. 1 (Nov. 1975):45–76; and Robert L. Heilbroner, *Marxism: For and Against* (New York: Norton, 1980), especially pp. 61–89.

6. The definition of health as ability to work is analyzed helpfully by E. Richard Brown, "Public Health in Imperialism: Early Rockefeller Programs at Home and Abroad," *American Journal of Public Health* 66 (1976):897–903, and *Rockefeller Medicine Men* (Berkeley: University of California Press, 1979), pp. 112–34. Of course, other influential definitions of health include: an absence of disease; functional capacity to perform basic activities of daily living; ability to function in various social roles; "a state of complete physical, mental, and social well-being, and not merely the absence of disease and infirmity" (the motto of the World Health Organization—see *International Dictionary of Medicine and Biology*, vol. 2 [New York: Wiley, 1986], p. 1276); and so forth. Notwithstanding such formal definitions, public policies and clinical procedures in practice have emphasized a vision of health as the capacity for productive work.

7. Brown, *Rockefeller Medicine Men*; Saul Franco-Agudelo, "The Rockefeller Foundation's Anti-Malarial Program in Latin America," *International Journal of Health Services* 13 (1983):51–57; P. J. Donaldson, "Foreign Intervention in Medical Education: A Case Study of the Rockefeller Foundation's Involvement in a Thai Medical School," in Vicente Navarro, ed., *Imperialism, Health and Medicine* (Farmingdale, N.Y.: Baywood, 1981). As shown by the examples of the Soviet Union and other countries of Eastern Europe, socialist nations also have tended to define health as the ability to work.

8. Sander Kelman, "The Social Nature of the Definition Problem in Health," *International Journal of Health Services* 5 (1975):625–42.

9. For a classic statement of this perspective, see M. C. Weinstein and W. B. Stason, "Foundations of Cost-Effectiveness Analysis for Health and Medical Practices," *New England Journal of Medicine* 296 (1977):716–21.

10. Friedrich Engels, *The Origin of the Family, Private Property and the State* (New York: International, 1942 [1891]).

11. The classic statement of Gramsci's position on ideology appears in Gramsci, *Prison Notebooks*, pp. 123–202, 375–77, 406–07.

12. Lukács' development of these themes appears in Georg Lukács, *History and Class Consciousness* (Cambridge: MIT Press, 1971), especially pp. 46–148, and *The Theory of the Novel* (Cambridge: MIT Press, 1971), pp. 112–43. A helpful interpretation of these materials is Fredric Jameson, "The Case for Georg Lukács," in *Marxism and Form* (Princeton: Princeton University Press, 1971). A convenient definition of reification appears in Tom Bottomore, et al., eds., *A Dictionary of Marxist Thought* (Cambridge: Harvard University Press, 1983), p. 411: "The act (or result of the act) of transforming human properties, relations and actions into properties, relations and actions of man-produced things which have become independent (and which are imagined as originally independent) of man and govern his life. Also transformation of human beings into thing-like beings which do not behave in a human way but according to the laws of the thing-world." For an extension of Lukács' perspectives to medicine, see Michael T. Taussig, "Reification and the Consciousness of the Patient," *Social Science & Medicine* 14B (1980):3–13: "By denying the human relations embodied in symptoms, signs, and therapy, we not only mystify them but we also reproduce a political ideology in the guise of a science of (apparently) 'real things'—biological and physical thinghood."

13. A statement of these themes appears in Althusser, "Ideology and Ideological State Apparatuses." For critiques of Althusser's positions, see n. 3 above.

14. Juergen Habermas, "Technology and Science as 'Ideology,'" in *Toward a Rational Society* (Boston: Beacon, 1970), p. 82.

15. Ibid., p. 111.

16. Juergen Habermas, *Communication and the Evolution of Society* (Boston: Beacon, 1979), pp. 119–20; other pertinent passages appear on pp. 1–68 and 130–77. Habermas deals with these themes also in *Knowledge and Human Interests* (Boston: Beacon, 1971), especially pp. 214–73 and 301–17; *Theory and Practice* (Boston: Beacon, 1974), pp. 1–40, 195–282; *Legitimation Crisis* (Boston: Beacon, 1975), especially pp. 33–96; and *The Theory of Communicative Action* (Boston: Beacon, 1985), vol. 1, *Reason and the Rationalization of Society*, pp. 273–337.

17. Early and still pertinent theoretical statements about medicalization include the following. Parsons argues that entry into the sick role becomes a "safety valve," regulated by doctors, that eases periodic strains in the family and at work: Talcott Parsons, *The Social System* (Glencoe: Free Press, 1951), pp. 297–321, 428–54. Relatively repressive institutions like prisons and the military, which I have observed, often expand access to the sick role to prevent more disruptive social protest: Howard Waitzkin, "Latent Functions of the Sick Role in Various Institutional Settings," *Social Science & Medicine* 5 (1971):45–75; Howard Waitzkin and Barbara Waterman, *The Exploitation of Illness in Capitalist Society* (Indianapolis: Bobbs-Merrill, 1974), pp. 36–65. Zola maintains that medicine is growing as an agency of social control because complex bureaucratic and technologic systems foster reliance on professional experts: Irving Kenneth Zola, "Medicine as an Institution of Social Control," *Sociological Review* 20 (1972):487–504, "In the Name of Health and Illness: On Some Sociopolitical Consequences of Medical Influence," *Social Science & Medicine* 9 (1975):83–87, and *Socio-Medical Inquiries* (Philadelphia: Temple University Press, 1983), pp. 243–96. As Freidson points out in his analysis of professional dominance, doctors may be more effective in enforcing societal norms than are other social control agents, partly due to the inherently hierarchical nature of the doctor-patient relationship; Eliot Freidson, *Profession of Medicine* (New York: Dodd, Mead, 1970), pp. 205–301, and *Professional Powers: A Study of the Institutionalization of Formal Knowledge* (Chicago: University of Chicago Press, 1986), pp. 1–19, 185–208. Regarding medical control of women, feminists such as Ehrenreich and English argue that medicine has regulated women's social relations, reproductive and sexual activities, family roles, and work aspirations: Barbara Ehrenreich and Deirdre English, *Complaints and Disorders: The Sexual Politics of Sickness* (Old Westbury, N.Y.: Feminist Press, 1973), and *For*

Her Own Good (New York: Anchor/Doubleday, 1978). Finally, several studies have documented how the medicalization of specific social problems—child abuse, hyperactivity, obesity, childbirth, aging, and so forth—has evolved historically: Renée C. Fox, "The Medicalization and Demedicalization of American Society," *Daedalus* 106 (1977):9–22; Peter Conrad, "The Discovery of Hyperkinesis: Notes on the Medicalization of Deviant Behavior," *Social Problems* 23 (1975):12–21; Peter Conrad and J. W. Schneider, *Deviance and Medicalization: From Badness to Sickness* (St. Louis: Mosby, 1980); P. E. S. Freund, *The Civilized Body* (Philadelphia: Temple University Press, 1982).

18. Michel Foucault, *Power/Knowledge: Selected Interviews and Other Writings* (New York: Pantheon, 1980). For a superb interpretation of the continuities and discontinuities between Marxism and Foucault's work, see Mark Poster, *Foucault, Marxism, and History* (New York: Basil Blackwell, 1984).

19. Michel Foucault, *The Birth of the Clinic: An Archaeology of Medical Perception* (New York: Vintage, 1975); *Discipline and Punish* (New York: Pantheon, 1977).

20. For instance, Foucault, *Discipline and Punish*, p. 200.

21. Michel Foucault, *The History of Sexuality*, vol. 1 (New York: Pantheon, 1978).

22. Ibid., pp. 101–02.

23. Poster, *Foucault, Marxism, and History*, pp. 131–32.

24. Foucault's analysis of professional control has stimulated other critical studies that are pertinent to social control in medicine. In particular, Donzelot's work on the "policing of families" has extended Foucault's perspectives to the professional regulation of family life. See Jacques Donzelot, *The Policing of Families* (New York: Pantheon, 1979). While not influenced to a great extent by Foucault, Lasch's historical studies of the family also shed light on the impact of professional control. See Christopher Lasch, *Haven in a Heartless World: The Family Besieged* (New York: Basic Books, 1979), especially pp. 97–110. The historical conditions that Donzelot and Lasch perceive are very similar to those outlined by Foucault: a widening involvement by professionals in the regulation of family life, and a connection between that regulation and the economic requirements of industrial society.

25. Grace Ziem, "Medical Education Since Flexner," *Health/PAC Bulletin* 76 (1977):8–14, 23. For pertinent studies of the interrelationships of race and class in the recruitment and career patterns of minorities in medicine, see Steven Shea and Mindy Thompson Fullilove, "Entry of Black and Other Minority Students into U.S. Medical Schools," *New England Journal of Medicine* 313 (1985):933–40; Stephen N. Keith, Robert M. Bell, August G. Swanson, and Albert P. Williams, "Effects of Affirmative Action in Medical Schools: A Study of the Class of 1975," *New England Journal of Medicine* 313 (1985):1519–25; and Robert Wood Johnson Foundation, *Special Report: The Foundation's Minority Medical Training Programs* (Princeton: The Foundation, 1987).

26. Murray Edelman reaches a similar conclusion about the "helping" rhetoric of the helping professions, in *Political Language: Words That Succeed and Policies That Fail* (New York: Academic Press, 1977), especially pp. 57–75.

27. The discussion that follows focuses on some theoretical implications of findings from sociolinguistics, conversation analysis, and discourse analysis. The methodologic problems of research techniques in these fields receive attention in chapter 4.

28. Studies in sociolinguistics have dealt extensively with social class, gender, and language use. A complete review of further sociolinguistic studies touching on these issues is beyond my scope here, but helpful examples include: Basil Bernstein, *Class, Codes and Control* (London: Routledge & Kegan Paul, 1971), vol. 1, *Theoretical Studies towards a Sociology of Language*; William Labov, *Sociolinguistic Patterns* (Philadelphia: University of Pennsylvania Press, 1972); William Labov and David Fanshel, *Therapeutic Discourse: Psychotherapy as Conversation* (New York: Academic Press, 1977); Sue Fisher and Alexandra Dundas Todd,

eds., *The Social Organization of Doctor-Patient Communication* (Washington, D.C.: Center for Applied Linguistics, 1983); Sue Fisher, *In the Patient's Best Interest* (New Brunswick, N.J.: Rutgers University Press, 1986); Peter Trudgill, *Sociolinguistics* (New York: Penguin, 1983). Some of my own theoretical work on these themes appears in Howard Waitzkin and John D. Stoeckle, "The Communication of Information About Illness: Clinical, Sociological, and Methodological Considerations," *Advances in Psychosomatic Medicine* 8 (1972):180–215, and "Information Control and the Micropolitics of Health Care," *Social Science & Medicine* 10 (1976):263–76. Reports of empirical findings concerning sociolinguistic barriers in medical encounters include Howard Waitzkin, "Doctor-Patient Communication: Clinical Implications of Social Scientific Research," *JAMA* 252 (1984):2441–46, and "Information Giving in Medical Care," *Journal of Health and Social Behavior* 26 (1985):81–101.

29. Candace West, *Routine Complications: Troubles with Talk between Doctors and Patients* (Bloomington: Indiana University Press, 1984), especially pp. 71–96. Other pertinent studies of doctors' interruptions and "dispreference" for patient-initiated questions are Richard M. Frankel, "Talking in Interviews: A Dispreference for Patient-Initiated Questions in Physician-Patient Encounters," in George Psathas, ed., *Interaction Competence* (New York: Irvington, 1986); Howard B. Beckman and Richard M. Frankel, "The Effect of Physician Behavior on the Collection of Data," *Annals of Internal Medicine* 101 (1984):692–96.

30. Elliot G. Mishler, *The Discourse of Medicine: Dialectics of Medical Interviews* (Norwood, N.J.: Ablex, 1984), especially chapters 3–5.

31. Jay Katz, *The Silent World of Doctor and Patient* (New York: Free Press, 1984).

32. Eric J. Cassell, *Talking with Patients*, 2 vols. (Cambridge: MIT Press, 1985). For a sample of my own hortatory suggestions about improving doctor-patient communication, see Waitzkin, "Doctor-Patient Communication: Clinical Implications of Social Scientific Research."

CHAPTER 3: A CRITICAL THEORY OF MEDICAL DISCOURSE

1. Let me immediately anticipate an objection that is doubtless already cropping up for certain theoretically minded readers. My approach will apply perspectives from both structuralism and post-structuralism to medical discourse. In searching for an underlying structure of medical discourse, I do not necessarily think of my orientation as structural*ist*. Nor do I argue that a certain structure manifests itself at all times and places. Later in this chapter, I say more about the self-imposed limits and historical specificity of this effort to look for underlying structure within medical discourse.

2. Waitzkin, "Information Giving in Medical Care."

3. In distinguishing between the spoken and written versions of the PI, I, of course, am taking some bearings from the extensive philosophic treatment of the distinction. While I am not arguing for the primacy of spoken language, there is no doubt that the spoken version of the medical encounter offers more meaningful material for critical interpretation than does the written medical record. For an influential discussion of spoken versus written language, see Jacques Derrida, *Of Grammatology* (Baltimore: Johns Hopkins University Press, 1976), especially pp. 1–140 and the translator's preface by Gayatri Chakravorty Spivak.

4. For studies on the wide differences between the spoken version of medical encounters and what doctors write about those encounters in the medical record, see A. Zuckerman, B. Starfield, C. Hochreiter, and B. Kovasznay, "Validating the Content of Pediatric Outpatient Medical Records by Means of Tape Recording Doctor-Patient Encounters," *Pediatrics* 56 (1975):407–11; Aaron V. Cicourel, "Text and Discourse," *Annual Review of Anthropology* 14 (1985):159–85; and Richard M. Frankel, "Some Observations on the Intersection of Speaking and Writing in Calls to a Poison Control Center," *Western Journal of Speech Communication* 53 (1989):195–226.

5. Harold C. Sox, Iris Margulies, and Carol Hill Sox, "Psychologically Mediated Effects of Diagnostic Tests," *New England Journal of Medicine* 95 (1981):680–85.

6. For pertinent observations of interruptions in medical encounters, see West, *Routine Complications*, pp. 56–70; Howard B. Beckman and Richard M. Frankel, "The Effect of Physician Behavior on the Collection of Data," *Annals of Internal Medicine* 101 (1984):325–29.

7. For a presentation of research on information giving, see Waitzkin, "Doctor-Patient Communication: Clinical Implications of Social Scientific Research," and "Information Giving in Medical Care."

8. John D. Stoeckle and J. Andrew Billings, "A History of History-Taking: The Medical Interview," *Journal of General Internal Medicine* 2 (1987):119–27.

9. Byron J. Good and Mary-Jo Delvecchio Good, "The Meaning of Symptoms: A Cultural Hermeneutic Model for Clinical Practice," in Leon Eisenberg and Arthur Kleinman, eds., *The Relevance of Social Science for Medicine* (Boston: Reidel, 1981); see also Arthur Kleinman, *The Illness Narratives* (New York: Basic Books, 1988), especially chapters 1 and 2.

10. Among many discussions of the effectiveness of modern medicine, see Waitzkin, *The Second Sickness*, pp. 3–43; Thomas McKeown, *The Role of Medicine: Dream, Mirage, or Nemesis?* (Princeton: Princeton University Press, 1979); Jack Hadley, *More Medical Care, Better Health? An Economic Analysis of Mortality* (Washington, D.C.: Urban Institute Press, 1982); Barbara Starfield, *The Effectiveness of Medical Care: Validating Clinical Wisdom* (Baltimore: Johns Hopkins University Press, 1985). For a valuable review of the physical examination's effectiveness, see S. K. Oboler and F. M. LaForce, "The Periodic Physical Examination in Asymptomatic Adults," *Annals of Internal Medicine* 110 (1989):214–26.

11. For critical accounts of discourse analysis and conversation analysis within medicine, and for more on the integration of macro and micro levels of analysis, see Aaron V. Cicourel, "Notes on the Integration of Micro- and Macro-Levels of Analysis," in Knorr-Cetina and Cicourel, *Advances in Social Theory and Methodology: Toward an Integration of Micro- and Macro-Sociologies*; West, *Routine Complications*, pp. 16–34; Mishler, *Discourse of Medicine*, pp. 17–57; and Fisher, *In the Patient's Best Interest*, pp. 131–85. I further consider the integration of micro and macro levels of analysis in chapter 2, and methodologic issues in sociolinguistics, conversation analysis, and discourse analysis in chapter 4.

12. Ferdinand de Saussure, *Course in General Linguistics*, trans. Roy Harris (La Salle, Ill.: Open Court, 1986 [1915]), especially pp. 11–20, 71–78.

13. A helpful collection of Jakobson's work appears in Roman Jakobson, *Verbal Art, Verbal Sign, Verbal Time* (Minneapolis: University of Minnesota Press, 1985), especially pp. 3–7, 28–33, 59–68.

14. Claude Lévi-Strauss, *Structural Anthropology* (Garden City, N.Y.: Anchor, 1967), especially pp. 202–28.

15. Pertinent sources include Claude Lévi-Strauss, *Tristes Tropiques* (New York: Criterion, 1961), and *The Raw and the Cooked* (New York: Harper & Row, 1969).

16. Lévi-Strauss, *Structural Anthropology*, pp. 181–201.

17. Derrida, for instance, has interpreted texts like love letters and art reviews, which bear little resemblance to what traditionally has been labeled literature even though they still involve mainly written materials; Jacques Derrida, *The Post Card: From Socrates to Freud and Beyond* (Chicago: University of Chicago Press, 1987), pp. 3–256, and *The Truth in Painting* (Chicago: University of Chicago Press, 1987), pp. 255–382. Similarly, Barthes has attended critically to photography, film, sports, and theater, in addition to more traditional written texts; see, for instance, Roland Barthes, *A Barthes Reader*, ed. Susan Sontag (New York: Hill and Wang, 1982), pp. 18–30, 74–88, 194–210, 317–33; and Barthes, *Image-Music-Text* (New York: Hill and Wang, 1977), pp. 79–124.

18. Terry Eagleton, *Literary Theory: An Introduction* (Minneapolis: University of Minnesota

Press, 1983), pp. 210–11; see also Fredric Jameson, *The Political Unconscious: Narrative as a Socially Symbolic Act* (Ithaca: Cornell University Press, 1981), pp. 297–99; Michael Ryan, *Marxism and Deconstruction: A Critical Articulation* (Baltimore: Johns Hopkins University Press, 1982), p. 221; Sumner, *Reading Ideologies*, pp. 207–45; John Frow, *Marxism and Literary History* (Cambridge: Harvard University Press, 1986), pp. 51–82; Richard Ohmann, *Politics of Letters* (Middletown, Conn.: Wesleyan University Press, 1987), pp. 135–211. For his development of Marxist-oriented social theory, Giddens also has adapted similar perspectives from literary criticism; see Anthony Giddens, "Action, Subjectivity, and the Constitution of Meaning," *Social Research* 53 (1986):529–45, and *The Constitution of Society* (Berkeley: University of California Press, 1984), pp. 110–61, 281–372.

19. Derrida, *Tympan*, in *Margins of Philosophy* (Chicago: University of Chicago Press, 1982), pp. xxiii–xxiv; *Of Grammatology*, pp. 141–64, and preface by Chakravorty Spivak, pp. lxxvi–lxxviii.

20. Jameson, *Political Unconscious*, pp. 80–83.

21. Terry Eagleton, *Criticism and Ideology* (London: Verso, 1978), pp. 69, 89.

22. For Bakhtin's treatment of context, social class, and ideologic elements in discourse, see especially M. M. Bakhtin, *The Dialogic Imagination* (Austin: University of Texas Press, 1981), pp. 270–300. Bakhtin extends his theoretical approach also in V. N. Volosinov (a pseudonym), *Marxism and the Philosophy of Language* (New York: Seminar Press, 1973), especially pp. 83–98. Jameson discusses these matters in *Political Unconscious*, pp. 83–89; for another application of this theoretical approach to class and discourse, see Jameson, *Marxism and Form*, especially pp. 182–205.

23. Jameson, *Political Unconscious*, p. 84.

24. See the discussion of "the language of medical encounters" in chapter 2.

25. For pertinent criticism of sexual ideology in discourse, see Sheila Rowbotham, *Hidden from History: Rediscovering Women in History from the Seventeenth Century to the Present* (New York: Pantheon, 1975), pp. 119–24, 152–56, and *Dreams and Dilemmas: Collected Writings* (London: Virago, 1983), pp. 207–14; Ryan, *Marxism and Deconstruction*, pp. 194–221; Eagleton, *Literary Theory*, p. 215; Greene and Kahn, *Making a Difference*. Critical theories of aging are currently more difficult to locate; examples include Ronald Blythe, *The View in Winter: Reflections on Old Age* (New York: Penguin, 1979), pp. 3–29; and Simone de Beauvoir, *Old Age* (London: Deutsch, Weidenfeld and Nicolson, 1972) and *Who Shall Die?* (New York: Springer, 1985). On ideologies of race, see, for instance, Angela Davis, *Women, Race and Class* (New York: Random House, 1981); Henry Louis Gates, Jr., ed., *Black Literature and Literary Theory* (New York: Methuen, 1984); Susan Willis, "Black Women Writers: Taking a Critical Perspective," in Greene and Kahn, *Making a Difference*; W. Lawrence Hogue, *Discourse and the Other: The Production of the Afro-American Text* (Durham, N.C.: Duke University Press, 1986).

26. Jameson, *Political Unconscious*, especially pp. 52–53, 266.

27. Similarly, Burawoy has clarified how the gratifications of "lived experience" in the labor process help achieve consent; see Burawoy, *Manufacturing Consent*, especially pp. 13–30, 193–203.

28. Jameson, *Political Unconscious*, p. 287. Certain philosophical underpinnings of this critique, of course, derive largely from the Frankfurt School; examples include Max Horkheimer and Theodor W. Adorno, "The Culture Industry: Enlightenment as Mass Deception," in *Dialectic of Enlightenment* (New York: Continuum, 1982), pp. 120–67; Herbert Marcuse, *One-Dimensional Man* (Boston: Beacon, 1964), especially chapters 1–7.

29. Eagleton, *Literary Theory*, pp. 186–87.

30. Eloquent statements of this calling appear in Jameson, *Political Unconscious*, pp. 296–99; and Eagleton, *Literary Theory*, pp. 214–17. From a different perspective, Walzer reaches a

complementary conclusion about the role of the socially engaged critic, in Michael Walzer, *Interpretation and Social Criticism* (Cambridge: Harvard University Press, 1987), pp. 35–66.

CHAPTER 4: ON METHOD

1. For a further development of the relationships between "micro-level" processes in medicine and "macro-level" structures of society, see chapter 2.

2. In developing these compromises, I have benefitted from the observations of Theron Britt (currently at the Department of English and Comparative Literature, University of California, Irvine), whose knowledge of critical theory in the humanities has helped a great deal in this project. At several points in the notes below, I present some of Britt's concerns that emerged from our dialogue about the compromises reached.

3. As defined in chapter 1, *medical discourse* here refers to the talk that doctors and patients exchange in their encounters. In limiting the focus to spoken discourse, I have chosen not to consider technical journals and books, conferences, conversations between doctors, and other instances of talk that a broader definition of medical discourse would encompass. A *text* is a written or spoken unit of language that is available for appraisal by one or more observers; here, the texts to be considered are transcribed recordings of spoken medical discourse in actual doctor-patient encounters. I also should emphasize here the difference between "writing down" and "reading" medical texts, which I discuss in later sections of this chapter.

4. Waitzkin and Stoeckle, "The Communication of Information About Illness: Clinical, Sociological, and Methodological Considerations."

5. Pertinent reviews of this literature appear in Howard Waitzkin, "Doctor-Patient Communication: Clinical Implications of Social Scientific Research"; Thomas S. Inui and William B. Carter, "Problems and Prospects for Health Services Research on Provider-Patient Communication," *Medical Care* 23 (1985):521–38; Debra L. Roter and Judith A. Hall, "Studies of Doctor-Patient Interaction," *Annual Review of Public Health* 10 (1989):163–80; Judith A. Hall, Debra L. Roter, and Nancy R. Katz, "Meta-Analysis of Correlates of Provider Behavior in Medical Encounters," *Medical Care* 26 (1988):657–75. My self-criticism of quantitative methodology here applies mainly to the techniques presented in Waitzkin, "Information Giving in Medical Care." Helpful critiques of quantitative methods used to study professional-client communication also appear in Mishler, *Discourse of Medicine: Dialectics of Medical Interviews*, chapter 2; Cicourel, "Notes on the Integration of Micro- and Macro-levels of Analysis"; Inui and Carter, "Problems and Prospects for Health Services Research"; and William B. Stiles, "Evaluating Medical Interview Process Components," *Medical Care* 27 (1989):212–20.

6. We used the following categories, by which we classified passages of recorded doctor-patient interactions: history taking, comments about the physical examination, further diagnostic tests, future visits, drugs or other treatment, general reassurance, silence, miscellaneous, and information about illness; Waitzkin, "Information Giving in Medical Care."

7. Some of our study's most startling findings came from a simple frequency distribution of data from time measures, rather than from the more complex, multivariate analysis that we performed according to customary social science expectations. Specifically, we found that doctors spent a remarkably small amount of time giving information to their patients—about 1.3 minutes on the average, in encounters lasting about 17 minutes each. On the other hand, doctors greatly overestimated the time that they spent giving information. In the questionnaires that we gave to the doctors after recording the encounters, doctors' mean estimate of time spent giving information in particular recording sessions was 8.9 minutes, which was 6.8 times greater than the mean time of 1.3 minutes that was observed. In short, doctors perceived that they spent much more time informing their patients than

they actually did. The frequency distributions also showed that doctors often underestimated their patients' informational needs. A measure of doctors' perception of patients' needs was derived from the discrepancy in responses to two items on the questionnaires that asked patients and doctors respectively how much information the patient desired. In fewer than one-third of the encounters did doctors correctly perceive patients' informational needs; in 6 percent doctors overestimated and in 65 percent they underestimated patients' desire for information. Thus, while doctors believed that they should take into account patients' unique characteristics in the informative process, they greatly misperceived patients' preferences. These simple quantitative findings generated amazingly wide attention in professional circles and in the mass media, much more so than the detailed multivariate results that we generated.

One multivariate finding that does deserve mention, here, however, is that doctors gave little information to patients with lower incomes or less education, as compared to patients with higher incomes or better education. This difference related to social class emerged, even though patients did not vary by class in their expressed desire for information communicated in terms that they could understand. We believed that the class differences in information giving probably derived from sociolinguistic patterns, also observed in other studies, by which working-class patients take less verbal initiative to obtain information through asking questions. See Waitzkin, "Information Giving in Medical Care."

8. Examples of quantitative content analysis include: Philip J. Stone, Dexter C. Dunphy, Marshall S. Smith, and Daniel M. Ogilvie, *The General Inquirer: A Computer Approach to Content Analysis* (Cambridge: MIT Press, 1966); Edward F. Kelly and Philip J. Stone, *Computer Recognition of English Word Senses* (New York: Elsevier, 1975); Karl Erik Rosengren, ed., *Advances in Content Analysis* (Beverly Hills: Sage, 1981); L. A. Gottschalk, F. Lolas, and L. L. Viney, eds., *Content Analysis of Verbal Behavior* (New York: Springer, 1986); Peter Abell, *The Syntax of Social Life: The Theory and Method of Comparative Narratives* (Oxford: Clarendon, 1987).

9. Claude Lévi-Strauss, *Structural Anthropology* (Garden City, N.Y.: Anchor, 1967), pp. 225–26. The poignant passage is quite revealing about Lévi-Strauss' optimism about quantification, an optimism that was either dashed or not much prioritized in his later work.

10. At this point, Theron Britt comments: "You might note that the 'qualitative''s inferiority stems from its relation to the true. Science defines the 'true' as that which is iterable over time and thus held to be timeless, but more importantly, that which *performs* in Lyotard's sense of *performativity* (Jean-François Lyotard, *The Postmodern Condition: A Report on Knowledge* [Minneapolis: University of Minnesota Press, 1984], pp. 41–60). . . . Paradoxically science measures the 'true' yet balks at the field of meaning. The moon's composition, for instance, can be accurately measured, but no scientist would attempt to analyze the meaning of the moon, or anything else. This is just another way of saying that the most important questions of human experience are not technical ones."

11. Howard Waitzkin and Barbara Waterman, *The Exploitation of Illness in Capitalist Society* (Indianapolis: Bobbs-Merrill, 1974), pp. 75–86; Howard Waitzkin, "Information Control and the Micropolitics of Health Care"; Jacqueline Wallen, Howard Waitzkin, and John D. Stoeckle, "Physician Stereotypes about Female Health and Illness: A Study of Patient's Sex and the Informative Process during Medical Interviews," *Women and Health* 4 (1979):135–46.

12. Howard Waitzkin, "Medicine, Superstructure, and Micropolitics," *Social Science & Medicine* 13A (1979):601–09.

13. Several references address these and other problems of qualitative methodology: Barney G. Glaser and Alselm L. Strauss, *The Discovery of Grounded Theory: Strategies for Qualitative Research* (Chicago: Aldine, 1967); Howard Schwartz, *Qualitative Sociology* (New York: Free Press, 1979); Jerome Kirk and Marc L. Miller, *Reliability and Validity in Qualitative*

Research (Beverly Hills, Calif.: Sage, 1986); Charles C. Ragin, *The Comparative Method: Moving beyond Qualitative and Quantitative Strategies* (Berkeley: University of California Press, 1987).

14. For more on the empirical grounding of theory in qualitative observations, see Glaser and Strauss, *Discovery of Grounded Theory;* David Silverman, *Communication and Medical Practice* (London: Sage, 1987), especially pp. 1–44.

15. Several excellent nonquantitative studies influenced by sociolinguistics, conversation analysis, and discourse analysis do not present very explicit ways to deal with these problems of bias in selection. See, for instance, the publications by Fisher, Frankel, Mishler, and West cited in chapter 2, nn. 28–30. Despite the common critique of bias in selection of observations, others argue that selectivity of interpretive categories and materials comprises the essence of good research. From this perspective, all research contains theoretical underpinnings, implicit or explicit, and creative accomplishment depends on the judicious selection of categories and materials. The latter perspective perhaps reaches its most drastic expression in post-structuralist techniques, which favor the selection for analysis, according to the analyst's conceptual leanings, of elements that are either absent or marginal within the materials under study. For pertinent discussions concerning the positive contributions of "bias" in scientific research, see Paul Feyerabend, *Against Method* (London: Verso, 1975); Jon Beckwith and Larry Miller, "Behind the Mask of Objective Science," *The Sciences* [New York Academy of Science] 16 (November/December 1976):16–31; Robert M. Young, "Evolutionary Biology and Ideology: Then and Now," in Watson Fuller, ed., *The Biological Revolution* (Garden City, N.Y.: Anchor, 1971); Thomas S. Kuhn, *The Essential Tension: Selected Studies in Scientific Tradition and Change* (Chicago: University of Chicago Press, 1977), especially chapters 11 and 13. Questions also arise about the fine line between creative selectivity and fraud in science: Barbara J. Culliton, "Coping with Fraud: the Darsee Case," *Science* 22 (1983):31–35; Arnold S. Relman, "Lessons from the Darsee Affair," *New England Journal of Medicine* 308 (1983):1415–17. For instances of interpretive emphasis on absent or marginal elements within post-structuralist criticism, see Derrida, *Of Grammatology,* and the translator's preface by Chakravorty Spivak, pp. lxxvi–lxxviii; and Derrida, *Tympan,* in *Margins of Philosophy.*

16. The self-criticism here focuses on Waitzkin, "Medicine, Superstructure, and Micropolitics."

17. For a helpful account of validity and reliability in qualitative research, see Kirk and Miller, *Reliability and Validity.*

18. Again, the pertinent studies in sociolinguistics and conversation analysis are referenced in chapter 2, nn. 28–30. Mishler has raised similar criticisms of interpretive practice in these fields; see Mishler, *Discourse of Medicine,* especially pp. 51–56.

　　In their pathbreaking work, Labov and Fanshel (*Therapeutic Discourse,* pp. 345–46) also have self-critically described the "paradox of microanalysis": "The more deeply we analyze the underlying speech actions that motivated these sequences of events, the further we remove ourselves from the conversation as it was actually experienced." To some extent, our own efforts to interpret elements of ideology, social control, and underlying structure in medical discourse also will manifest this same paradox, since these elements rarely reach the consciousness of the doctors and patients involved. Yet, I will argue, our interpretive approach does address in a more cogent way the linkages between medical discourse and the social context of medicine.

19. For influential views on interpretation in post-structuralist critical theory, see Derrida, *Of Grammatology,* especially pp. 27–93, and *The Post Card,* especially pp. 259–91. More recently, interpretive techniques in psychology and sociology have begun to adopt similar perspectives, using various criteria to evaluate the quality of subjective interpretation. Examples of such theories of interpretation include: Paul Ricouer, *Hermeneutics and the Human Sciences: Essays on Language* (New York: Cambridge University Press, 1981); Ricouer,

Lectures on Ideology and Utopia (New York: Columbia University Press, 1986); Anthony Giddens, *New Rules of Sociological Method: A Positive Critique of Interpretative Sociologies* (New York: Basic Books, 1976); Giddens, *The Constitution of Society: Outline of the Theory of Structuration* (Berkeley: University of California Press, 1984); Giddens, "Action, Subjectivity, and the Constitution of Meaning," *Social Research* 53 (1986):529–45; John B. Thompson, *Studies in the Theory of Ideology* (Berkeley: University of California Press, 1984).

Theron Britt summarizes some of the complaints that literary critics raise concerning social scientific criteria of interpretation: "As Derrida, Foucault and others have noted, however, concepts by the nature *qua* concepts cannot be empirical, and the generalized notion of the empirical itself is suspect. Concepts, rather than numbers, are necessarily mediated through the slippery passageway of language, which because of the nature of the sign, resists or undermines all efforts at quantification. . . . The 'same' text can produce equally competent but widely divergent readings or receptions from exactly the same 'data.' Standards are only appropriate when reader and writer share them; then one can judge a particular instance against a shared template. Luckily, our culture gives us many shared standards, but these common cultural paradigms are (as in this case) what are often in question."

20. This problem of presenting summaries of nonliterary texts actually reflects a more general presentational question in qualitative methods. In the social sciences, such methods usually include the presentation of a summary of the phenomenon under study. For instance, a qualitative study in anthropology (such as Lévi-Strauss' account of symbolic healing, mentioned in the last chapter) generally contains a detailed and extensive summary of pertinent observations collected during field work, before the writer interprets those observations (Lévi-Strauss, "The Effectiveness of Symbols," in *Structural Anthropology*). Similarly, qualitative research in sociology (such as Burawoy's study of ideologic consent in the workplace, cited in chapter 2) depends on the researcher's summarizing qualitative observations, based on which the interpretive analysis presumably flows (Burawoy, *Manufacturing Consent*). Although techniques of presentation vary widely in qualitative studies, an underlying assumption in such work is that the summary of observations offered by the writer conveys an accurate account of the observed reality.

Freud mentions the difficulties in making a summary of psychoanalytic interaction available for the reader. In his introduction to the famous case of Dora, Freud notes that the case record does not convey an exact transcription of his psychoanalytic encounters with Dora, but instead a trustworthy summary: "I have not yet succeeded in solving the problem of how to record for publication the history of a treatment of long duration. . . . [The] record is not absolutely—phonologically—exact, but it can claim to possess a high degree of trustworthiness. Nothing of any importance has been altered in it except in some places the order in which the explanations are given; and this has been done for the sake of presenting the case in a more connected form. . . . I have as a rule not reproduced the process of interpretation to which the patient's associations and communications had to be subjected, but only the result of that process" (Sigmund Freud, "Fragment of an Analysis of a Case of Hysteria," in *The Complete Psychological Works: Standard Edition*, trans. and ed. James Strachey [London: Hogarth, 1953 (1905)], vol. 7, pp. 10–11). Kleinman recently has repeated this dilemma of presenting clinical encounters in a readable form; Kleinman, *Illness Narratives*, pp. xiv–xv.

21. Waitzkin, "Medicine, Superstructure, and Micropolitics."

22. An influential sociolinguistic convention for transcribing conversation appears in Gail Jefferson, "Explanation of Transcript Notation," in Jim Schenkein, ed., *Studies in the Organization of Conversational Interaction* (New York: Academic Press, 1978), pp. xi–xvi. Modifications of this transcription scheme, applied to medical discourse, appear in West, *Routine Complications*, pp. xiii–xiv; and Mishler, *Discourse of Medicine*, pp. 91–93. For an example of concern with the margin in critical theory, see Derrida, *Tympan*. As noted in the last chapter,

calls for the application of critical theory to nonliterary texts, with few clues on how to do it, appear in the writings of critics such as Eagleton, Jameson, and Ryan; see chapter 3, n. 18.

23. For a helpful discussion of the problematic nature of transcription, see Mishler, *Discourse of Medicine*, pp. 28–35, 60–61. While Mishler describes his own transcription rules rather explicitly, he de-emphasizes the issues of training and quality assurance.

24. An example of this format appears in Howard Waitzkin, "The Micropolitics of Medicine: A Contextual Analysis," *International Journal of Health Services* 14 (1984):339–78.

25. For example, in Waitzkin, "Medicine, Superstructure, and Micropolitics."

26. For example, Waitzkin, *The Second Sickness*, pp. 137–83.

27. Mishler, *Discourse of Medicine*, pp. 95–135. The philosophic distinction between the pragmatics of narrative and the pragmatics of science also is pertinent to this clash of voices (Lyotard, *Postmodern Condition*, pp. 18–41). An anthropologic account of a similar clash of voices in primitive healing appears in Byron J. Good and Mary-Jo Delvecchio Good, "The Meaning of Symptoms: A Cultural Hermeneutic Model for Clinical Practice," in Leon Eisenberg and Arthur Kleinman, eds., *The Relevance of Social Science for Medicine* (Boston: Reidel, 1981). See also Kleinman, *Illness Narratives*, especially chapters 1 and 2. With a quite different theoretical slant, studies in "medical humanities" also have emphasized the importance of storytelling in medicine; for recent examples, see Howard Brody, *Stories of Sickness* (New Haven: Yale University Press, 1987), and Robert Coles, *The Call of Stories* (Boston: Houghton Mifflin, 1989).

28. Feyerabend, *Against Method*, pp. 23–28; Feyerabend develops an extensive philosophic justification for an anarchist approach in scientific methodology, based on his review of creative milestones in the history of science.

29. Sumner's criteria for a "common-sense" reading of ideology are similar. These criteria call for the reader's focusing on repetitions, assumptions, inconsistencies, absences of certain topics, and "general drift" within the text to be interpreted. See Sumner, *Reading Ideologies*, pp. 191–93.

30. Theron Britt offers the following reservations about the compromise of group process in interpretation: "Note that your reliance for validity on multiple interpreters is a consensus model, and hence liable to the appropriation by ideology, which is, if nothing else, maintained via consensus, not 'truth.' A sticky problem this one. . . . Your consensus model of interpretation might best be outlined by Stanley Fish in his by now classic, *Is There a Text in This Class?* (Cambridge: Harvard University Press, 1980). He supports a model of ungrounded interpretation that is based on a community of readers sharing the same assumptions of validity. In my opinion, however, there simply is no way that 'validity' can be achieved as long as by 'validity' we mean an approximation to an empirically real world. I follow Althusser (from Lacan) in seeing the 'real' as our imaginative construct mediated by the forces of ideology. The best we can do is to map ideology, but to do that we must of course pick a point of reference from which to begin, and picking that initial point is a process that finally does not answer to 'validity.'"

Among the possible responses to Britt's reservations, I want to emphasize the adequacy of a group process that encourages communication in good faith, without the dominance of a single individual. In the present project, for instance, Britt's own force of intellect has prevailed in many interpretations of specific texts.

31. Theron Britt also raises some misgivings about the negative case: "As I mentioned to you previously, the 'negative case' in my opinion is not really viable since ideology is at work in *all* discourse or in none; the ideology may change, be worthy of support or not, but is always there as a principle of structure to be replicated, worked against or whatever, as one values it. The 'negative case' can only be negation to a particular ideologic message. Your statement implies some form of value free encounter. Anyway, you can deal with this

issue at length in a later chapter." Here, Britt actually anticipates a later interpretation, which critically examines medical encounters in which evidence of ideologic language is not apparent.

32. Further details about the sampling procedure appear in Waitzkin, "Information Giving in Medical Care." We recorded these doctor-patient interactions during the mid- and late-1970s. While one might expect to see some changes in medical discourse resulting from events during the 1980s (AIDS, increased malpractice litigation, consumerism, corporate involvement in medicine, and so forth), I have continued to sample doctor-patient interaction in a nonrandom way and have found no major changes from the patterns that I report in later chapters, which do not focus on these newer developments. On the other hand, a follow-up study using similar methodologic criteria would be quite reasonable, if we can find the time and financial support to do it.

33. Mishler used a similar technique of sampling from our larger random sample, although he did not select randomly from the larger sample and checked only the gender of patients in the smaller sample that he constructed for in-depth analysis. Mishler's justification of his own procedures (presented in a note) is interesting and pertinent to the sampling decisions underlying this type of work (*Discourse of Medicine*, pp. 59–60): "Waitzkin and Stoeckle's original corpus of nearly 500 interviews included a stratified random sample of physicians in private and clinic sessions in Boston and Oakland [actually, the larger sample encompassed three counties in Massachusetts and California]. For the present study, a small series of about 25 tapes was selected initially from the larger sample. Male and female patients were equally represented in the series, and both single and multiple interviews of a patient with the same physician were included. The original tapes were sequentially ordered by code numbers assigned to physicians and each of their successive patients. The selection procedure was to choose the 'next' code number in the sequence where the interview met the criteria noted above until the cells were filled. Although this was not a random sampling procedure it ensured heterogeneity among the interviews and there was no reason to believe that the series was biased in a systematic way with reference to the original sample. The analyses presented here are based on a small number of interviews drawn from this series. Further, analyses are restricted to brief excerpts from the full interviews which exemplify issues of primary theoretical interest. This description of the procedure is intended to clarify the grounds on which the claim is made that the interviews examined in this study are 'typical' medical interviews. This claim does not rely on statistical criteria or rules for selecting a 'representative' sample. Rather, it rests on a shared understanding and recognition of these interviews as 'representative,' that is, as displays of normatively appropriate talk between patients and physicians."

An unexpected sadness that arose from our random sampling procedures involved a lack of minority and women physicians in the sample that we eventually assembled. During the mid to late 1970s, these sampling procedures accurately reflected the very small number of practicing internists who were members of minority groups or women. That is, as we sampled randomly from lists of practicing internists, the names of minority or female physicians simply did not appear. Yet a question obviously remains: Do minority or women physicians process contextual problems differently from the doctors who appeared in our sample?

In preparing this book, I have chosen to report only on the encounters that we selected randomly. Since one purpose here is to represent typical encounters between patients and primary-care internists, this decision seems reasonable. On the other hand, our research group also has done several nonrandom recordings of encounters involving both minority and women physicians. This approach recognizes that the proportion of women entering medicine has increased during recent years, even though the proportion of minorities has changed very little. When we have applied the interpretive techniques described below to these recordings, we actually have found, interestingly enough, no clear-cut differences in the patterns that we describe for encounters involving white male physicians. We will report more details about these comparisons in later publications.

One further question involves the possibility that sampling encounters in other primary-care specialties or in community-clinic settings would lead to alternative conclusions. For instance, practitioners of family medicine might deal with contextual issues in novel ways, or the values promoted by community-based clinics might encourage approaches different from those seen here. Again, we have done nonrandom recordings in family-practice and community-clinic settings and have not found striking variations. Still, the question of variability among specialties and practice settings, like that concerning gender and racial differences among practitioners, ought to be settled through additional research.

34. Examples of publications by other investigators deriving from this same data base of recordings include: Mishler, *Discourse of Medicine*; Marianne A. Paget, "On the Work of Talk: Studies in Misunderstanding," in Fisher and Todd, *Social Organization of Doctor-Patient Communication*; and Stephany Borges, "A Feminist Critique of Scientific Ideology: An Analysis of Two Doctor-Patient Encounters," in Sue Fisher and Alexandra Dundas Todd, eds., *Discourse and Institutional Analysis: Medicine, Education, and Law* (Norwood, N.J.: Ablex, 1986).

35. Eloquent discussions about the need for transcription rules and the types of compromises involved in selecting workable ones appear in Mishler, *Discourse of Medicine*, pp. 21–35, 59–64, and 91–93; and West, *Routine Complications*, pp. xiii–xiv and 42–46.

36. Althusser, "Ideology and Ideological State Apparatuses," in *Lenin and Philosophy and Other Essays*, p. 162. For further discussion and critique of Althusser's work on ideology, see chapter 2.

37. For more details, see: Howard Waitzkin, "Two-Class Medicine Returns to the United States: Impact of Medi-Cal Reform," *Lancet* 2 (1984):1144–46; Howard Waitzkin, Barbara V. Akin, Luis M. de la Maza, F. Allan Hubbell, Hooshang Meshkinpour, Lloyd Rucker, and Jerome S. Tobis, "Deciding Against Corporate Management of a State-Supported Academic Medical Center," *New England Journal of Medicine* 315 (1986):1299–1304; F. Allan Hubbell, Howard Waitzkin, Lloyd Rucker, Barbara V. Akin, and M. Gabriela Heide, "Financial Barriers to Medical Care: A Prospective Study in a University-Affiliated Community Clinic," *American Journal of the Medical Sciences* 297 (1989):158–62; Barbara V. Akin, Lloyd Rucker, F. Allan Hubbell, Ralph W. Cygan, and Howard Waitzkin, "Access to Medical Care in a Medically Indigent Population," *Journal of General Internal Medicine* 4 (1989):216–20; F. Allan Hubbell, Howard Waitzkin, Shiraz I. Mishra, and John Dombrink, "Evaluating Health Care Needs of the Poor: A Community-Oriented Approach," *American Journal of Medicine* 87 (1989):127–31; Vicki Mayster, Howard Waitzkin, F. Allan Hubbell, and Lloyd Rucker, "Local Advocacy for the Medically Indigent: Strategies and Accomplishments in One County," *JAMA* 263 (1990):262–68.

38. Theron Britt.

39. Stephany Borges and Constance Williams.

40. See the Preface for information on obtaining the transcripts. Designations of the encounters presented in the chapters that follow correspond to these original code numbers: Encounter 5A, 05/048; 5B, 03/027; 5C, 05/053; 6A, 09/094; 6B, 10/103; 6C, 09/092; 7A, 01/007; 7B, 05/055; 7C, 05/049; 8A, 10/101; 8B, 03/025; 8C, 06/062; 9A, 01/009; 10A, 01/002; 10B, 01/001; 10C, 06/061; 10D, 01/006.

CHAPTER 5: MEN, WORK, AND THE FAMILY

1. For details about the methods used, see chapter 4.

2. This summary repeats, now for the third time, the encounter that introduced chapter 1 and concluded chapter 3. The other summaries earlier matched with this one reappear

respectively, with fuller interpretation, in chapters 6 and 8. Preliminary interpretations of this transcript previously have appeared in Waitzkin, *The Second Sickness*, pp. 145–55, and "The Micropolitics of Medicine: A Contextual Analysis."

3. For more on ideologic dimensions of defining health as capacity to work, see chapter 2.

4. See chapter 2 for further discussion of Gramsci.

5. Regarding the post-structuralist focus on the "margins" of a text, see chapter 3.

6. Ross J. Baldessarini, "Drugs and the Treatment of Psychiatric Disorders," in Alfred Goodman Gilman, Louis S. Goodman, Theodore W. Rall, and Ferid Murad, eds., *The Pharmacological Basis of Therapeutics* (New York: Macmillan, 1985), pp. 387–445.

7. Lukács' analysis of reification receives attention in chapter 2.

8. For the pertinence of Foucault, see chapter 2.

9. The impact of scientific ideology in supporting such relations of dominance and subordination also recalls Habermas' treatment of this theme; see discussion in chapter 2.

10. See n. 3 above.

11. An occupational illness is usually defined as one that is caused or aggravated by a condition or exposure at work. For instance, see Linda Rosenstock and Mark R. Cullen, *Clinical Occupational Medicine* (Philadelphia: Saunders, 1986), p. 9.

12. For descriptions of jokes among doctors, see Charles L. Bosk, *Forgive and Remember: Managing Medical Failure* (Chicago: University of Chicago Press, 1979), pp. 75, 103–10; Marcia Millman, *The Unkindest Cut: Life in the Backrooms of Medicine* (New York: Morrow, 1977), especially pp. 61–87; Terry Mizrahi, *Getting Rid of Patients: Contradictions in the Socialization of Physicians* (New Brunswick, N.J.: Rutgers University Press, 1986), especially pp. 21–42. Regarding tension release through joking and other maneuvers in medical encounters, see Judith A. Hall, Debra L. Roter, and Nancy R. Katz, "Task Versus Socioemotional Behaviors in Physicians," *Medical Care* 25 (1987):399–412; Richard C. Wasserman and Thomas S. Inui, "Systematic Analysis of Clinician-Patient Interactions: A Critique of Recent Approaches with Suggestions for Future Research," *Medical Care* 21 (1983):279–93.

13. Richard Sennett and Jonathan Cobb, *The Hidden Injuries of Class* (New York: Vintage, 1972), especially pp. 3–50.

14. Waitzkin, *The Second Sickness*, pp. 8–18.

15. For a classic psychoanalytic discussion of anxiety's roots in psychic conflict, see Sigmund Freud, *A General Introduction to Psychoanalysis* (New York: Permabooks, 1953), pp. 400–418. Lacan extends this interpretation of anxiety to conflicts in language (Jacques Lacan, *Ecrits* [New York: Norton, 1977], especially pp. 292–324).

16. Gordon H. Williams and Eugene Braunwald, "Hypertensive Vascular Disease," in Eugene Braunwald, Kurt J. Isselbacher, Robert G. Petersdorf, Jean D. Wilson, Joseph B. Martin, and Anthony S. Fauci, eds., *Harrison's Principles of Internal Medicine* (New York: McGraw-Hill, 1987), p. 1024.

17. For studies on the frequency of emotional problems in primary care, see D. A. Regier, J. D. Burke, R. W. Manderscheid, and B. J. Burns, "The Chronically Mentally Ill in Primary Care," *Psychological Medicine* 15 (1985):265–73; Lloyd Rucker, Elizabeth B. Frye, and Ralph W. Cygan, "Feasibility and Usefulness of Depression Screening in Medical Outpatients," *Archives of Internal Medicine* 146 (1986):729–31; Douglas B. Kamerow, "Is Screening for Mental Health Problems Worthwhile in Family Practice? An Affirmative View," *Journal of Family Practice* 25 (1987):181–87; Greg Wilkinson, *Overview of Mental Health Practices in Primary Care Settings, with Recommendations for Further Research*, Department of Health and Human Services Pub. No. (ADM) 86-1467 (Washington, D.C.: U.S. Government Printing Office, 1986), pp. 4–15; Stephen F. Jencks, "Recognition of Mental Distress and Diagnosis of Mental Disorder in Primary Care," *JAMA* 253 (1985):1903–07; Julia E. Connelly and Alvin I.

Mushlin, "The Reasons Patients Request 'Checkups,'" *Journal of General Internal Medicine* 1 (1986):163–65.

18. Examples include: Marian R. Stuart and Joseph A. Lieberman, *The Fifteen Minute Hour: Applied Psychotherapy for the Primary Care Physician* (New York: Praeger, 1986); Steven L. Dubovsky and Michael P. Weissberg, *Clinical Psychiatry in Primary Care* (Baltimore: Williams, Wilkins, 1986).

19. For the problem of medicalization and its implications for social control, see chapter 2.

CHAPTER 6: WOMEN, WORK, AND THE FAMILY

1. Recent studies of the different utilization of medical services by men and women include: Tommy McLemore and James DeLosier, "1985 Summary: The National Ambulatory Care Survey," *NCHS Advance Data* (Hyattsville, Md.: National Center for Health Statistics [DHHS Publication No. (PHS) 87-1250], 1987), pp. 1–3; W. A. V. Clark, H. E. Freeman, R. Kane, and C. E. Lewis, "The Influence of Domestic Position on Health Status," *Social Science & Medicine* 24 (1987):501–06; P. D. Cleary, D. Mechanic, and J. R. Greenley, "Sex Differences in Medical Care Utilization: An Empirical Investigation," *Journal of Health & Social Behavior* 23 (1982): 106–19. For perspectives on feminist complaints about medicine from a general viewpoint, see Ellen Lewin and Virginia Olesen, eds., *Women, Health, and Healing* (New York: Tavistock, 1985); Ehrenreich and English, *For Her Own Good*; Judith Lorber, *Women Physicians: Careers, Status and Power* (New York: Tavistock, 1984); Regina Markell Morantz, Cynthia Stodola Pomerleau, and Carol Hansen Fenichel, eds., *In Her Own Words: Oral Histories of Women Physicians* (Westport, Conn.: Greenwood, 1982). Studies of communication between doctors and female patients include: Wallen, Waitzkin, and Stoeckle, "Physician Stereotypes about Female Health and Illness"; West, *Routine Complications*; Fisher, *In the Patient's Best Interest*. In this chapter, I am especially indebted to Stephany Borges, who developed a somewhat different interpretation of two encounters considered here, in "A Feminist Critique of Scientific Ideology: An Analysis of Two Doctor-Patient Encounters," and to Leslie Rabine for thoughtful suggestions and feedback.

2. Among the many outstanding examples of feminist scholarship that have appeared during the past two decades, several have proved very helpful in this chapter's interpretive approach: Kuhn and Wolpe, eds., *Feminism and Materialism*, especially pp. 1–41; Greene and Kahn, *Making a Difference*, especially pp. 1–36 and 59–112; Nancy Chodorow, *The Reproduction of Mothering: Psychoanalysis and the Sociology of Gender* (Berkeley: University of California Press, 1978); Dorothy Dinnerstein, *The Mermaid and the Minotaur: Sexual Arrangements and Human Malaise* (New York: Harper & Row, 1976); Luce Irigaray, *Speculum of the Other Woman* (Ithaca, N.Y.: Cornell University Press, 1985), especially pp. 13–25; Julia Kristeva, *The Kristeva Reader* (New York: Columbia University Press, 1986), especially pp. 238–71.

For my purposes here, Greene and Kahn's definition of ideology becomes quite pertinent (pp. 2–3): "The social construction of gender takes place through the workings of ideology. Ideology is that system of beliefs and assumptions—unconscious, unexamined, invisible—which represents 'the imaginary relationships of individuals to their real conditions of existence' (Althusser . . .); but it is also a system of practices that informs every aspect of daily life—the clothes we wear, the machines we invent, the pictures we paint, the words we use. . . . Ideology masks contradictions, offers partial truths in the interests of a false coherence, thereby obscuring the actual conditions of our existence and making people act in ways that may actually contradict their material interests."

Useful feminist studies of language, including medical discourse, include Robin Lakoff, *Language and Woman's Place* (New York: Harper & Row, 1975); Nancy Henley, *Body Politics: Power, Sex, and Nonverbal Communication* (Englewood Cliffs, N.J.: Prentice-Hall, 1977); West, *Routine Complications*; Alexandra D. Todd, *Intimate Adversaries* (Philadelphia: University of Pennsylvania Press, 1989); and Fisher, *In the Patient's Best Interest*.

3. For further details on the methodology of selecting and interpreting these transcripts, see chapter 4.

4. Professional surveillance of sexuality in Foucault's work receives attention in chapter 2. Feminists have pointed out the roots of hysterization in Freudian thought, as well as its influence on diagnostic thinking in obstetrics, gynecology, and other fields of medicine. For instance, see Juliet Mitchell, *Psychoanalysis and Feminism* (New York: Random House, 1975); Juliet Mitchell, "Introduction I," in Mitchell and Jacqueline Rose, eds., *Feminine Sexuality: Jacques Lacan and the "Ecole Freudienne"* (New York: Norton, 1982); Judith Kegan Gardiner, "Mind Mother: Psychoanalysis and Feminism," in Greene and Kahn, *Making a Difference*; G. J. Barker-Benfield, *The Horrors of the Half-Known Life: Male Attitudes toward Women and Sexuality in Nineteenth-Century America* (New York: Harper & Row, 1976), especially Part 2; Ehrenreich and English, *For Her Own Good*; Irigaray, *Speculum*; Kristeva, *Kristeva Reader*; Charles Bernheimer and Claire Kahane, eds., *In Dora's Case: Freud-Hysteria-Feminism* (New York: Columbia University Press, 1985). For Freud's classic statements, see Freud, "Fragment of an Analysis of a Case of Hysteria [Dora]" (1905), "Some Psychical Consequences of the Anatomical Distinction Between the Sexes" (1925), and "Female Sexuality" (1931), in *The Complete Psychological Works: Standard Edition*.

5. Lawrence L. Weed, *Medical Records, Medical Education, and Patient Care* (Cleveland: Press of Case Western Reserve University, 1970). For sympathetic critiques of problem-oriented records, see Stephen E. Goldfinger, "The Problem-Oriented Record: A Critique from a Believer," *New England Journal of Medicine* 288 (1973):606–08; Robert H. Fletcher, "Auditing Problem-Oriented Records and Traditional Records," *New England Journal of Medicine* 290 (1974):829–33.

6. Again, minor references to lines in the transcript that I have not excerpted here may be traced to the full transcripts in the microfilmed appendix; the preface gives details on acquisition.

7. Marcia Millman, *Such a Pretty Face: Being Fat in America* (New York: Norton, 1980); Susie Orbach, *Fat Is a Feminist Issue* (New York: Berkley, 1979); Kim Chernin, *The Hungry Self: Women, Eating and Identity* (New York: Times Books, 1985), and *The Obsession: Reflections on the Tyranny of Slenderness* (New York: Harper, 1982).

8. Thomas A. Wadden and Albert J. Stunkard, "Social and Psychological Consequences of Obesity," *Annals of Internal Medicine* 106 (1985):1062–67; James E. Mitchell, Harold C. Seim, Eduardo Colon, and Claire Pomeroy, "Medical Complications and Medical Management of Bulimia," *Annals of Internal Medicine* 107 (1987):71–77; Rudolph M. Bell, *Holy Anorexia* (Chicago: University of Chicago Press, 1985).

9. Childrearing as an activity that defines self within the social order has received wide critical attention among feminists. For a recent application of Lacan's theory of the phallus to this theme, see Greene and Kahn, *Making a Difference*, p. 9: "Only by accepting a definition of herself as the one who lacks a penis, and consenting to her role as childbearer (that is, reproducer of the phallus) in the marital exchange, does she take her place in the symbolic and social order." See review of Engels' discussion of the family's reproductive function in chapter 2.

10. When he offers himself as a resource, the doctor's tone on the tape is a bit reluctant. Theron Britt has commented on this passage as follows: "Yet that contextual history finally is used solely as a barometer of where further along the line of 'expertise' she is to be sent— i.e., to another health professional who specializes in such things."

11. Male-oriented devices in language to create order from the perceived disorder of women's experience also have attracted feminist criticism; for instance, see Greene and Kahn, *Making a Difference*, pp. 10, 22. The post-structuralist emphasis on the margins of discourse receives attention in chapter 3.

12. See chapter 5, nn. 17 and 18, for references on psychiatric problems in primary care.

13. In the case of Dora, Freud refers to the "housewife's psychosis" of Dora's mother, who was "an uncultivated woman and above all as a foolish one, who had concentrated all her interests upon domestic affairs, especially since her husband's illness and the estrangement to which it led. She presented the picture, in fact, of what might be called the 'housewife's psychosis.' She had no understanding of her children's more active interests, and was occupied all day long in cleaning the house with its furniture and utensils and in keeping them clean—to such an extent as to make it impossible to use or enjoy them." Presumably, certain elements of Dora's hysteria derived in part from her mother's enactment of the housewife role. See Sigmund Freud, "Fragment of an Analysis of a Case of Hysteria [Dora]," p. 20. I am indebted to Theron Britt for reminding me about this passage. For a classic feminist discussion of similar themes, see Betty Friedan, *The Feminine Mystique* (New York: Norton, 1963).

14. Michael Balint and others, *Treatment or Diagnosis: A Study of Repeat Prescriptions in General Practice* (Philadelphia: Lippincott, 1970).

15. Timothy E. Quill, "Somatization Disorder," *JAMA* 254 (1985):3075–79; Wayne Katon, Alfred O. Berg, Anthony J. Robins, and Steven Risse, "Depression—Medical Utilization and Somatization," *Western Journal of Medicine* 144 (1986):564–68; G. Richard Smith, Roberta A. Monson, and Debby C. Ray, "Patients with Multiple Unexplained Symptoms," *Archives of Internal Medicine* 146 (1986):69–72; G. Richard Smith, Roberta A. Monson, and Debby C. Ray, "Psychiatric Consultation in Somatization Disorder: A Randomized Controlled Study," *New England Journal of Medicine* 314 (1986):1407–13; Javier I. Escobar, Jacqueline M. Bolding, Richard L. Hough, Marvin Karno, M. Audrey Burnam, and Kenneth B. Wells, "Somatization in the Community: Relationship to Disability and Use of Services," *American Journal of Public Health* 77 (1987):837–40; and Craig Kaplan, Mack Lipkin, Jr., and Geoffrey H. Gordon, "Somatization in Primary Care: Patients with Unexplained and Vexing Symptoms," *Journal of General Internal Medicine* 3 (1988):177–90. For Freud's exposition of "conversion-hysteria," see, for instance, Sigmund Freud, *A General Introduction to Psychoanalysis* (New York: Permabooks, 1953), especially lectures 24 and 25; "Studies in Hysteria," in Freud, *Standard Edition* (with J. Breuer, 1895); and "Fragment of an Analysis of a Case of Hysteria [Dora]."

16. This summary repeats again an encounter that introduced chapter 1 and concluded chapter 3. Other summaries earlier matched with this one appear with more extensive interpretation in chapter 5 and chapter 8.

17. See n. 9 above for more on the family's reproductive function.

18. On the medical management of family violence, see, for instance, Kathleen M. White, Jane Snyder, Richard Bourne, and Eli H. Newberger, *Treating Family Violence in a Pediatric Hospital* (Rockville, Md.: Public Health Service [DHHS Publication No. (ADM) 87-1504], 1987); Stephen Ludwig, "Child Abuse and Neglect," in M. William Schwart, ed., *Principles and Practice of Clinical Pediatrics* (Chicago: Year Book Publishers, 1987); Richard J. Gelles, *Family Violence* (Newbury Park, Calif.: Sage, 1987).

19. For more on medicalization, see chapter 2 and accompanying notes.

CHAPTER 7: AGING

1. Within a now voluminous literature, the following sources give useful descriptions of the aging population and the growing role of geriatric medicine: Robert N. Butler, *Why Survive? Being Old in America* (New York: Harper & Row, 1975); Carroll L. Estes and others, *Political Economy, Health, and Aging* (Boston: Little, Brown, 1984); Meredith Minkler and Carroll L. Estes, eds., *Readings in the Political Economy of Aging* (Farmingdale, N.Y.: Baywood, 1984); John W. Rowe and Richard Besdine, *Geriatric Medicine* (Boston: Little, Brown, 1988); Chris-

tine K. Cassel and John R. Walsh, eds., *Geriatric Medicine* (New York: Springer, 1990). Many commentators have noted the inadequacy of social policies pertinent to the elderly; for instance, see Butler; Estes and others; Minkler and Estes; Nancy R. Zweibel and Christine K. Cassel, eds., *Clinical and Policy Issues in the Care of the Nursing Home Patient* (Philadelphia: Saunders, 1988). Controversial ethical dilemmas in the care of elderly patients have received attention in such sources as Daniel Callahan, *Setting Limits: Medical Goals in an Aging Society* (New York: Simon and Schuster, 1987); Diane E. Meier and Christine K. Cassel, "Nursing Home Placement and the Demented Patient: A Case Presentation and Ethical Analysis," *Annals of Internal Medicine* 104 (1986):98–105; Robert Steinbrook and Bernard Lo, "Artificial Feeding—Solid Ground, Not a Slippery Slope," *New England Journal of Medicine* 318 (1988):286–90; Eric B. Larson, Bernard Lo, and Mark E. Williams, "Evaluation and Care of Elderly Patients with Dementia," *Journal of General Internal Medicine* 1 (1986):116–26.

2. For descriptions and evaluations of multidisciplinary approaches in geriatrics, see Laurence Z. Rubenstein, Karen R. Josephson, G. Darryl Wieland, Patricia A. English, James A. Sayre, and Robert L. Kane, "Effectiveness of a Geriatric Evaluation Unit: A Randomized Clinical Trial," *New England Journal of Medicine* 311 (1984):1664–70; Arnold M. Epstein, Judith A. Hall, Richard Besdine, Edward Cumella, Jr., Michael Feldstein, Barbara J. McNeil, and John W. Rowe, "The Emergence of Geriatric Assessment Units: The 'New Technology of Geriatrics,'" *Annals of Internal Medicine* 106 (1987):299–303; and Arnold M. Epstein, Judith A. Hall, Richard Besdine, and others, "Consultative Geriatric Assessment for Ambulatory Patients: A Randomized Trial in a Health Maintenance Organization," *JAMA* 263 (1990): 538–44.

3. Descriptive studies of doctor-patient interaction involving elderly patients have only begun to emerge recently. Examples include Kathryn Rost and Debra Roter, "Predictors of Recall of Medication Regimens and Recommendations for Lifestyle Change in Elderly Patients," *Gerontologist* 27 (1987):510–15; Michele G. Greene, Ronald Adelman, Rita Charon, and Susie Hoffman, "Ageism in the Medical Encounter: An Exploratory Study of the Doctor-Elderly Patient Relationship," *Language & Communication* 6 (1986):113–24; Michele G. Greene, Susie Hoffman, Rita Charon, and Ronald Adelman, "Psychosocial Concerns in the Medical Encounter: A Comparison of the Interactions of Doctors with Their Old and Young Patients," *Gerontologist* 27 (1987):164–68; Marie R. Haug and Marcia G. Ory, "Doctor-Patient Relationships and Their Impact on Self Care of the Elderly," in B. Holstein, K. Dean, T. Hickey, and L. Coppard, eds., *Self Care and Health Behavior in Old Age* (Copenhagen: Croom Helm, 1986); Earle L. Snider, "The Elderly and Their Doctors," *Social Science & Medicine* 14A (1980):527–31; Barbara Bender Dreher, *Communication Skills for Working with Elders* (New York: Springer, 1987). For a useful review of this literature, see Marie R. Haug and Marcia G. Ory, "Issues in Elderly Patient-Provider Interactions," *Research on Aging* 9 (1987): 3–44. Fruitful readings of aging in literature include: Blythe, *The View in Winter*; Beauvoir, *Old Age* and *Who Shall Die?*; May Sarton, *As We Are Now: A Novel* (New York: Norton, 1973) and *At Seventy: A Journal* (New York: Norton, 1984); and Kathleen Woodward and Murray M. Schwartz, eds., *Memory and Desire: Aging—Literature—Psychoanalysis* (Bloomington: Indiana University Press, 1986).

4. In chapter 2, I discuss applications of Lukács' theory of reification to medical discourse.

5. My emphasis on superficially marginal elements of discourse again takes its bearings from a post-structuralist approach to textual reading, as noted in chapter 3.

6. During the late 1980s, Medicare has covered approximately 44 percent of senior citizen's medical bills, and elderly people currently pay more money out of pocket for health services (per capita, both in absolute dollars and expenses controlled for inflation) than before the passage of Medicare in 1965. For pertinent discussions of the limitations of public and private insurance for the elderly, see Minkler and Estes, *Political Economy of Aging*; Linda H. Aiken and Karl D. Bays, "The Medicare Debate—Round One," *New England Journal of*

Medicine 311 (1984):1196–1200; David Blumenthal, Mark Schlesinger, Pamela Brown Drumheller, and the Harvard Medicare Project, "The Future of Medicare," *New England Journal of Medicine* 314 (1986):722–28; Howard Waitzkin, "Why It's Time for a National Health Program in the United States," *Western Journal of Medicine* 150 (1989):101–07.

7. Andrew J. Silver, "Anorexia of Aging," in John E. Morley, ed., "Nutrition in the Elderly," *Annals of Internal Medicine* 109 (1988):890–904; John E. Morley and Andrew J. Silver, "Anorexia in the Elderly," *Neurobiology of Aging* 9 (1988):9–16.

8. In chapter 2, I apply Gramsci's theory of "hegemonic" ideology to medical discourse. Among the many discussions of individual responsibility as a dominant ideology in the United States, a useful account appears in Sennett and Cobb, *Hidden Injuries of Class*, pp. 3–50.

9. Regarding the prevalence, incidence, evaluation, and treatment of depression in the elderly, see Richard C. Veith and Murray A. Raskind, "The Neurobiology of Aging: Does It Predispose to Depression?" *Neurobiology of Aging* 9 (1988):101–17; Larry W. Thompson, Vincent Gong, Edmund Haskins, and Dolores Gallagher, "Assessment of Depression and Dementia during the Late Years," *Annual Review of Gerontology & Geriatrics* 7 (1987):295–324.

10. For this physician, a pattern of interaction with the wife of a depressed and relatively passive male patient occurred more than once in the sampled encounters. See also Encounter 5A in chapter 5 and its interpretation.

11. The contribution of alcohol to depression among the elderly is discussed in Nancy J. Osgood, "The Alcohol-Suicide Connection in Late Life," *Postgraduate Medicine* 81 (1987): 379–84.

12. We selected this second encounter that includes the same physician to convey some of the variability of medical discourse involving the elderly. For more details about the random sampling procedures and subsequent selection of encounters for interpretation, see chapter 4.

13. On oversedation as a side effect of major tranquilizers among the elderly, see Eric B. Larson, Walter A. Kukull, David Buchner, and Burton V. Reifler, "Adverse Drug Reactions Associated with Global Cognitive Impairment in Elderly Persons," *Annals of Internal Medicine* 107 (1987):169–73; Troy L. Thompson, Michael G. Moran, and Alan S. Nies, "Psychotropic Drug Use in the Elderly," *New England Journal of Medicine* 308 (1983):134–38, 194–99; Paul M. Helms, "Efficacy of Antipsychotics in the Treatment of the Behavioral Complications of Dementia," *Journal of the American Geriatrics Society* 33 (1985):206–09.

14. This doctor's desire for a vacation in the sun also comes up in Encounter 6B, where he advises the patient with suburban syndrome to head south for a long rest; see chapter 6.

15. Commenting on the ideology of individualism as it affects the elderly in the United States, Theron Britt notes: "From Emerson onward if not before when Danforth set foot on Plymouth, the role of the individual has been stressed—mind your own business. Yet . . . American life has been shot through with dependence on faceless bureaucracies and impersonal institutions. This contradiction is the heart of ideology in American's post-war life. . . . Here in the 'aging' chapter that contradiction appears most painfully in the form of those who are most in need of social support yet most socialized into not asking for it."

CHAPTER 8: SELF-DESTRUCTIVE BEHAVIOR AND OTHER VICES

1. Within the rapidly changing literature on AIDS, the following articles convey these points, as of the moment of this writing: Health and Public Policy Committee, American College of Physicians, "The Acquired Immunodeficiency Syndrome (AIDS) and Infection with the Human Immunodeficiency Virus (HIV)," *Annals of Internal Medicine* 108 (1988):460–69; Felix I. D. Konotey-Ahulu, "AIDS in Africa," *Lancet* 2 (1987):206–07; Daniel B. Hrdy, "Cultural Practices Contributing to the Transmission of Human Immunodeficiency Virus in

Africa," *Reviews of Infectious Diseases* 9 (1987):1109–19; Nzila Nzilambi, Kevin M. De Cock, Donald N. Forthal, and others, "The Prevalence of Infection with Human Immunodeficiency Virus over a 10-Year Period in Rural Zaire," *New England Journal of Medicine* 318 (1988):276–79; Charles W. Hunt, "AIDS and Capitalist Medicine," *Monthly Review* 39 (January 1988):11–25, and "Africa and AIDS: Dependent Development, Sexism, and Racism," *Monthly Review* 39 (February 1988):10–22.

2. For influential policy pronouncements on health promotion and disease prevention, see Julius B. Richmond, *Healthy People: The Surgeon General's Report on Health Promotion and Disease Prevention* (Washington, D.C.: U.S. Government Printing Office [DHEW (PHS) Publication No. 79-55071], 1979); National Center for Health Statistics, *Health, United States, 1989, and Prevention Profile* (Hyattsville, Md.: U.S. Department of Health and Human Services [DHHS Pub. No. (PHS) 90-1232], 1990). For critical appraisals of professional, corporate, and governmental policies on health promotion and disease prevention, see Nicole Lurie, Willard G. Manning, Christine Peterson, and others, "Preventive Care: Do We Practice What We Preach?" *American Journal of Public Health* 77 (1987):801–04; B. Woo, B. Woo, E. F. Cook, and others, "Screening Procedures in the Asymptomatic Adult: Comparison of Physicians' Recommendations, Patients' Desires, Published Guidelines, and Actual Practice," *JAMA* 254 (1985):1480–84; Kim Goldenberg, "Periodic Health Examination: Comparison of Residency Programs and National Recommendations," *Journal of General Internal Medicine* 1 (1986):282–86; "Should We Pay for Health Instead of Illness?" *The Internist* 27 (October 1986):5–18; Peter Conrad, "Worksite Health Promotion: The Social Context," *Social Science & Medicine* 26 (1988):485–89, and Sylvia Noble Tesh, *Hidden Arguments: Political Ideology and Disease Prevention Policy* (New Brunswick, N.J.: Rutgers University Press, 1988).

3. For estimates of the financial costs of self-destructive habits, see, for instance, David L. Parker, James M. Shultz, Lois Gertz, and others, "The Social and Economic Costs of Alcohol Abuse in Minnesota, 1983," *American Journal of Public Health* 77 (1987):982–86; Louis J. West, "Alcoholism," *Annals of Internal Medicine* 100 (1984):405–16; Merrill Singer, "Toward a Political-Economy of Alcoholism: The Missing Link in the Anthropology of Drinking," *Social Science & Medicine* 23 (1986):113–30; Jonathan E. Fielding, "Smoking: Health Effects and Control," *New England Journal of Medicine* 313 (1985):491–98, 555–61.

4. In chapter 2, I examine Foucault's account of professional surveillance and several theorists' views on the reproduction of dominant ideologies.

5. This summary repeats an encounter that introduced chapter 1 and concluded chapter 3; a more extensive interpretation follows.

6. Studies in sociolinguistics, outside the field of medical interaction, have found that repetitive questioning is a verbal style that both reflects and achieves interpersonal dominance. This encounter represents a rather extreme instance of the interrogatory format. For elaboration on this point and supporting references, see chapter 2 and accompanying notes.

7. Regarding the diffidence of working-class patients in asking questions, see also chapter 2.

8. Althusser, "Ideology and Ideological State Apparatuses," pp. 170–71. Althusser claims that ideology "interpellates," or "hails," individuals as subjects, and that this achievement becomes the distinguishing feature of "ideological state apparatuses." In chapter 2, I have discussed medicine as one of these apparatuses of ideologic reproduction.

   During the present medical encounter, the doctor's language interpellates the patient as a subject taking part in a web of social relationships. For this observation, I am indebted to Theron Britt, who writes: "In 'Lobster Pots,' the patient is a classic example, I think, of the Subject's being 'hailed.' Not only, as you rightly point out, is the doctor stressing an ideology that emphasizes moral rectitude and individual control, but he is also in that activity conspiring with his patient to produce him as a Subject with concrete role expectations; before the 'role' he is literally no one; after it he has an identity in relation to the power of the State, to the Family, and the doctor is assisting at his birth into the category of the Subject who has an identity (as opposed to an individual, who may or may not have an identity, but as soon as he is hailed—e.g., for drinking too much—he has concrete form in a web of rules and systemic injunction). It is not for laughs that Althusser reminds us that 'with the rise of bourgeois ideology, above all with the rise of legal ideology, the category of the subject (which may function under other names: e.g., as the soul in Plato, as God, etc.) is the constitutive category of all ideology.' "

9. For instance, basic textbooks of gastroenterology and otolaryngology do not mention such a connection within treatises on ear disease and hiccups; J. Edward Berk, ed., *Gastroenterology* (Philadelphia: Saunders, 1985), vol. 1, pp. 195–96; Marvin H. Sleisenger and John S. Fordtran, eds., *Gastrointestinal Disease: Pathophysiology, Diagnosis, Management* (Philadelphia: Saunders, 1989), p. 1959; Jerry Templer and William E. Davis, *Otolaryngology* (St. Louis: Ishiyaku, 1987), no reference to hiccups in index; David D. De Weese, William H. Saunders, David E. Schuller, and Alexander J. Schleuning II, *Otolaryngology* (St. Louis: Mosby, 1988), no reference to hiccups in index.

10. For further examples of this doctor's dark humor, see Encounter 5B (chapter 5).

11. That doctors frequently refer to their patients as symptoms or diagnoses rather than people has proven a consistent observation in studies of medical practice and training programs. For examples, see Mizrahi, *Getting Rid of Patients*, especially pp. 69–83.

12. In chapter 2, I apply Lukács' theory of reification to medical discourse. For a pertinent discussion of alcoholism as a disease, see J. Taylor Hays and W. Anderson Spickard, Jr., "Alcoholism: Early Diagnosis and Intervention," *Journal of General Internal Medicine* 2 (1987): 420–26.

13. Despite the common clinical opinion that it is difficult to stop more than one noxious habit at a time, little research substantiates this view. Further, the reasons *why* these consummatory behaviors co-occur remain unexplained. A review dealing with the co-occurrence of self-destructive habits appears in Joseph Istvan and Joseph D. Matarazzo, "Tobacco, Alcohol, and Caffeine Use: A Review," *Psychological Bulletin* 95 (1984):301–26.

14. I am indebted to Theron Britt for suggesting the framework of libidinal economy to interpret this passage.

15. The linkage of punishment and cure has a long history, and a corresponding critical interpretation. For instance, Foucault views this linkage as part of the professional surveillance of deviance; for more on this theme, see chapter 2. Similarly, Derrida describes the double nature of medicine and relates the paradox of poison/cure in Plato's *Phaedrus* (Jacques Derrida, *Dissemination* [Chicago: University of Chicago Press, 1981], pp. 70–71).

16. For further analysis of the traditional medical history, including the review of systems, see chapter 3.

17. Examples of research on socioemotional factors in hypertension include Joseph Eyer, "Hypertension as a Disease of Modern Society," *International Journal of Health Services* 5 (1975):539–58; Joan R. Bloom and Susan Monterossa, "Hypertension Labeling and Sense of Well-Being," *American Journal of Public Health* 71 (1981):1228–32; Sarah S. Knox, Tores Theorell, Jan Ch. Svensson, and Dick Waller, "The Relation of Social Support and Working Environment to Medical Variables Associated with Elevated Blood Pressure in Young Males: A Structural Model," *Social Science & Medicine* 21 (1985):525–31; Neil B. Shulman, Beverly Martinez, Donna Brogan, Albert A. Carr, and Carolyn G. Miles, "Financial Cost as an Obstacle in Hypertension Therapy," *American Journal of Public Health* 76 (1986):1105–08.

18. Such drugs do not typically appear within lists of causes and precipitants of hypertension that textbooks contain; see Alastair J. J. Wood and John A. Oates, "Adverse Reac-

tions to Drugs," in Braunwald, Isselbacher, Petersdorf, Wilson, Martin, and Fauci, eds., *Harrison's Principles of Internal Medicine,* p. 356. On the other hand, the medical literature does contain reports of occasional associations between the use of mind-altering drugs and blood pressure changes; for instance, see Elliot D. Sternberg, Lloyd Rucker, and Ralph W. Cygan, "Drug-Induced Hypertension," in J. I. Drayer, ed., *Drug Therapy in Hypertension* (New York: Marcel Dekker, 1987).

19. For discussions about the controversial health effects of physical conditioning, see Peter D. Wood, Marcia L. Stefanick, Darlene M. Dreon, and others, "Changes in Plasma Lipids and Lipoproteins in Overweight Men during Weight Loss through Dieting as Compared with Exercise," *New England Journal of Medicine* 319 (1988):1173–79; Henry Blackburn and David R. Jacobs, Jr., "Physical Activity and the Risk of Coronary Heart Disease," *New England Journal of Medicine* 319 (1988):1217–19; Victor Froelicher, *Exercise and the Heart* (New York: Year Book Medical Publishers, 1987); American College of Sports Medicine, *Guidelines for Exercise Testing and Prescription* (New York: Lea and Febiger, 1986). Regarding exercise as a nonpharmacologic treatment of hypertension with modest impact, see P. A. Ades, P. G. Gunther, C. P. Meacham, and others, "Hypertension, Exercise, and Beta-Adrenergic Blockade," *Annals of Internal Medicine* 109 (1988):629–34.

20. Waitzkin, *The Second Sickness,* pp. 230–38, and "Why It's Time for a National Health Program in the United States," pp. 101–107.

21. The following sources discuss the social history of medical policing: George Rosen, *From Medical Police to Social Medicine: Essays on the History of Health Care* (New York: Science History Publications, 1974); Johann Peter Frank, *A System of Complete Medical Police,* ed. Erna Lesky (Baltimore: Johns Hopkins University Press, 1976); Odin W. Anderson, *Syphilis and Society—Problems of Control in the United States, 1912–1964* (Chicago: Health Information Foundation, 1965). For more on professional surveillance and social control, see n. 4 above. Critiques of medical attempts to modify life-style include: Rob Crawford, "You Are Dangerous to Your Health," *International Journal of Health Services* 7 (1977):663–80; J. Warren Salmon, "Defining Health and Reorganizing Medicine," in Salmon, ed., *Alternative Medicines: Popular and Policy Perspectives* (New York: Tavistock, 1984); and Larry Sirott and Howard Waitzkin, "Holism and Self-Care: Can the Individual Succeed Where Society Fails?" in Victor W. Sidel and Ruth Sidel, eds., *Reforming Medicine: Lessons of the Last Quarter Century* (New York: Pantheon, 1984).

CHAPTER 9: TROUBLESOME EMOTIONS

1. On the expanding and sometimes difficult role of primary-care physicians in mediating patients' psychiatric problems, see chapter 5, nn. 17 and 18. Psychiatry's current movement toward more organic forms of diagnosis and treatment also tends to increase the involvement of primary-care physicians in patients' routine psychiatric difficulties. A helpful history of this transformation in psychiatry appears in Michael R. Trimble, *Biological Psychiatry* (New York: Wiley, 1988), especially pp. 1–53.

2. References on approaches in radical psychiatry appear in chapter 1, n. 3.

3. On the proportion of psychiatric problems in primary-care practice, see chapter 5, n. 17.

4. Regarding psychiatric manifestations of physical diseases, see American Psychiatric Association, *Diagnostic and Statistical Manual of Mental Disorders* (3d ed., rev.). (Washington, D.C.: The Association, 1987), pp. 97–163.

5. The following reference describes alternate-day steroid treatment: J. Blake Tyrrell and John D. Baxter, "Glucocorticoid Therapy," in Philip Felig and others, eds., *Endocrinology and Metabolism* (New York: McGraw-Hill, 1987), pp. 806–07.

6. On steroid-induced euphoria and other neuropsychiatric toxicities of glucocorticoids, see C. Gallant and P. Kenny, "Oral Glucocorticoids and Their Complications," *Journal of the*

American Academy of Dermatology 14 (1986):161–77; J. Blake Tyrrell and Peter H. Forsham, "Glucocorticoids and Adrenal Androgens," in Francis S. Greenspan and Peter H. Forsham, eds., *Basic and Clinical Endocrinology* (Los Altos, Calif.: Lange, 1986).

7. Lukács' theory of reification and its pertinence to medical discourse receives attention in chapter 2.

8. The debate here between the patient and doctor, who offer psychoanalytic versus organic interpretations of psychologic symptoms, also mirrors a hot debate within psychiatry itself; see also n. 1 above for a pertinent reference.

9. Regarding the improvement of psychologic toxicity after discontinuation of corticosteroids, see Gallant and Kenny, "Oral Glucocorticoids and Their Complications."

10. For more on the ideology of individualism and its relation to aging, see chapter 7 and accompanying notes.

11. Here, after Althusser, ideologic elements again "interpellate" the participants as subjects, each with a set of expectations attached to his or her social roles. Regarding ideology's interpellation of the subject, see chapter 2, chapter 8, and the notes that accompany them.

12. Details of the sampling procedure appear in chapter 4.

CHAPTER 10: THE NEGATIVE CASE

1. For details about the sampling procedures, see chapter 4.

2. Chapter 4 offers a discussion of these methodologic compromises.

3. For convenience, I have arranged the encounters that follow in a sequence of the life cycle, with the youngest patient first and the oldest last. This order conveys my preliminary view that the reasons why contextual issues do not enter medical discourse change at different ages.

4. This perspective receives critical attention in chapter 8.

5. Chapter 6 and its notes discuss the ideology of weight control that affects women.

6. From informal observations, I have concluded that the checking of weight frequently creates anxiety among women as patients and that the preference for shoelessness during this procedure is common.

7. On eating disorders associated with cultural standards of weight, see n. 7 of chapter 6.

8. For statistics on marijuana use by adolescents, see Thomas N. Robinson, Joel D. Killen, Barr Taylor, and others, "Perspectives on Adolescent Substance Use: A Defined Population Study," *JAMA* 258 (1987):2072–76.

CHAPTER 11: CHANGING DISCOURSE, CHANGING CONTEXT

1. Karl Marx, "Theses on Feuerbach," in Karl Marx and Friedrich Engels, *Basic Writings on Politics and Philosophy,* edited by Lewis S. Feuer (Garden City, N.Y.: Anchor, 1959), p. 245.

2. For eloquent statements of these themes, see Jameson, *Political Unconscious,* pp. 281–99; and Eagleton, *Literary Theory,* pp. 194–217.

3. In previous work, I have discussed the limits of health reform within the context of capitalist society and also have set forth some priorities for "nonreformist" reform leading to basic change in patterns of economic and political power. See Howard Waitzkin and Barbara Waterman, *The Exploitation of Illness in Capitalist Society* (Indianapolis and New York: Bobbs-Merrill, 1974), pp. 108–16; and Waitzkin, *The Second Sickness,* pp. 214–38. Critiques of the current health-care system and proposals for a national health program appear in Waitzkin, "Why It's Time for a National Health Program in the United States"; and Working Group on Program Design, Physicians for a National Health Program, "A National Health Program for the United States: A Physicians' Proposal," *New England Journal of Medicine* 320 (1989):102–08.

4. The following discussion is based on Howard Waitzkin, "Latent Functions of the Sick Role in Various Institutional Settings," *Social Science and Medicine* 5 (1971):45–75; and Mark Field, *Doctor and Patient in Soviet Russia* (Cambridge: Harvard University Press, 1957).

5. Regarding recent health-care reform proposals in the Soviet Union, a comprehensive discussion appears in Harry Nelson, "Soviet Goal: Resuscitate Health Care," *Los Angeles Times*, May 15, 1988, p. I–1. Other sympathetic yet critical accounts of Soviet medicine include Vicente Navarro, *Social Security and Medicine in the USSR: A Marxist Critique* (Lexington, Mass.: Lexington Books, 1977); and Victor W. Sidel and Ruth Sidel, *A Healthy State* (New York: Pantheon, 1983), pp. 176–208. Among the many critiques of Soviet psychiatry, a resume appears in Alexander Podrabinek, "Soviet Psychiatry: A Message from Moscow," *New York Review of Books* 35 (December 8, 1988):40–42. For discussions of medicine in Eastern Europe, see Waitzkin and Waterman, pp. 109–11; E. R. Weinerman, *Social Medicine in Eastern Europe* (Cambridge: Harvard University Press, 1969); and Bob Deacon, "Medical Care and Health under State Socialism," *International Journal of Health Services* 14 (1984):453–80.

6. For descriptions of Chinese medicine during and after the Cultural Revolution, see Joshua S. Horn, *Away with All Pests: An English Surgeon in People's China* (New York: Monthly Review Press, 1969); Ruth Sidel and Victor W. Sidel, *The Health of China* (Boston: Beacon, 1982); and Robert S. Hsu, "The Barefoot Doctors of the People's Republic of China—Some Problems," *New England Journal of Medicine* 291 (1974):124–27.

7. Regarding changes after the Chinese Cultural Revolution, the following sources present useful observations: Sidel and Sidel, *The Health of China*; David Mechanic and Arthur Kleinman, "Ambulatory Medical Care in the People's Republic of China: An Exploratory Study," *American Journal of Public Health* 70 (1980):62–66; William C. Hsiao, "Transformation of Health Care in China," *New England Journal of Medicine* 310 (1984):932–36; Jeffrey P. Koplan, Alan R. Hinman, Robert L. Parker, Gong You-Long, and Yang Ming-Ding, "The Barefoot Doctor: Shanghai County Revisited," *American Journal of Public Health* 75 (1985): 768–70; Arthur Kleinman, *Social Origins of Distress and Disease: Depression, Neurasthenia, and Pain in Modern China* (New Haven: Yale University Press, 1986).

8. The following discussion summarizes my own research observations in Cuba during April–May 1979 and November 1988, as well as published material appearing in Howard Waitzkin, "Health Policy and Social Change: A Comparative History of Chile and Cuba," *Social Problems* 31 (1983):235–48; José A. Fernandez Sacasas and Julio Lopez Benitez, "El Profesor en la Comunidad [The Professor in the Community]," *Revista Cubana de Administración de Salud* 2 (1976):1–9; Ross Danielson, "Medicine in the Community: The Ideology and Substance of Community Medicine in Socialist Cuba," *Social Science & Medicine* 15C (1981): 239–47 and *Cuban Medicine* (New Brunswick, N.J.: Transaction Books, 1979); Sally Guttmacher and Ross Danielson, "Changes in Cuban Health Care: An Argument against Technological Pessimism," *International Journal of Health Services* 7 (1977):383–400; Vicente Navarro, "Health, Health Services, and Health Planning in Cuba," *International Journal of Health Services* 2 (1972):397–432, and "Health Services in Cuba: An Initial Appraisal," *New England Journal of Medicine* 287 (1972):954–59; J. Bellerin Muñoz, "El modelo cubano de atención primaria de salud [The Cuban Model of Primary Health Care]," *Revista de Enfermería* 9 (1986):54–59; C. Ordóñez Carceller, "El Futuro de la Atención Primaria [The Future of Primary Care]," *Educación Médica y Salud* 19 (1985):74–84.

9. In addition to the sources in the last note, see, for instance: Robert Ubell, "Cuba's Great Leap," *Nature* 302 (1983):745–48, and "High-Tech Medicine in the Caribbean: 25 Years of Cuban Health Care," *New England Journal of Medicine* 309 (1983):1468–72; S. de Brun and R. H. Elling, "Cuba and the Philippines: Contrasting Cases in World-System Analysis," *International Journal of Health Services* 17 (1987):681–701.

10. I observed the cases that follow during research visits to community-based family medicine practices affiliated with two polyclinics (Policlínico Comunitario Docente Wilfredo

Pérez Pérez and Policlínico Lawton) in the San Miguel de Padron and Lawton municipalities of the city of Havana, Cuba, during November 1988. Because the visits to the local primary-care practices were impromptu and unscheduled, I have no reason to believe that the encounters observed were atypical. Transcripts and video recordings of the encounters are available on request.

11. Theron Britt has commented perceptively on the ideology of individualism, as it pertains to the differences between Cuba and the United States: "What characterizes the Cuban model as fundamentally different is not, as one would suppose, that it takes into account the social context. That is a significant difference, but not the most important. What is really at stake in the Cuban model is a more fundamental and pervasive problem—that is, what is the purpose of the health-care system? In our health-care system in the United States the goal as revealed in medical discourse is to fit the individual into the system through a concentration on the individual problem apart from its context. The ideology of individualism serves, then, a larger systemic goal of producing consensus by undermining the possibilities for alternatives. The Cuban model begins at another point of departure and fits the system to the needs of the individual, by focusing on the larger context as productive of the conditions within which individual problems arise. This Cuban model flies in the face of American wisdom, but it paradoxically pays more attention to the needs of the individual than does our own. We exalt the individual, but trap him/her in large and impersonal forces by ignoring their effects, and the result is poorer health care. Our usual image of socialist countries is that they exalt the collectivity and forget the individual, serving the needs of the bureaucracy rather than of the citizenry. But the Cuban model shows that, though this certainly can happen, it is not a structural necessity of collective action that the individual be forgotten."

12. For instance, the following discussions contain pertinent suggestions for changes in doctor-patient communication: Waitzkin, "Doctor-Patient Communication"; Mack Lipkin, Jr., Timothy E. Quill, and Rudolph J. Napodano, "The Medical Interview: A Core Curriculum for Residencies in Internal Medicine," *Annals of Internal Medicine* 100 (1984):277–84; Samuel M. Putnam, William B. Stiles, Mary Casey Jacob, and Sherman A. James, "Teaching the Medical Interview: An Intervention Study," *Journal of General Internal Medicine* 3 (1988): 38–47; John D. Stoeckle, ed., *Encounters between Patients and Doctors* (Cambridge: MIT Press, 1987); Elliot G. Mishler, Jack A. Clark, Joseph Ingelfinger, and Michael P. Simon, "The Language of Attentive Patient Care: A Comparison of Two Medical Interviews," *Journal of General Internal Medicine* 4 (1989):325–35; Kleinman, *Illness Narratives*; Katz, *Silent World of Doctor and Patient*; Eric J. Cassell, *Talking with Patients*.

13. For further discussion of these and related trends, see Waitzkin, *The Second Sickness*, pp. 3–43, 50–51, and "Information Giving in Medical Care."

14. Additional development of the themes that follow appears in Waitzkin, *The Second Sickness*, pp. 185–238; and Vicente Navarro, "Radicalism, Marxism, and Medicine," *International Journal of Health Services* 13 (1983):179–202.

15. From my own clinical experience, I have found that making decisions about how best to introduce such strategies with particular patients becomes quite challenging. Consultation with similarly minded coworkers proves valuable in these decisions.

16. For an appraisal of these attempts to link medical care with wider social change, see Waitzkin, *The Second Sickness*, pp. 125–36, and "Community-Based Health Care: Contradictions and Challenges," *Annals of Internal Medicine* 98 (1983):235–42.

INDEX

305

Personal issues. *See* Contextual issues
Physical, camp, case of: summary of en-
counter, 233; bureaucratic goals of, 233–
35; marijuana use, 235; weight issues
and, 235–36; athletics and, 236–37
Physical examination: in medical encounters, 30
Policing functions of medical role, 209
Polypharmacy, and emotional problems,
80–81
Post-structuralism, 36–37, 40, 59, 61
Prevention: and self-destructive behavior,
8, 177–78, 204, 207, 208–10, 299*n*2; in
Cuba, 266–67
Professional discourse, xiv, 9, 20–21, 41.
See also Medical discourse
Professional social control: history of, 19–
21; of self-destructive behavior, 177–78,
186–88, 194, 201–10; professional sur-
veillance and, 177–78, 186–88, 194, 204–
10, 259; theoretical view of, 282*n*24. *See
also* Social control
Psychological distress. *See* Emotional distress
Psychotropic medications, 80–81, 126–29,
162–63, 168–71

Qualitative research methods, 53–61
Quantitative research methods, 50–53, 60
Questioning, 24, 179–80, 299*n*6

Race, as basis of dominance and subor-
dination, 39–40
"Radical psychiatry" movement, 279*n*3
Reification, 15–16, 81, 137, 194, 217, 227,
229, 281*n*12
Repressive state apparatuses (RSAS), 16–17
Research method. *See* Method
Rest, occupational barriers to, 86–88. *See
also* Leisure
RSAS. *See* Repressive state apparatuses

Sampling procedures, 61, 63, 64–65, 291–
92*n*33
Saussure, Ferdinand de, 35
Scientific ideology, 18–19
Scientific language, 60–61
Scientific legitimation, 18–19
Scientific medicine, 18, 19, 265
Self-destructive behavior: as contextual
problem in medical discourse, 7; marital
conflict and, 116–17; and prevention,

177–78; professional surveillance of,
177–78, 186–88, 194, 204–10; smoking,
drinking and sex, 178–200; moral control
and medical technique, 186–88; ideology
and structure in encounters, 188–90,
197–200, 206–8; drugs and other recreational activities, 200–208; co-occurrence
of, 300*n*13. *See also* Alcohol use and
abuse; Smoking; Sexuality; Substance
use and abuse
Sexuality, 7, 20–21, 186–87, 196–97
Sexually transmitted diseases, 237–40
Sign: in structural linguistics, 35
Smoking, 116, 182–83, 187–90, 195–200
Social change, 41–42, 262. *See also* Medical
discourse, change in
Social class: class consciousness, 15–16; of
doctors, 22, 265; language use among,
24; Marxist theory of, 38–39; and ideology of work, 91; benefits of, 243, 248,
255–56; domination and, 260; and accessibility of health care in Cuba, 266
Social context. *See* Contextual issues
Social control: and barriers to doctor-
patient communication, xiv; definition
of, 7, 19; in medical encounters, 7–10,
24, 231–32; Gramsci's view of, 15; Althusser's view of, 16–17; history of professional, 19–21; unintentionality of
medical, 21–23; medical, 21–23, 40–42,
47; exclusions from doctor-patient communication, 24; masked by gratifications
of medical encounters, 41; and method
of study of medical discourse, 49, 53, 54;
and control of information, 54; qualitative studies of, 57; in case of disability
certification, 78–79; of self-destructive
behavior, 177–78, 186–88, 194, 201–10;
professional surveillance and, 177–78,
186–88, 194, 204–10, 259; avoidance of,
273. *See also* Professional social control
Social intervention. *See* Contextual intervention
Social issues. *See* Contextual issues
Social oppression, 260
Sociolinguistics, xv, 24–26, 55, 65, 282–
83*n*28, 288*n*18, 289–90*n*22, 299*n*6
Sociological imagination, 11
"Somatization" disorder, 130
South Africa, Republic of, 6, 261
Soviet bloc, medical discourse in, 263–64,
288*n*7

"Strategies of containment," 40
Stress, in work and family life, 93–104. *See also* Emotional distress
Structuralism, 33–36, 40, 59, 61
Structural linguistics, 35
Substance use and abuse: as contextual issue, 7; and role expectations affecting men, 44–45; marital conflict and, 116–17; aging and, 163–64; men and, 183–90, 193–95, 198–99; recreational drugs, 201–3, 235; marijuana use, 235
Suburban syndrome, case of: summary of encounter, 123; many complaints of patient, 123–24; discussion of, 124–26; rest and tranquilization for, 126–29; physical versus psychosocial aspects of, 129–31; context and tone of encounter, 131–32; ideology and structure of encounter, 132–34
Suicide, 118–19, 221
Summaries of nonliterary text, 56–57, 289n20
Sumner, Colin, 290n29

Text: definition of, 37, 286n2; presentation of medical discourse as, 56–59. *See also* Method
Textual absence, 37, 38
Textual analysis, 33–37, 59, 284n17
Therapeutic plan, 31–32
Tobacco. *See* Smoking
Tranquilizers, 79–81, 126–29, 298n13
Transcription: summary of transcripts, 56–57; of medical discourse, 56–59; standardized rules of, 62, 65, 66–67; reliability of, 62, 65, 67–68; presentation of transcripts for publication, 63, 70; sociolinguistic convention for, 289–90n22
Troublesome emotions. *See* Emotional distress
Truth, 287n9

Venereal diseases, 237–40

Video recordings, 61–62, 65
Vision: and aging, 144–48
"Voice of medicine," 25, 39
"Voice of the lifeworld," 25, 39, 47

Walzer, Michael, 285–86n30
Weight, 114, 116, 154–55, 235–36, 246–47, 302n6
West, Candace, 24, 67
Women: Marxist theory concerning, 14–15; family life and, 14–15, 43–44, 107, 109–112, 123–34, 141–42, 222–26, 227; case of marital conflict, 108–22; work and, 109–12, 141–42, 245–46; female problems and, 112–13; weight issues and, 114, 116; depression and, 115–19, 218–22; alcohol use, 116–17; smoking, 116–17; and case of suburban syndrome, 123–34; and housewife syndrome, 125, 296n13; and case of physical difficulties with housework, 134–40; and husband's work, 138–39; passivity and, 141; aging and, 144–58; and emotional manifestations of physical disease, 214–29; and middle age without stress, 240–48; medical control of, 281–82n17; childbearing and, 295n9
Work: as contextual issue, 6–7; health as ability to work, 13–14, 17, 84, 280nn6–7; Marxist theory of, 13–15; case of disability certification and, 76–83; and return to uncertain employment, 76–83; men and, 76–106, 138–39, 180–81, 198; in case of occupational illness, 83–92, 293n11; pain and, 84–86; ideologies of, 90–91; success in, and stress in the family, 93–104; women and, 107, 109–12, 141–42, 245–46; and case of physical difficulties in housework, 134–40. *See also* Economic production

Zola, Irving Kenneth, 281n17